Language Disorders in Speakers of Chinese

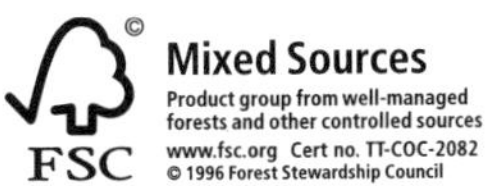

COMMUNICATION DISORDERS ACROSS LANGUAGES
Series Editors: Dr Nicole Müller and Dr Martin Ball, *University of Louisiana at Lafayette, USA*

While the majority of work in communication disorders has focused on English, there has been a growing trend in recent years for the publication of information on languages other than English. However, much of this is scattered through a large number of journals in the field of speech pathology/communication disorders, and therefore, not always readily available to the practitioner, researcher and student. It is the aim of this series to bring together into book form surveys of existing studies on specific languages, together with new materials for the language(s) in question. We also envisage a series of companion volumes dedicated to issues related to the cross-linguistic study of communication disorders. The series will not include English (as so much work is readily available), but will cover a wide number of other languages (usually separately, though sometimes two or more similar languages may be grouped together where warranted by the amount of published work currently available). We envisage being able to solicit volumes on languages such as Norwegian, Swedish, Finnish, German, Dutch, French, Italian, Spanish, Russian, Croatian, Japanese, Cantonese, Mandarin, Thai, North Indian languages in the UK context, Celtic languages, Arabic and Hebrew among others.

Full details of all the books in this series and of all our other publications can be found on http://www.multilingual-matters.com, or by writing to Multilingual Matters, St Nicholas House, 31-34 High Street, Bristol BS1 2AW, UK.

COMMUNICATION DISORDERS ACROSS LANGUAGES
Series Editors: Dr Nicole Müller and Dr Martin Ball,
University of Louisiana at Lafayette, USA

Language Disorders in Speakers of Chinese

Edited by
Sam-Po Law, Brendan S. Weekes and Anita M-Y. Wong

MULTILINGUAL MATTERS
Bristol • Buffalo • Toronto

Library of Congress Cataloging in Publication Data
A catalog record for this book is available from the Library of Congress.
Language Disorders in Speakers of Chinese
Edited by Sam-Po Law, Brendan Weekes, and Anita M-Y. Wong.
Communication Disorders Across Languages
Includes bibliographical references.
1. Language disorders–China.
I. Law, Sam-po. II. Weekes, Brendan. III. Wong, Anita M-Y. IV. Series.
[DNLM: 1. Language Disorders–therapy–China. 2. Speech Disorders–therapy–China.
3. Language Therapy–methods–China. WL 340.2 L2865 2008]
RC423.L339 2008
362.196'85500951–dc22 2008026641

British Library Cataloguing in Publication Data
A catalogue entry for this book is available from the British Library.

ISBN-13: 978-1-84769-116-3 (hbk)
ISBN-13: 978-1-84769-115-6 (pbk)

Multilingual Matters
UK: St Nicholas House, 31-34 High Street, Bristol BS1 2AW, UK.
USA: UTP, 2250 Military Road, Tonawanda, NY 14150, USA.
Canada: UTP, 5201 Dufferin Street, North York, Ontario M3H 5T8, Canada.

Typeset by Datapage International Ltd.
Printed and bound in Great Britain by the Cromwell Press Ltd.

Contents

Contributors

Yanchao Bi, State Key Laboratory of Cognitive Neuroscience & Learning, Beijing Normal University, Beijing 100875, China (ybi@bnu.edu.cn).

Hintat Cheung, Graduate Institute of Linguistics, National Taiwan University, 1, Section 4, Roosevelt Road, Taipei 106, Taiwan (hintat@ntu.edu.tw).

Karen Chiu, Speech Therapy Department, Tung Wah Hospital, 12 Po Yan Street, Sheung Wan, Hong Kong (chiumy@ha.org.hk).

Paul Fletcher, Department of Speech & Hearing Sciences, College of Medicine & Health, Brookfield Health Sciences Complex, University College Cork, College Road, Cork, Ireland (p.fletcher@ucc.ie).

Roxana S-Y. Fung, Department of Chinese and Bilingual Studies, The Hong Kong Polytechnic University, Hunghom, Kowloon, Hong Kong (ctsyfung@polyu.edu.hk).

Zaizhu Han, State Key Laboratory of Cognitive Neuroscience & Learning, Beijing Normal University, Beijing 100875, China (zzhhan@bnu.edu.cn).

Thomas Klee, School of Education, Communication & Language Sciences and Institute of Health & Society, Newcastle University, King George VI Building, Queen Victoria Road, Newcastle upon Tyne, NE1 7RU, United Kingdom (thomas.klee@newcastle.ac.uk).

Kathrin Klingebiel, Department of Psychology, University of Sussex, Falmer, BN1 9QN, United Kingdom (k.a.m.klingebiel@sussex.ac.uk).

Anthony Pak-Hin Kong, Department of Communication Sciences and Disorders, University of Central Florida, HPA-2 101Z, PO Box 162215, Orlando, FL 32816-2215, USA (pkong@mail.ucf.edu).

Sam-Po Law, Division of Speech & Hearing Sciences and Center of Communication Disorders, University of Hong Kong, 5/F, Prince Philip Dental Hospital, 34 Hospital Road, Hong Kong (splaw@hkucc.hku.hk).

Laurence B. Leonard, Speech, Language, and Hearing Sciences, 500 Oval Drive, Heavilon Hall, Purdue University, West Lafayette, IN 47907, USA (xdxl@purdue.edu).

Jie Liang, College of Foreign Languages, Xinjiang Normal University, Xinyi Road 102, 830054 Urumqi, Xinjiang, China (j_liang@xjnu.edu.cn / liangjie56@163.net).

Jerome L. Packard, Department of East Asian Languages & Cultures, 2090 Foreign Languages Building, University of Illinois, Urbana, IL 61801, USA (jpackar@uiuc.edu).

Hua Shu, School of Psychology, Beijing Normal University, Beijing, China (shuh@bnu.edu.cn).

Stephanie F. Stokes, School of Education, Communication & Language Sciences and Institute of Health & Society, Newcastle University, King George VI Building, Queen Victoria Road, Newcastle upon Tyne, NE1 7RU, United Kingdom (s.stoke@newcastle.ac.uk).

I Fan Su, Department of Psychology, University of Sussex, Falmer, BN1 9QN, United Kingdom (i.f.su@sussex.ac.uk).

Brendan S. Weekes, Department of Psychology, University of Sussex, Falmer, BN1 9QN, United Kingdom (b.s.weekes@sussex.ac.uk).

Anita M-Y. Wong, Division of Speech & Hearing Sciences and Center of Communication Disorders, University of Hong Kong, 5/F, Prince Philip Dental Hospital, 34 Hospital Road, Hong Kong (amywong@hkusua.hku.hk).

Elva Wong, Tung Wah Group of Hospitals Kwan Fong Kai Chi School, 28 Nam Shan Chuen Road, Tai Hang Tung, Kowloon, Hong Kong (elvapig@gmail.com).

Winsy Wong, Division of Speech & Hearing Sciences and Center of Communication Disorders, University of Hong Kong, 5/F, Prince Philip Dental Hospital, 34 Hospital Road, Hong Kong (winsywg@graduate.hku.hk).

Sina Wu, Chinese Language and Literature School, Beijing Foreign Studies University, Beijing 100089, China (wusina@bfsu.edu.cn).

Wengang Yin, Institute of Psychology, Chinese Academy of Science, Datun Road 10A, Chaoyang District, Beijing 100101, China (wengang3@hotmail.com).

Olivia Yeung, Division of Speech & Hearing Sciences and Center of Communication Disorders, University of Hong Kong, 5/F, Prince Philip Dental Hospital, 34 Hospital Road, Hong Kong (h0021212@graduate.hku.hk).

Hua Zhu, Department of Applied Linguistics, Birkbeck, University of London, 43 Gordon Square, Bloomsbury, London, WC1H OPD, United Kingdom (zhu.hua@bbk.ac.uk).

Preface

Research in language disorders among children and adults of European languages and alphabetic scripts have undoubtedly demonstrated the value of these data in informing theories of the normal cognitive system underlying language comprehension and production. More significantly, observations of individuals with language disorders offer researchers unique opportunities, such as selective impairment to language processes or specific difficulties with certain grammatical components, to investigate issues that cannot otherwise be examined. Studies of language disorders have also been instrumental in the rapid development of evidence-based clinical research in recent decades, resulting in sophisticated diagnostic tools and treatment approaches. These advances in the basic science of communication disorders allow clinicians, educators and policy makers to make informed decisions about intervention and to proceed with treatment using the scientist-practitioner model.

Research interest in language impairments in Chinese, a language spoken by one fifth of the world's population, can be traced back to the 1930s. The importance of investigating languages with written and spoken forms that are vastly different from European languages, such as Chinese, need not be further highlighted, as evidenced by many volumes of publications on psycholinguistic studies of East-Asian languages. Yet, despite the significant advances made in basic research investigating Chinese speakers with language difficulties in the past two decades, this body of work has not received the attention that it deserves. The need for a book devoted entirely to the study of Chinese language disorders is not only academic, but also practical. Stroke is a leading cause of death and disability in China. Recent surveys have revealed age- and sex-standardized prevalence rates of about 7% among people over 65 years of age in many Chinese communities. It is estimated that about 38% of acute cases of focal brain damage to the left hemisphere lead to different degrees of language impairments that are both long lasting and devastating. Likewise, studies have shown that about 12% to 14% of five-year-old children speak and/or understand language at levels below age expectations, and most of these children continue to lag behind in spoken language and perform below age levels in reading at school age.

This book fills a gap in the field and represents the latest research in Chinese language disorders in children and adults by more than 20 scholars from Hong Kong, Mainland China, Taiwan, the United Kingdom and the USA. It features single case and group studies addressing theoretical and clinical issues relevant to understanding specific language impairment in children, developmental dyslexia, phonological impairment in children and adults, acquired dyslexia and dysgraphia, deficits in word and narrative production in adults and the relationship between memory and language impairment. While the focus of most chapters is on monolingual speakers, our volume concludes with a study of language impairments in bilingual speakers who are largely neglected in the research literature.

Chapter 1

Characteristics of Chinese in Relation to Language Disorders

ROXANA S-Y. FUNG

Introduction

The Chinese language, or group of related languages, is the most widely spoken language in the world. Over a billion people, about one sixth of the world's population, speak some form(s) of Chinese as their native language. The spoken forms of the Chinese language exhibit a high degree of diversity to such an extent that its geographical variants may not be mutually intelligible. However, the Chinese language is still regarded as a single language by the Chinese people mainly due to the same written form shared by all the geographical variants. There are seven major geographical dialect groups (each with many subdialects): (1) Mandarin (which has over 870 million speakers living across the Northern, Central and Western regions of China), (2) Wu (speakers of which are most commonly found in Jiangsu and Zhejiang including Shanghai), (3) Xiang (in Hunan), (4) Gan (in Jiangxi), (5) Yue (in Guangdong), (6) Min (in Fujian), and (7) Kejia (in Guangdong and other Southern Chinese provinces). The standardised form of modern spoken Chinese in Mainland China as well as in Taiwan is Putonghua (also referred to as Mandarin)[1] of which the phonology is based mainly on Beijing Mandarin and the grammar loosely on the subdialects of Northern China. Cantonese, which has over 110 million speakers, is the most influential variety of Chinese other than Mandarin (Matthews & Yip, 1994). It is the standardised form of the Yue dialect group spoken in the Southern Chinese provinces of Guangdong, Guangxi, Hong Kong and Macau, as well as in many overseas Chinese communities in Singapore, Malaysia and in the Western world. Thus, most studies of Chinese language disorders involve mainly Mandarin or Cantonese speakers.

It is traditionally believed that Chinese dialects differ from each other mostly in matters of pronunciation and vocabulary and they exhibit the greatest degree of uniformity in matters of grammar. Thus, Chao (1968) claimed that there was practically one universal Chinese grammar. However, more and more recent studies question the validity of this long-held claim. In light of the topics of other chapters in this book, this chapter will not discuss in detail the grammatical differences between

Mandarin and Cantonese. Rather, it aims to highlight some characteristics of these two dialects that are related to language difficulties that have been investigated by contributors of this volume. The brief review here will provide the readers with sufficient background on the grammar of Mandarin and Cantonese and the Chinese writing system to appreciate the findings and analyses presented in subsequent chapters. Readers who are interested in learning more detailed accounts of these two dialects may consult Chao (1968) for Mandarin grammar, Matthews and Yip (1994) for Cantonese grammar and Liu (2001) for descriptions of significant typological differences between these two Chinese variants.

Phonology

Phonologically, Mandarin has 22 consonants and 12 vowels, whereas Cantonese has 17 consonants and 11 vowels. An overview of the phonological inventories of Mandarin and Cantonese is shown in Table 1.1. Note that *Hanyu Pinyin* is adopted as the standard romanisation of Mandarin, whereas *Jyutping*, developed by the Linguistic Society of Hong Kong, is adopted as that of Cantonese in this book.

Compared with other languages, such as English, the syllabic structure of Chinese is relatively simple. A syllable in Chinese is usually depicted by the following form: (C)V(C). Consonant clusters are not

Table 1.1 Segmental inventories of Mandarin and Cantonese phonetic value (left) and romanisation equivalents (right)

	Mandarin	*Cantonese*
Syllable-initial consonants shared by both dialects	b[p], d[t], g[k], p[p^h], t[t^h], k[k^h], z[ts], c[ts^h], s[s], f[f], m[n], n[n], l[l]	b[p], d[t], g[k], p[p^h], t[t^h], k[k^h], z[ts], c[ts^h], s[s], f[f], m[m], n[n], l[l]
Syllable-initial consonants unique to individual dialects	zh[tʂ], ch[$tʂ^h$], sh[ʂ], j[tɕ], q[$tɕ^h$], x[ɕ], r[ɹ], h[x]	gw[kw], kw[kw^h], ng[ŋ], h[h]
Syllable-final consonants shared by both dialects	ng[ŋ], n[n]	ng[ŋ], n[n]
Syllable-final consonants unique to individual dialects	–	m[m], p[p], t[t], k[k]
Vowels shared by both dialects	i[i], ü[y], u[u], e[e], e[ɛ], a[a], o[o]	i[i], yu[y], u[u], e[e], e[ɛ], aa[a], o[o]
Vowels unique to individual dialects	i[ɿ], i[ʅ], a[ɑ], e[ə], e[ɤ]	eo[ø], oe[œ], a[ɐ], o[ɔ]

permitted in a Chinese syllable. The tone and the nuclear vowel (or vocalic segment) are the two obligatory elements in a syllable, whereas the syllable-initial and syllable-final consonants are optional. In Mandarin, all consonants in the inventory except [ŋ] can be the onset of a syllable. However, the coda is restricted to [n] and [ŋ] only. The syllable nucleus can be a monophthong such as [a], a diphthong such as [ai] or a triphthong such as [uai]. In Cantonese, all consonants in the inventory can be the onset of a syllable. It has a rich coda inventory compared with Mandarin. In addition to the nasal consonants [m], [n] and [ŋ], unreleased oral stops [p], [t], [k] can also be the coda of a syllable. The nucleus is usually a monophthong such as [a] or a diphthong such as [ai]. In addition, the two nasal sonorants [m] and [ŋ] can serve as the nucleus and form a syllable totally on their own.

Chinese is a tone language that employs pitch change to contrast lexical meanings. All geographical variants of Chinese are tonal, but they differ in the number of tones they have. As shown in Table 1.2, Mandarin has four basic tones and one neutral tone, whereas Cantonese has six distinct tones without the occurrence of neutral tone.

The neutral tone in Mandarin, also referred to as the fifth tone or the zero tone, is the reduced form of any full-fledged tone. It is produced in a lighter, shorter and less stressed manner. The exact pitch of the neutral tone depends almost entirely on the tone carried by the syllable preceding it. Many grammatical words/morphemes in Mandarin have been assigned the neutral tone.

In Mandarin, tone sandhi takes place in connected speech. A syllable has one of the tones when it stands alone, but the same syllable may take on a different tone without a change of meaning when followed by another syllable. The most important tone sandhi in Mandarin involves the juxtaposition of two third tone syllables. The dipping third tone

Table 1.2 Tones of Mandarin and Cantonese

Mandarin			*Cantonese*		
Tone No.	*Description*	*Pitch*	*Tone No.*	*Description*	*Pitch*
1	High level	55	1	High level	55
2	High rising	35	2	High rising	35
3	Dipping	214	3	Mid level	33
4	High falling	51	4	Low falling	21/11
5/0	Neutral		5	Low rising	23
			6	Low level	22

changes to a rising second tone when followed by another third tone. Although there are tone changes in Cantonese, they are not tone sandhi as in Mandarin. Tone changes in Cantonese are not triggered by phonological environments, but are motivated by a number of morphological and semantic factors. For example, the noun 皮 *pei* means 'skin' when pronounced in the fourth tone, its citation form, but 'leather' when pronounced in the second tone, the changed tone.

As Packard (1993) points out, the set of possible syllable structures in Chinese is small given the structural simplicity and a small inventory of phonemes. There are only about 1200 and 1600 distinct syllables in Mandarin and Cantonese, respectively, even taking into account different tones in the two dialects. Almost all syllables are possible words and the occurrence of homophones is extensive in Chinese.

The phonological development of normally and atypically developing Mandarin-speaking children is presented in Chapter 2 by Zhu. The author explains the unique developmental patterns observed by taking an approach combining two concepts, phonological saliency and phonological template. A new paradigm for cross-linguistic research in speech disorders is also introduced. Focusing on lexical tone perception, in Chapter 9 Liang studies tone impairments in Mandarin adult speakers subsequent to brain injury. Questions concerning whether phonological encoding is modality-specific or not and whether the nature of tone disruption is related to structural deficits or processing limitations are addressed.

Grammar

The word

Chinese is often referred to as an analytic language[2] because it possesses very little inflectional or derivational morphology. Additionally, Chinese is often described as an isolating language.[3] However, this description applies to Classical Chinese but not modern Chinese. Classical Chinese is a perfect example of an isolating language because most words in Classical Chinese consist of one single morpheme and each morpheme corresponds to one single syllable. Whereas morphemes in modern Chinese are predominately monosyllabic, most words are no longer monosyllabic. Content words, such as nouns, verbs and adjectives in modern Chinese are largely disyllabic and bimorphemic. There are three main means by which words are formed in Chinese: affixation, reduplication and compounding. As there are few inflectional or derivational affixes in Chinese, compounding is the most productive means of word formation in modern Chinese. It is a process of forming a single new word by combining two or more morphemes. By studying the internal composition of Chinese compound words, five major types of syntactic/semantic relation between the component morphemes are identified. These are listed and illustrated in Table 1.3.

It should be noted that the internal relation of a compound is not always clear because some compounds are fully lexicalised and their meanings are not predictable from their components. For example, it is not clear how the meaning of the adjective 大方 *da4 fang1* 'generous' is related to the two component morphemes 'big' and 'square'. Hence, the internal relation of this adjective cannot be determined.

Given the paucity of inflectional morphology, there is no change in word form in Chinese to mark person, gender, case, number (obligatorily expressed only for pronouns), tense or mood. Moreover, there is no formal distinction between a finite and an infinite verb. Chinese also lacks formal markers for parts-of-speech. To assign part-of-speech to a word on the basis of its surface form only is not an easy task. A sharp

Table 1.3 Compound words in Mandarin

Syntactic relation	***Examples***
Juxtapositional	保守 *bao3shou3* (adjective) keep-maintain juxtaposed-juxtaposed 'conservative'
Modificational	黑心 *hei1xin1* (adjective) black-heart modifier-modified 'malicious'
Predicational	海嘯 *hai3xiao4* (noun) sea-scream subject-predicate 'tsunami'
Governmental	關心 *guan1xin1* (verb) close-heart verb-object 'care about'
Complemental	提高 *ti2gau1* (verb) move-high verb-complement 'promote'

distinction between nouns, verbs and adjectives, in particular, is difficult to draw. For instance, 代表 *dai4biao3* is a noun in 我們的代表 *wo3men0 de0 dai4biao3* 'our representative', but a verb in 代表我們 *dai4biao3 wo3men0* 'represent us'. Furthermore, the noun 科學 *ke1xue3* 'science' shares the exact same surface form with its derived adjective as in 很科學 *hen3 ke1xue3* 'very scientific'. However, despite the absence of overt markers, many Chinese grammarians have tried to define Chinese parts-of-speech on the basis of syntactic distribution. A word is considered a noun if it can be modified by a demonstrative/numeral measure phrase, but cannot be negated by the adverb 不 *bu4* 'not'. On the contrary, adjectives and verbs are words that can be negated by *bu4*. Adjectives are further distinguished from verbs by another adverb 很 *hen3* 'very'. Most adjectives can be modified by *hen3*, but verbs proper cannot. Although there is a group of verbs denoting psychological activities that can be modified by *hen3*, they are all transitive. That is to say, psychological verbs can take an object noun phrase (NP) but adjectives cannot.

The productivity of compounding in Chinese and the extent of homophony in the language render compound words an ideal context for investigating the relationship between morphological deficits and developmental dyslexia. This is examined by Wu, Packard and Shu in Chapter 7. Despite the fact that distinctions among major word classes, such as nouns and verbs, in Chinese cannot be made as clearly as in Indo–European languages, dissociation in production between these grammatical classes has nonetheless been reported. Case studies of double dissociation of selective impairment to nouns versus verbs are reviewed in Chapter 10 by Han and Bi. Furthermore, given that compound words of one form class can be composed of components of a different word class, as illustrated by the examples in Table 1.3, Han and Bi also examine previous reports of grammatical class deficits at the sublexical level.

Classifiers

Many languages have measure words for noun phrases. Taking English as an example, there is a group of measure words that express the length, weight and volume of an object, such as 'a pint of beer, two pounds of oranges', and there is another group of measure words that are used for objects denoted by uncountable nouns, such as 'two pieces of paper, a flock of sheep'. Unlike those in English and other languages, measure words in Chinese go with all kinds of nouns when the nouns are modified by numerals or demonstratives.[4] Measure words in Chinese are also referred to as classifiers[5] because they have an additional feature of expressing the conceptual classification of the referent of a noun along with some features that are salient to the speaker, such as size, shape and so on. For example, the classifier 條 *tiao2* in Mandarin is used for objects that are long and narrow in shape, such as threads and dogs, and 張 *zhang1* for objects that spread out with a flat surface, such as paper and tables. In contemporary Mandarin, there is a strong tendency to use a general classifier 個 *ge4* for all nouns, whether animate or inanimate.

Each Chinese dialect has its own classifier system. The choice of classifiers for individual nouns is particular to each dialect. Compared to Mandarin, Cantonese has a greater number of classifiers and there is no general classifier in this dialect.

Aspect markers

Like a number of other East Asian languages, Chinese is an aspect language and not a tense language (Norman, 1988). Tense is not grammaticalised in Chinese as there are no distinctions in verb form to indicate past, present or future tense. Temporal relations in Chinese are expressed by time words and contextual factors. On the contrary, the Chinese language has a rich system of aspect. Aspect is concerned with how a speaker presents a situation through different viewpoints, whether an action is completed or not, whether it is in progress or not, or whether a state has occurred or not. There are various grammatical means to express aspect in Chinese, including aspect markers (a group of bound morphemes most of which behave like verbal affixes), verb reduplication and verbal particles. Focusing on aspect markers, the perfective aspect for instance, which denotes some actions that have taken place, is expressed by the verbal suffix 了 *le0* in Mandarin.

(1) 我買了很多書
wo3 mai3le0 hen3 duo1 shu1
I buy-ASP[6] very many book
'I bought a lot of books'

(2) 明天下了課我們去游泳
ming2tian1 xia4-le0 ke4 wo3men0 qu4 you2yong3
tomorrow down-ASP lesson we go swim
'We'll go to swim after class tomorrow'

As illustrated by (2), the perfective aspect does not relate to past tense as it may refer to events in the future. In fact, the occurrence of the perfective aspect marker 了 *le0* in some past events may be ungrammatical.

(3) 這是我昨天買/*買了的書
*zhe4 shi4 wo3 zuo2tian1 mai3/*mai3le0 de0 shu1*
this is I yesterday buy POSS book
'This is the book I bought yesterday'

Table 1.4 Major aspect markers and verbal particles indicating aspects in Mandarin and Cantonese

Type	*Mandarin*	*Cantonese*
Perfective	了: verb-*le0*	咗: verb-*zo2*
Progressive	在: *zai4*-verb	喺度: *hai2dou6*-verb
	着: verb-*zhe0*	緊: verb-*gan2*
Durative/continuous	着: verb-*zhe0*	住: verb-*zyu6*
Experiential	過: verb-*guo4*	過: verb-*gwo3*
Delimitative	一: verb-*yi1*-verb; verb-verb	下: verb-*haa5*
Habitual	–	開: verb-*hoi1*
Adversative/habitual	–	親: verb-*can1*
Beginning	起／起來:	起／起嚟／起上嚟:
	verb-*qi3*/*qi3lai2*	verb-*hei2*/*hei2lei4*/*hei2soeng5lei4*

Source: Adapted from Matthews and Yip (1994: 198)

The aspect system and the usage of individual aspects in different dialects of Chinese may differ substantially from that of Mandarin. Cantonese, for instance, has a more complex aspectual system. It has a larger number of aspect-related morphemes that are unique to Cantonese. The approximate correspondence of the most commonly found aspects in Cantonese to those in Mandarin is shown in Table 1.4.

While most aspect markers in Mandarin carry the unstressed neutral tone, all aspect makers in Cantonese bear the full-fledged tone, similar to lexical items of other grammatical classes in the language.

Finally, it must be pointed out that it may not be necessary for aspect in both dialects to be marked by grammatical means, as aspect can also be expressed by lexical meanings or in context. For instance, the perfective marker is optional in (4) because the perfective aspect can be expressed by the verb with its resultative complement.

(4) 我收到／了一封信
wo3 shou1dao4/le0 yi1 feng1 xin4
I receive-arrive one CL letter
'I received a letter'

Chinese sentences

Sentence-hood or clause-hood in the Chinese language is not as straightforward as in other languages. In most Indo–European languages, a full sentence is characterised by the presence of a subject formed by a noun phrase and a predicate formed by a finite verb. However, neither the subject NP nor the predicate verb is obligatory in a Chinese sentence. The subject position in a Chinese sentence can be filled by an adjective as in (5a), a verb phrase (VP) as in (5b) or even left empty as in (6).

(5a) 乾淨是很重要的
gan1jing4 shi4 hen3 zhong4yao4 de0
clean is very important SFP
'To be clean is very important'

(5b) 做運動是很重要的
zuo4 yun4dong4 shi4 hen3 zhong4yao4 de0
do exercise is very important
'Doing exercise is very important'

(6) 下雨了
xia4 yu3 le0
down rain SFP
'It is raining'

Similarly, the predicate in a Chinese sentence may not involve any verbal element. The adjectival predicate in (7a) and the nominal predicate in (7b) are simply juxtaposed with their subjects without any linking verbs. Furthermore, an NP itself without any predicate can stand alone as a formal Chinese sentence as in (8).

(7a) 她很漂亮
ta1 hen3 piao4liang4
she very pretty
'She is very pretty'

(7b) 今天星期三
jin1tian1 xing1qi1san1
today Wednesday
'Today is Wednesday'

(8) 我媽媽呢?
wo3 ma1ma0 ne0
I mother SFP
'Where is my mother?'

By now it should become apparent that minor sentences, i.e. irregular sentences not in the form of subject-predicate, are quite common in written Chinese. In fact, it has been claimed that minor sentences are more common than major sentences, i.e. full sentences in the form of subject-predicate, in Chinese (Chao, 1968; Cheung, 2007; Norman, 1988).

Many Chinese grammarians have also remarked that the grammatical relation between the subject and predicate in Chinese is very loose. A subject in a Chinese sentence does not have an independent thematic role and it may stand in a number of different semantic relations with the predicate. For example, the subject may be the agent of a transitive verb in the predicate as in (9) or the patient of the action as in (10).

(9) 我買了車
wo3 mai3le0 che1
I buy-ASP car
'I bought a car'

(10) 車買了
che1 mai3le0
car buy-ASP
'The car, (I) have bought it'

Hence, the grammatical meaning of subject and predicate has been defined as that of 'topic' and 'comment' in Chinese grammar.[7] As a topic, the subject in a Chinese sentence is that about which something is said. Due to the importance of topic rather than subject, in its grammar, Mandarin is often referred to as a topic-prominent language.[8]

The basic word order in a Chinese sentence is generally recognised as subject-verb-object (SVO). However, it is observed that Mandarin exhibits more features of subject-object-verb (SOV) than other dialects, through topicalisation. For instance, Mandarin may pose the object 'clothes' before the verb 'wash' to make it the secondary topic of the sentence:

(11) 他衣服洗了
ta1 yi1fu0 xi3 le0
he clothes wash-ASP
'He washed the clothes'.

Complex sentences

As mentioned earlier, sentence-hood and clause-hood in Chinese is not as transparent as in English and there is no formal distinction between finite and infinite verbs in Chinese. As a consequence, the boundary between simple sentences and complex sentences in Chinese cannot be easily identified. A Chinese sentence may look quite 'complex' on the surface form. Verb stacking is a common feature in Chinese grammar in which two or more verbs or verb phrases are often strung together in a sentence. The inventory of complex sentences has long been a tricky area in Chinese grammar. Many Chinese linguists depart from the Western grammatical tradition of defining a clause by the presence of a verb and analyse the following seemingly complex sentences as simple sentences. Taking into account that the subject serves as a topic in Chinese sentences and is not restricted to NP only, there are good reasons to analyse (12) as a simple sentence with the subject position filled by the clause 'he leaves'.

(12) [他走]是很可惜
[ta1 zou3] shi4 hen3 ke3xi1
[he leave] is very pity
'His leaving is a real pity'

Pivotal constructions are also classified as simple sentences in traditional Chinese grammar. A pivotal construction, as illustrated by (13), is characterised by the dual role of the NP 'he' which occurs between two verbs. It serves as the object of the first verb 'invite' and the subject of the second verb 'come'.

(13) 我請他來
wo3 qing3 ta1 lai2
I invite he come
'I invite him to come'

No matter which approach one may adopt in theoretical linguistics to analyse these complicated constructions, it is interesting to study how these sentences are processed psychologically.

Passive

Being an analytic language, Chinese depends heavily on context rather than grammatical form to express the passive voice. There are various forms of passive sentences in Chinese, both marked and unmarked. The most frequently used passive form is the unmarked one. It is a simple topic-comment sentence that does not employ any formal grammatical marker at all.

(14) 杯子洗了
bei1zi0 xi3le0
cups wash-ASP
'Those cups were washed'

As the subject in a Chinese sentence can be either the agent or the patient of the action denoted by the verb in the predicate, ambiguity may occur if the subject noun phrase is animate:

(15) 雞不吃了
ji1 bu4 chi1le0
chicken no eat-ASP
'The chicken stops eating/(We) do not eat chicken'

The less commonly used passive sentences are the marked ones, where an overt passive marker similar to 'by' in English is employed to introduce the agent of the action in the sentences. The marked passive sentences in Chinese are restricted to specific situations: when the patient is considered by the speaker to be affected by the action, which often caused undesirable outcomes. Typical examples of passive markers of adversity are 被 *bei4* in Mandarin and 畀 *bei2* in Cantonese.[9]

(16) 他被警察打傷了
ta1 bei4 jing3cha2 da2shang1le0 (Mandarin)
佢畀警察打傷咗
keoi5 bei2 ging2caat3 daa2 soeng1zo2 (Cantonese)
he BEI police beat injure-ASP
'He was wounded by the police'

Unlike English, the '*bei* + noun' phrase in Chinese precedes the verb. Compared with its active counterpart, the passive sentence has undergone a word order change. It changes from the SVO order, agent-action-patient, in the active sentence to SOV order, patient-agent-action, in the passive. The word order change in passive sentences is believed to be motivated by pragmatic factors. From the point of view of information structure, the sentence-final position is a position reserved for focused or prominent elements of a sentence. By fronting the patient and agent in a passive sentence, the verb denoting the action and its consequence on the patient can occupy the sentence-final position and, hence, be able to receive focus.

Questions

There are various ways to form questions in Chinese. The simplest one is to raise the intonation of a declarative sentence to form an echo question, as in English and many languages. However, there are also other grammatical constructions to explicitly mark an utterance as a question. They include particle questions, disjunctive questions and wh-questions. Unlike English, none of the question forms involve the inversion of word order.

Particle questions are yes–no questions formed by adding a sentence-final particle to a declarative sentence. While 嗎 *ma0* is the exclusive question particle in Mandarin as in (17), 啊 *aa4* and 咩 *me1* are the two question particles in Cantonese as in (18):

(17) 你去嗎? (Mandarin)
ni3 qu4 ma0
you go SFP
'Are you going?'

(18a) 你去啊? (Cantonese)
nei5 heoi3 aa4
you go SFP
'Are you going?'

(18b) 你去咩? (Cantonese)
nei5 heoi3 me1
you go SFP
'Are you going?' (with stronger sense of surprise)

Disjunctive questions present the respondent with a choice of two or more possible answers. There are two types of disjunctive questions in Chinese. The first type is marked by the conjunction, 還是 *hai3shi4* in Mandarin and 定係/定 *ding6hai6/din*g6 in Cantonese.

(19) 你去美國還是英國? (Mandarin)
ni3 qu4 mei3guo2 hai3shi4 ying1guo2
你去美國定係/定英國? (Cantonese)
nei5 heoi3 mei5gwok3 ding6hai6/ding6 jing1gwok3
you go US or Britain
'Are you going to the US or Britain?'

The second type of disjunctive questions is marked by the A-not-A form. It juxtaposes the affirmative form and the negative counterpart of the lexeme in question for the respondent to choose from. The lexeme can either be an adjective, a lexical or a modal verb. It poses to the respondent: Is A the case or not? The answer is expected to be A or not-A. The negation morpheme is 不 *bu4* in Mandarin and 唔 *m4* in Cantonese:

(20) 你去不去 ? (Mandarin)
ni3 qu4-bu0-qu4?
你去唔去 ? (Cantonese)
nei5 heoi3-m4-heoi3?
you go not go
'Are you going or not?'

In Cantonese, the affirmative part is always monosyllabic even if the lexeme is disyllabic. Thus, in the case of disyllabic lexemes, only the first syllable of the lexeme is repeated. Compare:

(21) 你清楚不清楚 ? (Mandarin)
ni3 qing1chu0-bu0-qing1chu0
你清唔清楚 ? (Cantonese)
nei5 cing1-m4-cing1co2
you clear not clear
'Are you clear or not?'

Wh-questions are used to seek specific information. The wh-word, i.e. the question word, remains in the sentence at the position where the required information would be provided in the corresponding statement.

(22) 你吃甚麼？(Mandarin)
ni3 chi1 shen2me0
你食乜嘢？(Cantonese)
nei5 sik6 mat1je5
you eat what
'What do you eat?'

(23) 誰說的？
shei2 shuo1 de0 (Mandarin)
邊個講呀？
bin1go3 gong2 aa3 (Cantonese)
who say SFP
'Who said so?'

Previous sections describe the end state characteristics of some grammatical structures in Chinese. There has been a fair amount of work investigating how typical children learn these structures (see Lee, 1996 for review). Researchers have also begun to ask which of these structures might trip up children with language disorders, and why. Classifiers, aspect markers and complex sentences are examined in Cheung's study of two Mandarin-speaking children with specific language impairment (SLI). This is reported in Chapter 3. In Chapter 5, Fletcher, Leonard, Stokes and Wong review their work on Cantonese-speaking children with SLI, with a particular focus on aspect markers, wh-questions and passives. Deficits in grammatical morphology are well-documented in English-speaking children with SLI. Therefore, it is of interest to ask whether Chinese-speaking children with SLI also have problems with the few grammatical markers in the language they need to learn. Cantonese wh-words remain *in situ* and they do not need to move to the initial subject position, as is the case with English wh-questions. Does this make wh-questions less of a problem for Cantonese-speaking children with SLI? Answers to this question certainly contribute to the evaluation of current explanatory accounts of SLI. Wong and Stokes in Chapter 4 describe the development of A-not-A questions in a group of Cantonese-speaking children with SLI, and compare these findings with their earlier work on typical children. There are no parallels to Chinese A-not-A questions in English, and as Wong and Stokes pointed out, the nature of these questions leads us to consider additional factors for future investigations of language development in typical children and children with SLI.

The Chinese Orthographic System

The Chinese writing system is generally considered logographic in nature. Virtually all Chinese characters are monosyllabic, and the great majority of them represent morphemes; hence, the Chinese script is also described as a morphosyllabic system. Chinese characters are made up of spatial arrangements of strokes, which combine to form larger units called radicals. Radicals may further combine to form complex characters. At present, there are two co-existing Chinese scripts. Traditional characters are used in Hong Kong and Taiwan, whereas simplified characters are used in Mainland China. The Writing Reform to simplify traditional characters started around the middle of the 1950s. An official list of over 2000 simplified characters was issued in 1964 by the Chinese Committee on Writing Reform. The implementation of teaching these simplified characters took place a little later (Hannas, 1997). The characteristics of characters discussed later apply to both the traditional and simplified scripts.

Over 80% of all characters are so-called phonetic compounds, containing a signific radical and a phonetic radical. The signific radical provides a clue to the meaning of the character, whereas the phonetic radical provides a cue to its pronunciation. For instance, the character 湖 *hu2* 'lake' has a signific radical (three dots) on the left meaning 'water/liquid' and a phonetic radical 胡 on the right whose pronunciation *hu2* is the same as the character, making it a regular character. Although Chinese is a lexical tone language, tones are not marked orthographically. In modern day usage, about 26% of phonetic compounds in Mandarin are regular characters (Zhu, 1987). Xing (2002) also reported that approximately 25% of characters taught in elementary schools are regular. Law (1997) surveyed more than 12,000 phonetic compounds listed in a Cantonese dictionary and found that about 34% of the entries are identical in sound (including tone) to their phonetic radical. Regarding the structure of a character, in addition to the left–right configuration (e.g. 河), which accounts for 72% of the 1491 phonetic compounds examined by Shu *et al.* (2003), a phonetic compound may have a top–bottom structure (e.g. 箕), which is found in 18% of the complex characters. Moreover, Shu *et al.* report that the phonetic radical of horizontally structured phonetic compounds appears on the right 90% of the time, while the phonetic radical of characters with a vertical structure is equally likely to appear at the top or the bottom.

Although the phonetic radical can be said to supply phonological information on the sound of the character containing it, it must be emphasised that the situation is somewhat more complex. That is, it is not always possible to arrive at the correct pronunciation of such a character based on the phonetic radical for several reasons: (1) although in the majority of phonetic compounds, the phonetic radical appears on the right, it may occupy other positions of a character, e.g. the phonetic radical 其 *qi2* in 棋 *qi2*, 期 *qi1*, 基 *ji1* and 箕 *ji1*; (2) a character may contain more than one pronounceable constituent, e.g. 棋 (木 *muk4* and

其 *qi2*), 期 (其 *qi2* and 月 *yue4*); and (3) the phonetic radical is more often than not an unreliable cue according to the statistics in Mandarin and Cantonese just presented.

The description thus far has revealed a crucial difference between the Chinese script and alphabetic writing systems. Unlike alphabetic scripts where letters are associated with individual phonemes, there are no elements within a character that correspond to phonemes. The mapping between a character and its sound is at the level of a syllable. Given this divergence in form-sound mapping between Chinese and alphabetic systems, questions naturally arise about how the morpho-syllabic nature of Chinese characters may affect literacy development in children, or how it may constrain the architecture of the cognitive system supporting the recognition and production of written and spoken Chinese words and the structures of form representations. The former question is addressed in terms of the role of morphological awareness in reading development and in distinguishing subtypes of developmental dyslexia by Wu, Packard and Shu in Chapter 7. The issue is also considered in Chapter 8 by Klingebiel and Weekes, in a review of previous studies investigating how the nature of phonological awareness at the levels of phonemes, syllables and tones (in the case of Chinese) may help predict the development of reading across scripts. The authors also propose a model of literacy development in Chinese based on their discussion. Different theories of character naming have been put forth given the unique logograph-syllable meaning relationship in Chinese. In Chapter 11, Weekes, Su and Yin evaluate two particular frameworks, the triangular and lexical constituency models, in terms of how they account for reading error production by brain-injured adults with acquired dyslexia. In the last chapter of this volume, Weekes and Su further explore for the first time manifestation of reading disorders in Chinese–Mongolian bilingual and biscriptal individuals, and examine how the interaction between the representations of a logographic script and an alphabetic system may impact on the form of reading deficits.

Other Topics

In addition to the aforementioned chapters reporting studies motivated by linguistic and orthographic characteristics unique to the Chinese language, the remaining chapters address topics of significant clinical and theoretical values. Two chapters are concerned with clinical assessment. Klee, Wong, Stokes, Fletcher and Leonard in Chapter 6 present the findings of a survey of standardised tests of children with speech and language difficulties in Hong Kong and discuss their implications for evidence-based practice in clinical assessment. Kong and Law in Chapter 14 describe an objective measure, the first of its kind, for evaluating narrative production of Cantonese aphasic speakers, and illustrate the procedures involved in the validation of an assessment tool. Two chapters are related to word-finding difficulties in adult aphasic speakers, the most pervasive and persistent disorder experienced by virtually all language-impaired individuals. In Chapter 12, Law, Weekes, Yeung and Chiu examine, for the first time, the contribution of the age at which a word is learned (age-of-acquisition or AoA), among other variables that have been previously studied, toward predicting word retrieval success. The authors also consider the nature of the effects on lexical phonological and semantic representations. A treatment study of anomia employing a semantically based protocol is reported in Chapter 15 by Law, W. Wong and E. Wong. The application of the same therapy to anomic individuals with different underlying deficits allows the researchers to hypothesise about the factors that may predict treatment outcomes, a step toward a better understanding of the relationship between language therapies and impairments. In Chapter 13, W. Wong and Law present a study with the aim of resolving conflicting findings in the literature from individuals with semantic dementia, specifically the effects of integrity of semantic knowledge on verbal recall. The differential performance of two brain-injured participants with different degrees of impairment to temporarily retain semantic information sheds light on the situation, and thus highlights the potential theoretical contribution and significance of data from aphasic individuals.

Notes

1. The English term 'Mandarin' refers to the standard official language of Chinese as well as the largest dialect group that the standard language is based on. In this book, this term is used interchangeably with Putonghua, which refers only to the standard official language of Chinese.
2. An analytic language is a language where syntax and meaning are shaped more by the use of particles and word order rather than by inflection.
3. An isolating language is a language in which almost every word consists of a single morpheme.
4. A demonstrative can modify a noun without a measure word in Mandarin, but not in Cantonese.
5. They are also known as sortal classifiers in Erbaugh (2006).
6. Abbreviations of grammatical markers used: ASP, aspect marker; POSS, possessive marker, SFP, sentence-final particles.
7. The distinction of subject and topic has long been one of the most debated issues in the study of Chinese grammar. Detailed discussion can be found in Tsao (1979), Jiang (1991) and Shi (2000).
8. Liu (2001) demonstrates that Mandarin is more topic-prominent than Cantonese.
9. However, the adversity flavour of *bei* has been neutralised in modern writings. This phenomenon can be attributed to the influence of English.

References

Chao, Y.R. (1968) *A Grammar of Spoken Chinese.* Berkeley, CA: University of California Press.

Cheung, H-N. (2007) *A Grammar of Cantonese as Spoken in Hong Kong* (rev. edn). Hong Kong: The Chinese University Press. (In Chinese.)

Erbaugh, M. (2006) Chinese classifiers: Their use and acquisition. In P. Li, L.H. Tan, E. Bates and O. Tzeng (eds) *The Handbook of East Asian Psycholinguistics: Volume 1 Chinese* (pp. 39–51). Cambridge: Cambridge University Press.

Hannas, W.M. (1997) *Asia's Orthographic Dilemma.* Honolulu, HI: University of Hawaii Press.

Jiang, Z-X. (1991) Some aspects of the syntax of topic and subject in Chinese. Dissertation, University of Chicago.

Law, S.P. (1997) The role of the phonetic radical in constructing Chinese logographs: Data from Cantonese colloquial characters. Poster session presented at the 8th International Conference on Cognitive Processing of Asian Languages & Symposium on Brain, Cognition, and Communication, Nagoya, Japan, December.

Lee, T.H-T. (1996) Theoretical issues in language development and Chinese child language. In C.T.J. Huang and Y.H.A. Li (eds) *New Horizons in Chinese Linguistics* (pp. 293–356). Dordrecht: Kluwer Academic.

Liu, D-Q. (2001) The typological characteristics of Cantonese syntax. *Asia Pacific Journal of Language in Education* 2, 1–27. (In Chinese.)

Matthews, S. and Yip, V. (1994) *Cantonese: A Comprehensive Grammar.* London: Routledge.

Norman, J. (1988) *Chinese.* New York: Cambridge University Press.

Packard, J.L. (1993) *A Linguistic Investigation of Aphasic Chinese Speech.* Dordrecht and Boston, MA: Kluwer Academic.

Shi, D-X. (2000) Topic and topic-comment constructions in Mandarin Chinese. *Language* 76, 383–408.

Shu, H., Chen, X., Andersen, R.C., Wu, N. and Xuan, Y. (2003) Properties of school Chinese: Implications for learning to read. *Child Development* 74, 27–47.

Tsao, F-F. (1979) *A Functional Study of Topic in Chinese: The First Step Towards Discourse Analysis.* Taipei: Student Book Co.

Xing, H. (2002) Analysis of phonetics in semantic-phonetic compound characters in elementary school textbooks and a self-organizing connectionist model of character acquisition in Chinese. Unpublished PhD thesis, Beijing Normal University.

Zhu, Y.P. (1987) Analysis of cueing functions of the phonetic in modern Chinese. Unpublished manuscript, East China Normal University.

Chapter 2

The Role of Phonological Saliency and Phonological Template in Typically and Atypically Developing Phonology: Evidence from Putonghua-speaking Children

HUA ZHU

Setting the Scene: Approaches in Cross-linguistic Studies

Cross-linguistic studies of phonological development have increased in the last 20 years. Most studies have taken a 'comparative' approach, whereby a researcher compares one language with another (in most cases English is used as the baseline), formulates hypotheses about the language under study and tests the applicability of theories or models usually developed in the context of English. Some of the more important concepts that are compared in these studies are 'markedness' and 'feature theory'.

Studies of this kind are valuable in that they can identify commonalities and differences in the developmental patterns across languages and provide baseline information for clinical diagnosis. For example, Zhu and Dodd (2006) compared the error patterns of monolingual speakers of English, German, Putonghua, Cantonese, Maltese, Colloquial Egyptian Arabic and Turkish, and bilingual speakers of Spanish/English, Cantonese/English, Pakistani heritage language/English, Welsh/English, Arabic/English and Cantonese/English. They found that children, despite their language backgrounds, tend to use an unmarked feature to replace a marked feature. This is evident in the error pattern of deaspiration (using unaspirated sounds to replace aspirated sounds) in Putonghua- and Cantonese-speaking monolingual children and Putonghua/Cantonese-speaking bilingual children, and in the occurrence of the error pattern of deaffrication (i.e. using fricatives to replace affricates) in English-, German-, Cantonese-, Maltese- and Turkish-speaking monolingual children and Cantonese/English, Putonghua/Cantonese and Pakistani heritage language/English-speaking bilingual children. The commonalities lend strong support to the existence of 'developmental universals'.

A small number of recent studies have adopted a different approach, referred to as an explore and discover approach, in which a researcher explores the role of language-specific features in the process of acquisition and develops language-specific terms to interpret findings. These studies are sensitive to language-specific features and are thus capable of explaining language-specific developmental patterns for which theories or concepts developed on the basis of English cannot account. Following this approach, the concept of phonological saliency (PS), which will be elaborated in the following section, was developed to account for the unique characteristics in the developmental phonology of Putonghua-speaking children (Zhu, 2002b; Zhu & Dodd, 2000b).

In order to advance the field of cross-linguistic research, there is a need to integrate these two different approaches. This chapter will examine in detail two theoretical concepts, i.e. PS and phonological template (PT), using data from Putonghua speakers. PS was originally developed in the context of Putonghua, while PT was initially defined as nascent phonological systems or systematic adaptation of the adult form to explain the developmental pattern of English-speaking children (Macken, 1979; Vihman, 2001). Analysis of the Putonghua data in this chapter will show how these concepts work together to account for the unique developmental patterns associated with Putonghua-speaking children and the underlying deficits observed in speech disorders.

Putonghua Phonology

One major challenge facing clinical studies across languages is the categorisation of the language under study. It is often the case that the linguistic system of languages other than English is understudied and labels or terminologies that have been developed in the English context may not be suitable for other languages. Further to the introduction to Chinese phonology in the second section in Chapter 1, it should also be noted that Putonghua has pitch variation within an entire utterance, i.e. intonation. The main intonational patterns include falling (which is typically used to express confirmation, exclamation, etc.), rising (used in questions, calling for attention, etc.), flat (used in statements, description and ordinary conversation) and curved (expressing complicated emotion, exaggeration, surprise, etc.). Intonation is realised mainly on the tail, not on the head or the nucleus of an utterance. Table 2.1 gives an overview of a Putonghua syllable, on which discussion in the rest of this chapter is based.

Overview of Findings on Normally Developing and Disordered Phonology

In order to assess and diagnose the nature and severity of disordered speech and language, we need to know as much as we can about the

Table 2.1 An overview of a Putonghua syllable

Syllable structure	*$C_{0-1}V$ C_{0-1}+tone*
Lexical tones	T1 high level T2 rising T3 falling-rising T4 high falling
Syllable-initial consonants	p, pʰ, t, tʰ, k, kʰ m, n f, s, ɕ, x, ʂ l, ɹ ts, tsʰ, tɕ, tɕʰ, tʂ, tʂʰ
Syllable-initial clusters	None
Syllable-final consonants	n, ŋ
Vowels	i, y, u, ɤ, o, ᴀ, ɛ,ə,ɚ ae, ei, ɑo, ou, ia, iɛ, ua, uo, yɛ iɑo, iou, uae, uei

normal developmental patterns. This would subsequently permit a systematic study of abnormal development.

Normally developing phonology

A number of studies have examined the order of acquisition of phonemes, tones and error patterns among Putonghua-speaking monolingual children. These findings are briefly summarised next (for a more detailed review, see Zhu, 2002b).

(1) In terms of order of acquisition of different syllable components, tones are acquired first, then syllable-final consonants and vowels, and syllable-initial consonants are acquired last[1].
(2) Syllable structure: core syllables CV and reduplicated core syllables CVCVCV are dominant in children's early speech with the error pattern of final consonant deletion being a very common process (Chen & Kent, 2005; Zhu & Dodd, 2000b). The syllable structures of V and CVC develop later.
(3) Early acquisition of tones: tone errors are very rare beyond two years of age. Among four tones, high level/high falling tones emerge (a feature is considered to have emerged when it is produced correctly at least once in the speech) first, while falling-rising tones are the last to emerge (Clumeck, 1980; Zhu, 2002b).
(4) Vowels: simple vowels emerge early, while triphthongs and diphthongs are prone to systematic errors among young children.

(5) Consonants: phonetic acquisition of the 21 syllable-initial consonants is nearly complete by 3;6 (year;month), while most children can use syllable-initial consonants correctly on two thirds of occasions with the exception of four affricates and one retroflex fricative by 4;6.
(6) Error patterns: similar to English-speaking children, Putonghua-speaking young children have a tendency to produce structural and systemic simplifications in their production. However, there are also cross-linguistic differences in the error patterns. For example, syllable-initial consonant deletion and backing are evident in the speech of normally developing Putonghua-speaking children, but atypical in the error patterns of English-speaking children.

Adding to the growing body of research on monolingual children, some studies have been carried out on the phonological development of multilingual children acquiring Putonghua simultaneously with other languages. So and Leung (2006) and Law and So (2006) explored the phonological development of both Putonghua and Cantonese among Putonghua/Cantonese-speaking bilingual children. Both studies reported that language dominance plays a role in bilingual children's phonological development. Yang and Zhu (in press) examined the phonological development of trilingual children acquiring Putonghua, Taiwanese and Spanish, and argued that language input and the extent of language use influence the way that phonology is acquired across languages.

Pollock *et al.* (2003) compared speech and language development in English in two English/Putonghua-speaking bilingual children adopted from China by US families. They argue that the differences between these two children can be attributed to the age at the time of adoption, quality and quantity of prelinguistic vocalisations and general cognitive abilities. These studies not only identify some unique features associated with the phonological acquisition of Putonghua among children learning other language(s), but also uncover influential factors in the process of phonological acquisition in general.

Disordered phonology of Putonghua-speaking children

Prevalence figures regarding developmental speech disorder in English-speaking children range from 3% to 10% (Gierut, 1998) and almost 70% of children attending paediatric speech-language therapy clinics have speech disorder not language disorder (Weiss *et al.*, 1987). Speech disorders, if left untreated, can have serious immediate and long-term consequences for the children involved. A phonological disorder may impede the development of other language skills such as syntax, morphology, lexicon and literacy, and have adverse effect on the children's psychosocial development (Leonard, 1995). Even though these children can recover spontaneously with age to a certain extent (Zhu & Dodd, 2000a), they tend to have poor performance on a range of speech, reading, spelling and phoneme awareness tasks even during adolescence and adulthood (Lewis & Freebairn, 1992).

Despite this, in China 'speech disorder' is rarely known in nurseries and schools. It is reported that professionals working with children tend to associate low speech intelligibility with laziness and believe that children will 'grow out of' the problem given time. The lack of awareness of speech disorder among health and teaching professionals is by no means incidental. It is also reflected in the poor provision of speech therapy service in China and sometimes inappropriate diagnosis and subsequent treatment of children with speech difficulties. Speech therapy resources are still to be developed in China and where resources are available, priority is given to hearing impairment. It is reported that among the several speech and hearing clinics newly opened in China, almost all of them are aimed at providing audiological service for the hearing impaired (Cheng, 2001). The lack of understanding of the nature of speech difficulties often leads to clinical misdiagnosis. Xu and Ha (1992) reported that children with speech difficulties in some clinics had been unanimously misdiagnosed as having a short frenum and their unintelligible speech did not improve after the frenum had been cut. A number of studies have investigated the disordered phonology of Putonghua-speaking children with speech disorder. Zhu and Dodd (2000c) examined the phonological systems of 33 Putonghua-speaking children with functional speech disorder. Compared with normal development, disordered phonology is characterised by persisting developmental error patterns, unusual error types, restricted phonetic and phonemic inventories, systematic sound or syllable preference and, in some children, inconsistent production of the same words. The existence of these characteristics allows the classification of four subgroups of articulation disorder, delayed development, consistent disorder and inconsistent disorder following Dodd's (1995/2006) classification system of phonological disorder. These are:

(1) Articulation disorder: consistent distortion of a phone either in isolation or in any phonetic context. For example, in the data reported by Zhu and Dodd (2000c), a girl aged 7;6 has difficulty articulating /s/ both in word contexts and in isolation. She tends to substituted [θ], a non-Mandarin phoneme, for /s/. There is no apparent organic cause for her impairment; there is no anatomical anomaly and she passes oro-motor, hearing and visual-motor integration (VMI) screening tests.

(2) Delayed phonological development: defined as the use of consistent error patterns that are inappropriate for the child's chronological age, but appropriate for a younger child. The delayed error patterns reported in Zhu and Dodd's (2000c) study include consonant assimilation, syllable-initial deletion, fronting, stopping, affrication, X-velarisation and gliding. These error patterns do not occur among more than 10% of the children of the same age band in the normative data, but are frequently used by more than 10% of children in a younger age band.

(3) Consistent disorder: defined as the use of consistent error patterns that are atypical of normal phonological development (e.g. deleting all syllable-initial consonants, marking consonant clusters with a bilabial fricative in the English context). A range of unusual error patterns are used by the Putonghua-speaking children diagnosed with consistent phonological disorder in Zhu and Dodd's data (2000c). They are syllable-final consonant addition, replacing the syllable-final velar /ŋ/ with alveolar nasal [n], substituting alveolar and retroflex affricates for the velar stop [k] and vice versa, reducing affricates to fricatives at the same place of articulation.

(4) Inconsistent disorder: defined as variable pronunciation of the same words or phonological features (e.g. /ɕyon2 mɑo1/熊貓 in Putonghua is realised as [ia mɑo], [in mɑo], or [tʌ mɑo][2]). Variation due to alternation between a normal developmental error and a correct production is not counted as inconsistent production.

The individual profiles of the Putonghua-speaking children with functional speech disorder suggest that children differ significantly in terms of the size of phonetic and phoneme inventories, types of error pattern and degree of inconsistency. However, these children also exhibit some similarities. Firstly, despite the diversity of error types, the Putonghua-speaking children with speech disorder seldom make tonal errors; only a very small percentage of the children make vowel errors and use delayed processes affecting syllable-final consonants. Most errors affect syllable-initial consonants. Secondly, certain sounds (e.g. velar stops /k/ and /kʰ/, retroflexes and affricates) are often absent from disordered phoneme inventories in Putonghua-speaking children. It is not surprising that children with speech acquisition difficulties have problems with sounds such as retroflexes and affricates, as normally developing children also have difficulties with these sounds. This is evident both in late acquisition of these sounds and high frequency of fronting and backing processes in the normative sample. However, velar stops /k/ and /kʰ/ are exceptional. While 90% of children in the normative sample have mastered the stops by 3;6 years, 13 (39%) of the children with speech disorder in the sample were found unable to use velar stops, e.g. /k/ and /k^h/ either phonologically or phonetically correctly (Zhu & Dodd, 2000c).

Impaired phonology is also known to be characteristic of the communication profiles of hearing-impaired children. Zhu and Dodd (2001) reported a longitudinal case study of a Putonghua-speaking child with severe prelingual hearing impairment between the age of 3;5 and 4;5. The analysis of his single-word speech showed that he had complete syllable-final consonants and vowel repertories. His acquisition of tones was within normal range. However, he had difficulties with syllable-initial consonants. There were several illegal phones present in his speech and his phonemic inventory was restricted to a small number of phonemes. He also frequently used a syllable-initial consonant deletion process, and delayed and unusual error patterns were evident in his speech. Compared with his single-word spontaneous speech, his connected speech had lower intelligibility with a frequent occurrence of glottal stops between syllables and repetitions.

Despite these findings, there are still gaps in our knowledge about Putonghua-speaking children with speech disorder. Cheng (2004) reviewed the speech and language issues in assessing children from Asian–Pacific backgrounds, including attitudes towards disability and treatment methods, child-rearing practices and social cultural norms in conversation and practice. Many of these issues are relevant to Chinese-speaking children. Zhu (2002a) identified three areas that need urgent attention from researchers. First of all, there is a lack of normative data that is sensitive to sociolinguistic factors, such as gender, socioeconomic background, dialects and bilingual conditions. Secondly, there is also a lack of standardised speech and language tests that can profile the child's speech and language impairments and inform diagnosis and intervention. Thirdly, treatment efficacy studies are needed to examine the effect of different treatment approaches on Putonghua-speaking children who are acquiring a language with many characteristics different from English. To sum up, the research findings on both normally and atypically developing phonology of Putonghua-speaking children indicate that there are similarities and differences between the Putonghua-speaking children and children acquiring the phonology of other languages. The next section will seek to interpret these existing similarities and differences by examining the concepts of PS and PT.

Theoretical Account

The role of PS

One unique feature in the phonological acquisition of Putonghua-speaking children lies in the order of acquisition of syllable components.

It is evident in both normally and atypically developing phonology that among four Putonghua syllable components, tones are acquired earliest and are most resistant to impairment; vowels also emerge early and are very resistant to impairment; syllable-final consonants are acquired earlier than syllable-initial consonants and are less subject to impairment than syllable-initial consonants; and finally, syllable-initial consonants are the last component to be acquired and are also vulnerable to impairment.

To account for the order of acquisition of syllable components in a tonal language such as Putonghua, Zhu (2002b) proposed a syllable-based, language-specific concept, i.e. PS. PS is determined and affected by:

(1) The status of a component in the syllable structure, especially whether it is compulsory or optional; a compulsory component is more salient than an optional one.
(2) The capacity of a component to differentiate lexical meaning in a syllable; a component which is more capable of distinguishing lexical information is more salient than one which carries less lexical information.
(3) The number of permissible choices within a component in the syllable structure, e.g. 21 syllable-initial consonants would be considered *less* salient compared to four tonal contrasts.

Accordingly, in Putonghua, tones have the highest saliency: it is compulsory for every syllable; change of tones would result in a different lexical meaning; and there are only four alternative choices. The high saliency value carried by tones explains why tones are acquired earliest and are least subject to impairment among the four syllable components. Syllable-final consonants have lower saliency value than tones because they are an optional syllable component. However, they have a higher saliency value than syllable-initial consonants because there are only two syllable-final consonants (i.e. /n, ŋ/). Similar to syllable-final consonants, vowels, being a compulsory syllable component, have a higher saliency value than syllable-initial consonants. Syllable-initial consonants have the lowest saliency: their presence in a syllable is optional and there is a range of 21 syllable-initial phonemes that can be used. The rankings are backed up by empirical findings showing that syllable-final consonants and vowels are acquired earlier and are less subject to impairment compared with syllable-initial consonants.

The role of PS in the acquisition of various syllable components is also supported by empirical findings in other languages such as Cantonese, where data are available in a comparable format. Although both syllable-initial and syllable-final consonants are optional to a syllable, there are more permissible choices at syllable-initial position than syllable-final (17 syllable-initial consonants compared with six syllable-final consonants) and therefore syllable-final position has higher PS than syllable-initial position. This explains the order of acquisition of syllable components reported in So and Dodd (1995) and So (2006).

The role of PTs

The review in the third section highlights many unique patterns evident in the process of phonological acquisition of Putonghua-speaking children. While PS is successful in interpreting some phenomena, there are many other patterns that are unexplained. For example, some children have a preference for a particular type of syllable structure or a sound in their production; some children tend to make errors at the syllable level by deleting either syllable-initial or -final or using the same sounds across two adjacent syllables. Similar patterns are reported in the speech of children speaking other languages. To account for these phenomena, some researchers, based on English data, propose that in acquiring phonology, children construct PTs, i.e. nascent phonological systems or systematic adaptations of the adult form (Vihman, 2001). PTs are believed to be the chief organising principle that allows the child's flexible use of syllable deletion, harmony (a sound becomes more similar to an adjacent sound) and metathesis (a sound swaps with an adjacent sound) (Macken, 1979). Evidence from English suggests that PTs emerge at the early stage of phonological acquisition (Vihman), and disappears gradually as the child is slowly expanding his or her range of phonological gestures (Macken). However, given significant individual variation in children's acquisition, we do not know about the universality of PTs, i.e. whether it is a necessary stage for *all* children acquiring a language, including normally developing children and children with speech difficulties. Nor do we know about the language-specific features of PTs.

In order to explore these issues, Zhu and Li (2002) examined longitudinal data from four normally developing Putonghua-speaking children who were about one years old at the beginning of data collection. They found that PTs operate both at syllabic and subsyllable levels. At the syllabic level, a CV syllable structure seems to be dominant in the children's production, with many words in the syllable shape of CV. In addition, evidence for the use of subsyllable templates is also found in some children's speech, though individual variations and preference may play a greater role. While no dominant PTs can be observed in the speech of two children in their study (i.e. Z.J. & H.Y.), PTs seem to begin operating after the four-word point in the other two children's speech, plays an active role at 15- and 25-word point, and then disappears/expands into adult phonology when production begins to be

Table 2.2 Phonological templates identified at syllable and subsyllable level

Subjects	*Stage*	*Template*	*Example*	*Other patterns*
J.J.	15 words	$C_{anterior}V$	kua: pᴀ tɕitɕioʊ: titioʊ tsaitɕiɛn: taitiɛ	Frequent reduplication
Z.J.	15/25 words	None observed		Initial consonant deletion
H.Y.		None observed		
Z.W.	15 words	$(C_{anterior})V$ (C)		
	25 words	(t)ᴀ (t)iᴀ (t)uᴀ	ɕiɑŋ: tᴀ sɑŋ: iᴀ tu: tᴀ	

more rule-governed and more sensitive to the target words at 50-word point.[3]

Other similarities exist between these two children. Both children use a template of $C_{anterior}V$ at 15-word point and they tend to produce an anterior consonant in front of vowels, e.g. [pa] for /kua1/瓜; [taitiɛ] for /tsae4 tɕiɛn4/再見. Table 2.2 summarises the PTs identified both at the syllable and subsyllable levels.

In summary, the successful application of the concept of PTs to Putonghua data lends support to the validity of the concept. However, it also highlights individual and language variations in terms of the specific templates that are used across languages and the stages in which templates occur and expand into adult forms.

A case study of a child with disordered speech

In the previous sections, we demonstrated how PS and PT account for different patterns associated with the phonological development of normally developing Putonghua-speaking children. In this section, we describe a case study of a child diagnosed with a phonological disorder in Putonghua to demonstrate how PS and PTs can work together in interpreting the disordered speech of atypically developing children.

In a study on the phonological systems of Putonghua-speaking children with functional speech disorders, Zhu and Dodd (2000c) profiled the speech of 33 children who were initially referred to the researchers by their nursery or school teachers and later diagnosed as having functional speech disorders. L.C. is one of the 33 children, whose case history and phonology is summarised next.

Case history of L.C. (3;7 boy)

L.C. is from Beijing and is the only child in his family. He attends nursery five days a week. He was referred to the researchers by his nursery teacher because of difficulties 'being understood'. His language comprehension, as reported by his nursery teacher, was within the normal range. The screening tests (including pure tone audiometry, oromotor examination, VMI test) found no abnormalities with his hearing, oral structure or learning abilities. His phonology was assessed using a picture-naming and description task (Phonological Assessment of Chinese; Zhu, 2002b).

L.C.'s phonological profile

His overall speech was characterised by poor intelligibility and high inconsistency. His percentage of consonants in error (PCE) was very high and is 8.88 standard deviations below the average PCE of normally developing children. There were a number of deviant substitutions that are very uncommon in normally developing children. For example, [p] for /k/; [t] for [ɕ]; [l] for /ʂ/. His inconsistency rating, which compares the productions of the same words, is 76%, the highest among the group of children diagnosed with speech disorder. For example, in his speech, /ɕin1/心 realised as [iŋ], [tia] or [tin]; /ts^{h}ae4/菜 realised as [sae], [xae], [t^{h}ia] or [tsuo]; and /ɕyoŋ2 mɑo1/熊貓 realised as [ia mɑo], [in mɑo] or [tᴀ mɑo]. Due to the frequent variable productions, he was diagnosed as having an inconsistent disorder (Dodd, 1995/2006).

Compared with normally developing children of the same age, L.C. has much smaller phonetic and phonemic inventories. While 75% of normally developing children are able to articulate all the sounds in Putonghua at least once correctly, L.C. is unable to produce 11 phones (/t^{h}, k, k^{h}, p^{h}, s, tɕ^{h}, ʂ, tʂ, tʂ^{h}, ts, ts^{h}/). There are 15 phonemes (/t^{h}, x, ɕ, k, k^{h}, p^{h}, l, s, tɕ, tɕ^{h}, ʂ, tʂ, tʂ^{h}, ts, ts^{h}/) missing from his phonemic inventory and he is able to use only seven phonemes correctly.

L.C. has a restricted syllable structure and most of his words are in the shape of either vowel (V) or consonant-vowel (CV). Reduplications frequently occur in his speech: substituting [tia], [tɕia] or [tɕa] for a large number of different syllables while retaining the original tones (e.g 燈/təŋ1/[tia1]; 床/tʂ^{h}uɑŋ2/[tia2]; 裙子/tɕ^{h}yn2 tsi0/[tɕia2 tɕᴀ0]). In addition, assimilation occurs frequently in his speech. Adjacent syllables in his speech very often share the same initial consonant and sometimes the same vowel (e.g. 香蕉/ɕiɑŋ1 tɕiɑo1/[tiɑ tiɑo]; 男孩/nᴀn2 xae2/[nia nia]; 再見/tsae4 tɕiɛn4/[tʂa tʂiɑŋ]).

Interpretation

The characteristics associated with L.C.'s disordered speech can be explained by the concept of PS and PTs. There are two PTs evident in his speech: one at subsyllable level and the other at the syllabic level. A template of $C_{[t,\ tɕ]}\ V_{[a,\ ia]}$ is operating at the subsyllable level: L.C. replaces a large number of different syllables with [tia], [tɕia] or [tɕᴀ]. The second one is at the syllabic level: he has a very restricted syllable shape-V and CV. Consequently, assimilations across the syllables occur and syllable reduplications frequently take place.

As discussed earlier, PTs tend to occur in the early stage of speech development and gradually expand or mature to approximate the adult system. The templates, which were found at the 15- or 25-word point of two normally developing children, begin to disappear at the 50-word point well before the children turn two years of age. However, in L.C.'s case, his PT seems to be 'frozen' at the age of 3;7. A similar PT is used by one of the normally developing children at an early stage. This seems to suggest that if a child's PTs 'fossilise' at a particular point in the normal process of development, s/he will experience delay or disorder.

Despite the serious phonological difficulties, L.C.'s tone production remains intact. While his productions are restricted to words conforming to PTs and result in a range of errors both with consonants and vowels, he is able to use tones correctly for target words. As we argued earlier, tones in Putonghua have the highest PS value. Consequently, the prosodic level is apparently the most resistant to impairment.

Conclusion

This chapter examines the applicability of two key concepts (i.e. PS and PT) in the context of Putonghua. The case study of a child diagnosed with inconsistent speech disorder demonstrates how these two key concepts can work together to interpret unique features associated with Putonghua-speaking children. Specifically, it shows that while both typically and atypically developing children will be constrained by PS in their phonological development, the fossilisation of PTs may result in 'delay' or 'disorder' in the phonological system.

By illustrating how the two key concepts, developed on the basis of different languages, can work together, the chapter proposes a new paradigm in cross-linguistic studies, i.e. an integrated approach. It is important to test the applicability or universality of a theory or model developed in a particular language in other languages. It is equally important, and perhaps more imperative given the paucity of theories or models developed in this approach, to explore the role of language-specific features in developmental patterns and develop language-specific concepts or models to understand speech-related language problems in Chinese.

Notes

1. Initial consonants are present in children's productions before (and more frequently than) final consonants, but they are not produced accurately until after the final consonants have become accurate.
2. /ʌ/ is a phonetic symbol representing a low central vowel that often occurs in Putonghua open syllables.
3. 4-, 15- and 25-word points, as defined in Vihman (1996), are production points where the child spontaneously attempts to produce at least 4, 15 or 25 different adult word types.

References

Chen, L.M. and Kent, R. (2005) Consonant-vowel co-occurrence patterns in Mandarin-learning infants. *Journal of Child Language* 32, 507–534.

Cheng, L.L.R. (2001) Educating speech-language pathologists to work in multicultural populations. An Asian-Pacific perspective. *Speech and Hearing Review* 2, 192–213.

Cheng, L.L.R. (2004) Speech and language issues in children from Asian-Pacific backgrounds. In R. Kent (ed.) *The MIT Encyclopedia of Communication Disorder* (pp. 167–169). Cambridge, MA: The MIT Press.

Clumeck, H. (1980) The acquisition of tone. In G. Yeni-Komshian, J. Kavanagh and C. Ferguson (eds) *Child Phonology 1* (pp. 257–276). New York: Academic Press.

Dodd, B. (1995/2006) *Differential Diagnosis and Treatment of Children with Speech Disorder.* London: Whurr.

Gierut, J. (1998) Treatment efficacy: Functional phonological disorders in children. *Journal of Speech, Language and Hearing Research* 41, S85–100.

Law, N. and So, L.K.H. (2006) Relations of the phonological development of children bilingual in Cantonese and Putonghua to the language dominance in their acquisition setting. *International Journal of Bilingualism* 10, 405–428.

Leonard, L. (1995) Phonological impairment. In P. Fletcher and B. MacWhinney (eds) *The Handbook of Child Language* (pp. 572–602). Cambridge, MA: Blackwell.

Lewis, B.A. and Freebairn, L. (1992) Residual effects of preschool phonology disorders in grade school, adolescence, and adulthood. *Journal of Speech, Language and Hearing Research* 35, 819–831.

Macken, M.A. (1979) Developmental reorganisation of phonology: A hierarchy of basic units of acquisition. *Lingua* 49, 11–49.

Pollock, K., Price, J. and Fulmer, K. (2003) Speech-language acquisition in children adopted from China: A longitudinal investigation of two children. *Journal of Multilingual Communication Disorders* 1, 184–193.

So, L.K.H. (2006) Cantonese phonological development: Normal and disordered. In H. Zhu and B. Dodd (eds) *Phonological Development and Disorders in Children: A Multilingual Perspective* (pp. 109–134). Clevedon: Multilingual Matters.

So, L.K.H. and Dodd, B. (1995) The acquisition of phonology by Cantonese-speaking children. *Journal of Child Language* 22, 473–495.

So, L.K.H. and Leung, C.S.S. (2006) Phonological development of Cantonese-Putonghua bilingual children. In H. Zhu and B. Dodd (eds) *Phonological*

Development and Disorders in Children: A Multilingual Perspective (pp. 413–428). Clevedon: Multilingual Matters.

Vihman, M. (1996) *Phonological Development*. Oxford: Blackwell.

Vihman, M. (2001) Early word patterns or 'templates': Monolingual and bilingual children. Paper presented at the 3rd International Symposium on Bilingualism, University of the West of England, Bristol, April.

Weiss, C., Gordon, M. and Lillywhite, H. (1987) *Clinical Management of Articulatory and Phonological Disorders*. Baltimore, MD: Williams and Wilkins.

Xu, F. and Ha, P.A. (1992) Articulation disorders among speakers of Mandarin Chinese. *American Journal of Speech-Language Pathology* 1, 15–16.

Yang, H.Y. and Zhu, H. (in press) The phonological development of a trilingual child: facts and factors. *International Journal of Bilingualism.*

Zhu, H. (2002a) Mandarin-speaking children with developmental speech disorders. *Speech and Hearing Review* 3, 245–276.

Zhu, H. (2002b) *Phonological Development in Specific Contexts: Studies of Chinese-speaking Children*. Clevedon: Multilingual Matters.

Zhu, H. and Dodd, B. (2000a) Development and change in the phonology of Putonghua-speaking children with speech difficulties. *Clinical Linguistics and Phonetics* 14, 351–368.

Zhu, H. and Dodd, B. (2000b) The phonological acquisition of Putonghua (Modern Standard Chinese). *Journal of Child Language* 27, 3–42.

Zhu, H. and Dodd, B. (2000c) Putonghua (Modern Standard Chinese)-speaking children with speech disorder. *Clinical Linguistics & Phonetics* 14, 165–191.

Zhu, H. and Dodd, B. (2001) Phonological development of a Putonghua-speaking child with prelingual hearing impairment: A longitudinal case study. *Asia Pacific Journal of Speech Language and Hearing* 6, 197–213.

Zhu, H. and Dodd, B. (eds) (2006) *Phonological Development and Disorders in Children: A Multilingual Perspective*. Clevedon: Multilingual Matters.

Zhu, H. and Li, W. (2002) Phonological templates: Evidence from Chinese-speaking children. Poster session presented at the 23rd Annual Symposium on Research in Child Language Disorders and the 9th Congress International Association for the Study of Child Language, Madison, July.

Chapter 3

Grammatical Characteristics of Mandarin-speaking Children with Specific Language Impairment

HINTAT CHEUNG

Introduction

Children with specific language impairment (SLI) have unexplained difficulties in acquiring their mother tongue (Bishop, 1997). Their problems are not caused by any known factors, such as mental retardation, hearing impairment, social isolation or emotional disturbance. One of the hallmarks of English-speaking children with SLI is their low percentages of grammatical morpheme usage, such as past tense *-ed* and third person singular *-s*, when compared with language-matched controls. Various hypotheses have been proposed to account for such deficits. The 'extended optional infinitives', based on a modular view of language, suggests that SLI children suffer from a specific deficit in their underlying linguistic knowledge (Rice *et al.*, 1995). Other researchers argue that these children suffer from various limitations in language processing, such as a deficit in processing auditory stimuli that are brief in duration and are presented with short intervals (Tallal & Piercy, 1973), or a smaller phonological working memory that is measured by their performance in repeating nonwords (Gathercole & Baddeley, 1990). Since part of this debate is formulated around the acquisition of inflectional morphemes, language data from Chinese SLI children will bring a new perspective to the issue because inflectional morphology does not play a role in the development of grammar for Chinese. Without the pressure of building inflectional paradigms for verbs, Chinese SLI children should face different types of difficulties in the process of language acquisition. It will also be of interest to examine the accountability of these problems with theories mainly developed from English SLI data. While reports on the linguistic problems of Mandarin-speaking children with SLI (MSLI) are virtually nonexistent, several SLI studies have been implemented in the Cantonese-speaking population. It has been reported that Cantonese-speaking children with SLI are inferior to the language-matched children (Stokes & Fletcher, 2000) as well as age-peers (Stokes & Fletcher, 2003) in using aspectual forms. Their performance in passive constructions was below age-matched controls, but was better than language-matched peers (Leonard *et al.*, 2006). Previously, Wong and colleagues also reported that Cantonese-speaking children with SLI were outperformed by both language- and age-matched controls in their usage of who-object questions, but these three groups did not differ from each other in the use of who-subject questions (Wong *et al.*, 2004). Their vocabulary and MLU were also below age expectancy (Klee *et al.*, 2004) and displayed qualitative differences in using classifiers (Stokes & So, 1997). As Mandarin is very similar to Cantonese in terms of its grammatical structure, it is expected that MSLI children will also exhibit the same qualities in the previously mentioned linguistic areas. However, it is likewise possible that MSLI children are affected in other areas that have not yet been examined, some that may have specific ties to Mandarin.

As a pioneer study, the grammatical characteristics of two MSLI children will be explored in the present work. Spontaneous language samples collected from two seven-year-olds with MSLI will be examined and two research questions will be asked:

(1) Given that there is little inflectional morphology in Mandarin, what aspects of the grammatical system do Mandarin-speaking children with SLI suffer?
(2) Does their language resemble younger, typically developing children?

Scope of Investigation

As very little is known about the grammatical development of Mandarin-speaking children with SLI, the present study is largely built upon understandings for typically developing children. Several grammatical structures, which are possible indicators of grammatical capacity in elaborating nouns, verbs and clauses, are identified in children. At the noun phrase level, the use of a classifier is selected. In Mandarin, classifiers are optional most of the time except when a numeral word which is larger than one is expressed. For example, if a child says 兩杯子 *liang3 bei1zi5* 'two cups' instead of 兩個杯子 *liang3 ge5 bei1zi5* 'two classifier (CL) cups', all native speakers will be able to detect the error of omission. As for verbs, although the use of aspect markers is optional in Chinese, they have been examined for the purpose of comparing research findings between SLI children in Cantonese and English (Stokes & Fletcher, 2000, 2003). Finally, the use of complex sentences is selected as an index of grammatical development at the clause level. Complex sentences are used by Chinese children as early as age two (Hsu, 1986). Such speedy mastery in complex sentences contrasts sharply with the grammatical development in English. Therefore, the possibility of Mandarin-speaking children with SLI being spared from disability in this regard when they do not need inflectional morphology will be examined. Descriptions of these grammatical components are provided in the next three sections.

Noun: Classifiers

Structurally speaking, a noun classifier in Mandarin is placed between a numeral and a noun, such as 件 *jian4* in the noun phrase 一件衣服 *yi2 jian4 yi1fu1* 'one CL clothes'. Five types of classifiers are distinguished with respect to the denoted semantic content, including measure, kind, sortal, collective and event classifiers (Erbaugh, 2006). Measure classifiers are related to the quantity of the head noun. For example, 里 *li3* 'mile' in 一里路 *yi4 li3 lu4* 'one mile of road' refers to the length of the road. Kind classifiers are commonly used to highlight certain unspecified classifying principles that are involved, such as 種 *zhong3* 'kind' in 一種牛 *yi4 zhong3 niu2* 'one kind of ox'. Collective classifiers describe arrangement of objects, such as 疊 *die2* for 'a pile of'. Sortal classifiers focus on the shape of the object. In Mandarin, paper is usually used with the sortal classifier 張 *zhang1*, as in 一張紙 *yi4 zhang1 zhi3* 'a sheet of paper', when the flatness of the object is denoted. In reference to a pile of paper, the collective classifier 疊 *die2*, as in 一疊廢紙 *yi4 die2 fei4zhi3* 'a pile of discarded-paper' will be used. Event classifiers focus on the activity, such as 場 *chang3* 'showing' in 一場電影 *yi4 chang3 dian4ying2* 'a showing of movie'. Of all the classifiers, 個 *ge5* is the most common and it is also referred to as a general classifier for most semantically empty cases. For this reason, Myers (2000) argued that 個 *ge5* is the default in the classifier selection process. Since the use of sortal, collective, event and measure classifiers are subject to selection restrictions imposed by their head nouns, they are also called specific classifiers.

Erbaugh (1992) reported that Mandarin-speaking children rarely used specific classifiers before 2;6 (year;month) and the few occurring instances are lexical, with reference to a single object instead of an object category. Cheung and Fon (2002) reported that 11 different specific classifiers were used by a boy between 2;1 and 2;4, of which nine were used without head nouns. Hu (1993) found that children at age four started making overgeneralization errors, such as using 枝 *zhi1*, which denotes long and rigid objects, with belts, ties and jackets. In an experimental study, Hsu (2004) taught classifiers to a group of six-year-old children with language disorders. She found that children from the language disorder group produced more general classifiers than the control group (67% versus 42%) and some of them omitted the classifiers that were needed, a construction error not found in the controls.

In this study, the use of general classifiers and specific classifiers are tabulated in children. In addition, the combination of demonstrative

這 *zhe4* 'this' and general classifier 個 *ge5* is treated separately because 這個 *zhe4-ge5* is often used as a deictic pronoun and sometimes as a filler. If the two MSLI children had problems in lexical access, they may use 這個 *zhe4-ge5* to complete the lexical gap.

Aspect markers

Mandarin has no markers for tense although it has markers for aspects. In most Chinese grammar books, four aspect markers are identified: perfective 了 *le5*, progressive 在 *zai4*, durative 著 *zhe5* and experiential 過 *guo4* (see Table 3.1). Lin (1986) pointed out that verb reduplications, which encompass diminutive readings and the results component of the resultative verb compounds, e.g. 起來 *qi3lai2* 'start' in the compound word 打起來 *da3qi3lai2* 'start to fight', should also be included in the Mandarin aspectual system. However, since these markers have a rather low frequency of use in the language samples, a simple four-element aspect system serves the purpose for this study.

Another point for clarification on the aspectual system of Mandarin Chinese is the grammatical status of the form 了 *le5*. A sentence ending with the form 了 *le5* can be interpreted as a marker to highlight the 'current relevance' of the statement (Li & Thompson, 1981) and it is also called a sentence-final particle (SFP). This form of 了 *le5* can also have a

Table 3.1 Aspect markers in Mandarin

Type	*Marker*	*Example*
Perfective	*-le5*	我 戴 了 帽子 *wo3 dai4 le5 mao4zi5* I put-on ASP hat 'I have put on a hat'
Progressive	*zai4-*	我 在 戴 帽子 *wo3 zai4 dai4 mao4zi5* I ASP wear hat 'I am putting on a hat'
Durative	*-zhe5*	我 戴 著 帽子 *wo3 dai4 zhe5 mao3zi5* I wear ASP hat 'I wear a hat'
Experiential	*-guo4*	我 戴 過 帽子 *wo3 dai4 guo4 mao4zi5* I wear ASP hat 'I have put on a hat (before)'

Note. ASP, aspect marker

perfective reading when it follows a verb. For example, in the sentence 旗子拿下來了 *qi2zi5 na2 xia4lai2 le5* 'the flag has already been taken down', 了 *le5* has two functions. It is a perfective marker of the verb phrase 拿下來 *na2 xia4lai2* 'bring down' and a sentence-final particle that highlights the relevance of the statement. Erbaugh (1992: 426) pointed out that 'every *le* in the Taibei sample before MLU 2.5 is ambiguous. All are both verb and sentence final'. As a matter of fact, all the 了 *le*s found in the present study are placed right after verbs and most of them are both verb-final and utterance-final.

Of the four aspect markers, perfective 了 *le5* is reported as the first one used by Mandarin-speaking children (Erbaugh, 1992; Lin, 1986). Progressive 在 *zai4* and durative 著 *zhe5* usually emerge a month or two later. Experiential 過 *guo4* is the last one to be acquired. Associations are also found between grammatical aspect (aspect markers) and lexical aspect (verb semantics) in children's comprehension and production. Perfective aspect markers were better understood with telic verbs than with other verbs, such as process verbs (Li & Bowerman, 1998). In recent studies of the aspect system of Cantonese-speaking children with SLI (CSLI), CSLI children were found to be less productive in using aspect markers (Stokes & Fletcher, 2003) and were less likely to produce perfective and imperfective markers in contexts where these markers were favored by language controls (Fletcher *et al.*, 2005).

Complex sentence

A complex sentence consists of one independent clause and one or more dependent clauses. Li and Thompson (1981: 594) identified four types of sentences in Mandarin Chinese that contained two or more verb phrases with respect to conveyed meanings.[1] These four types of sentences can be reorganized into five groups when their structures are taken into consideration (see Table 3.2). Group (1) is serial verb construction. Serial verb constructions are single-clause sentences with two verb phrases. These two verb phrases share the initial noun phrase as their common subject. Group (2) is pivotal construction. The defining property for a pivotal construction is a noun phrase between the first verb and the second verb. This noun phrase serves as the grammatical object of the first verb as well as the grammatical subject of the second verb. For example, in the sentence 我請他過來 *wo3 qing3 ta1 guo4lai2* 'I invite him to come over', the second noun *ta1* 'he/him' is the object of the verb 請 *qing3* 'invite' and the subject of 過來 *guo4lai2* 'come over'. In some situations, a pivotal construction resembles a serial verb construction on the surface form when the first verb phrase of a serial verb construction contains an oblique object, such as 他去圖書館借書 *ta1 qü4 tu2shu1guan3 jie4 shu1* 'go to the library to borrow a book'. Structurally speaking, a

Table 3.2 Serial verb construction and complex sentences in Mandarin

Sentence type	*Example*
(1) Serial verb construction	穿 襪子 去 游泳 *chuan1 wa4zi5 qu4 you2yong3* wear sock go swimming 'He wore his socks and went swimming' (Howard 6;11)
(2) Pivotal construction	讓 我 修理 這個 *rang4 wo3 xiu1li3 zhe4ge5* let me fix this 'Let me fix this' (Howard 7;1)
(3) Clausal object	不 爱 睡 午覺 *Bu2 ai4 shui4 wu3-jiao4* NEG like sleep afternoon-sleep '(I) don't like taking a nap in the afternoon' (Ann 6;9)
(4) Clausal subject	這裡 用 正方形 才 可以 用 *zhe4li3 yong4 zheng4fang1xing2 cai2 ke3yi3 yong4* here use square only can use 'Placing a square here (you) can make it' (Ann 6;9)
(5) Descriptive clause	我 有 一 個 朋友 很 會 唱歌 *wo3 you3 yi2 ge4 peng2you3 hen3 hui4 chang4ge1* I have one CL friend very able sing 'I have a friend who can sing very well'

Note. NEG, negation

pivotal construction is a complex sentence while a serial verb construction is not. Yet, serial verb constructions are included in this analysis because in comparing the children's use of serial verb constructions with pivotal constructions, some understanding may be gained of their grammatical capacities in deriving proper clausal structures.

Group (3) is clausal object and Group (4) is clausal subject. These two groups of sentences involve embedding structures in different syntactic positions. On the structural side, they are complex sentences and both involve similar kinds of linguistic knowledge in constructing clausal embedding structures. However, on the processing side, they differ in their memory demands. In languages with subject-verb-object (SVO) word order, such as English, sentences with clausal subjects are more demanding in memory load than those with clausal objects (Cheung & Kemper, 1992). The embedding structure of a clausal subject leads to a heavier memory load because in the time that it takes to produce a clausal subject, the anticipated verb phrase that will be articulated is held in the memory, waiting for the completion of the embedded structure. Such demand in memory does not apply to clausal objects because they maintain a postverbal position and often are positioned at the end of the sentence. Comparing the acquisition of these two types of complex sentences, the role of memory capacity in children's acquisition of Mandarin grammar may be apparent.

Group (5) is descriptive clause. It is a rather unusual sentence type in Mandarin and structurally complex. Since younger children do not produce this type of sentence, it will not be reported in the subsequent analyses. Aside from that, conjoined clauses are not included because Chinese children often omit connectors and it is an arbitrary decision to label any two clauses that are semantically related as conjoined clauses. Such analysis should be deferred until there are clarifications on methodology.

In the literature of language development, there have not been any systematic studies on the development of complex sentences in Chinese, as commented by Lee (1996). Hsu (1986) reported that Mandarin-speaking children produced complex sentences, such as 我要爬給媽媽看 *wo3 yao4 pa2 gei3 ma1ma1 kan4* 'I want to let Mama see me crawling' as early as 2;0. Erbaugh (1992) also reported that children as young as 2;5 produced pivotal constructions, such as 姐姐帶我去上學 *jie3jie3 dai4 wo3 qu4 shang4xue2* 'older sister take me/I go enter school'. Lu (2003) adopted Li and Thompson's (1981) classification of serial verb constructions and examined language samples elicited from eight first or second graders with reading disabilities. She found that children with reading disabilities produced fewer serial verb constructions than their age-matched peers.

Method

Language samples

In this study, spontaneous language samples from two MSLI children and two typically developing children were analyzed. The two MSLI children were followed for 18 months in a longitudinal study (Cheung, 2000) and five language samples from each child were extracted from the larger corpus. Language samples of the two typically developing children were collected by the author in an earlier study (Cheung, 1998). These samples came from free-play sessions that were approximately 60 minutes in length. The mean number of utterances contained in these samples is 344, with a range of 179–612. MLU scores of all 20 language samples were computed according to Cheung's (1998) guidelines, which is adopted from Brown's (1973) rules for calculating MLU in English. In each sample, the first 100 utterances were analyzed with words as the basic counting unit. Compound words such as 茶杯 *cha2bei1* 'tea-cup' and proper names were counted as single words. Utterances

Table 3.3 Background of the children with SLI and their controls

Name	*Ann (SLI)*	*Howard (SLI)*	*GI (TD)*	*JC (TD)*
Sex	Female	Male	Male	Female
Age range	6;8–7;1	6;11–7;5	2;5–2;10	2;5–2;9
WPPSI-R PIQ	85	87	NA	NA
VIQ	51	61	NA	NA
TPLD – Receptive (Percentile)	2	2	NA	NA
TPLD – Expressive (Percentile)	9	2	NA	NA
PPVT (Percentile)	2	4	NA	NA
MLU range	2.22–2.55	2.08–2.27	2.04–2.30	1.97–2.37
Mean MLU	2.44	2.20	2.30	2.10

with unintelligible words were excluded. These MLU scores provided the basis for matching the two MSLI children with the two typically developing children (see Table 3.3).

In addition to MLU scores, the personal backgrounds of the two SLI children are also provided, which may help provide a complete picture, especially due to a lack of other reports on MSLI children.

Participants

The first MSLI child is a girl, Ann. Ann lives in central Taiwan and she was 6;8 when the study began. Ann has one elder brother and no family history of mental illness. Her first word was produced at 1;6, but after that, she had very little progress and stayed at the single-word stage until age four. At age six, she was evaluated at the Chang Hua Christian Hospital and her scores in the expressive subtest for the Test on Preschool Language Development (TPLD; Lin & Lin, 1993), a locally developed Chinese language assessment tool, was at the 9th percentile. In the receptive subtest, it was at the 2nd percentile. She had a very limited receptive vocabulary, with a performance at the 2nd percentile in the Chinese version of the Peabody Picture Vocabulary Test – Revised (PPVT-R; Lu & Liu, 1998). Her performance IQ in the Chinese version of the Wechsler Preschool and Primary Scale of Intelligence – Revised Edition (WPPSI-R; Chen, 1997) was 85 and verbal IQ was 51. Ann had been passive during most observation sessions and rarely initiated conversations.

The second MSLI child is a boy, Howard. He also resided in central Taiwan and was the third and youngest child in the family. He had one elder sister and one elder brother. Nobody in his family has any history of language impairment. He was about seven years old when the study began. Developmentally, it was reported that he did not babble as much as his older siblings. His first word was produced when he was 12 months old. He was initially diagnosed with autism due to his poor communication skills, lack of eye contact and repetitive behaviors, such as repeating certain rhymes excessively. By age three, these symptoms gradually disappeared, leaving poor language skill as the remaining problem. He was then reclassified as having SLI at Chang Hua Christian Hospital when he was six years old. During the reclassification process, he was given a full-scale evaluation and scored at the 2nd percentile in TPLD for both receptive and expressive subtests. His performance was at the 4th percentile in the Chinese version of PPVT-R (Lu & Liu, 1998). On the other hand, he had a score of 87 in the performance subtests of the Chinese version of WPPSI-R (Chen, 1997) and a score of 61 in the verbal subtests. For most observation sessions, Howard actively initiated conversation topics and play events. His social activities did not seem to be affected by his language problem.

Language samples from the two typically developing children were also collected at their homes. These two typically developing children, GI and JC, were in their third year of development during the periods of observation. They did not have any reported deficits in hearing or other disabilities. Since these observations were originally conducted for a different purpose, no standardized language tests were administered. Based on their MLU scores, these two children were considered typically developing. The test scores and MLU scores of the subjects are listed in Table 3.3.

Results

According to the current understanding of typically developing children, three grammatical components in Mandarin, namely, classifiers, aspect markers and complex sentences, were selected for the analyses. The assumption is that these components could reflect certain specific properties in the language and may help characterize the grammatical deficits in MSLI children. Results for each of these grammatical components are presented in the next three sections.

Noun: Classifiers

In this study, the children's use of general and specific classifiers is tabulated. For reasons stated earlier, 這個 *zhe4-ge5*, which is formed by the demonstrative 這 *zhe4* 'this' and the general classifier 個 *ge5*, is counted as a special unit. Besides, nouns that cannot be used with classifiers, such as proper names (e.g. 星期一 *xing1qi2yi1* 'Monday') and kinship terms, are subtracted from the pool of the nouns in the data set. All 'classifiable nouns' are then used to compute a classifier-to-noun ratio. Results for the use of classifiers are listed in Table 3.4.

During the five observation sessions, Ann produced 54 tokens of classifiers, including 32 general classifiers and 22 specific classifiers. Howard had 91 classifiers, with 16 being general and 75 being specific. All of these classifiers were correctly used with numerals, which was quite different from Hsu's (2004) experimental study, which elicited some omission errors (such as 兩(具)電話 *liang2 (jü4) dian4hua4* 'two telephone'). When computed with classifiable nouns, Ann was found to produce one classifier for every nine nouns and Howard one for every 10 nouns. These ratios are slightly higher than the two MLU-matched controls, which was about one classifier for 11 to 12 nouns. Moreover, Ann used nine types of specific classifiers and Howard had 10, which were also close to the two language-matched peers' (10 types for GI and seven types for JC).

Of the 17 specific classifiers listed in Table 3.5, four were used by all four subjects and all are sortal classifiers. Five of them are only found in the language samples of the MLU controls: 斤 *jin1-meat*, 朵 *duo3-flower*, 點 *dian3-rice*, 包 *bao1-cookie*, 罐 *guan4-milk*, and there are also five classifiers that are used by MSLI children, but not by the two MLU controls: 條 *tiao2-worm*, 顆 *ke1-star*, 間 *jian1-room*, 盤 *pan2-fruit*, 組 *zu3-toy*. When the classifier repertoires of the two groups are compared, it is found that children with SLI had only one measure classifier while the MLU controls had four. It seems that measure classifiers are probably

Table 3.4 Use of classifiers in the two children with SLI and their controls

	Ann (SLI)	*Howard (SLI)*	*GI (TD)*	*JC (TD)*
Token of general classifiers	32	16	42	8
Token of specific classifiers	22	75	25	28
Total	54	91	67	36
Number of classifiable nouns	485	905	735	439
Classifier to noun ratio	01:09.0	01:09.9	01:11.0	01:12.2
Type of specific classifiers	9	10	10	7
這個 *zhe4-ge5*	110	503	148	112
Number of errors	4	8	5	0

Table 3.5 Types of specific classifiers used by the four children

Classifier -noun	*Types*	*Ann (SLI)*	*Howard (SLI)*	*GI (TD)*	*JC (TD)*
本 *ben3* -book	S	√̲	√	√	√
隻 *zhi1* -dog	S	√	√	√	√
台 *tai2* -TV	S	√̲	√	√	√
件 *jian4* -clothes	S	√̲	√̲	√	√
張 *zhang1* -paper	S	√	√̲		√
杯 *bei1* -cup	M		√̲	√	√
條 *tiao2* -worm	S	√̲	√̲		
顆 *ke1* -star	S	√̲	√̲		
種 *zhong3* -color	K	√		√	
間 *jian1* -room	S	√̲			
盤 *pan2* -fruit	C	√			
組 *zu3* -toy	C		√		
朵 *duo3* -flower	S				√
斤 *jin1* -meat	M			√	
點 *dian3* -rice	M			√	
罐 *guan4* -milk	M			√	
包 *bao1* -cookie	C			√	
Total		10	9	10	7

Note. Type: S, sortal classifier; C, collective classifier; M, measure classifier; K, kind classifier; √̲, classifiers produced in one session in which most of the conversations are developed around some toys

somewhat more difficult because they are not related to the appearance or other visual properties of the referents. However, there needs to be awareness of the fact that only one of the MLU controls, GI, produced all of the measure classifiers. Since the examined language samples were quite limited, it is difficult to estimate the possible range of individual variations therefore, they should be re-examined for future research.

In addition to limited use of measure classifiers, the two MSLI children showed drastic variations in their productivity during the five observation sessions. When each of the sessions was scrutinized, it was found that Ann and Howard produced more than five new classifiers in one single session. For that session, some toys were brought in, which allowed the child to use clay to create objects of different shapes. Of the 10 types of specific classifiers that Ann had ever produced, five of them were found only in that specific session. Howard also used five types of specific classifiers that were not found in other sessions. The following conversation between Ann and the investigators is an example of the ways that classifiers were elicited with the toys:

Genie (GEN) and Yang (YAN) played with ANN (SLI subject)

GEN:	安安	會	不	會	做？
	an1an1	*hui4*	*bu2*	*hui4*	*zuo4*
	Ann	can	NEG	can	do
	'Can Ann do this?'				

GEN:	做	一	顆	球
	zuo4	*yi4*	*ke1*	*qiu2*
	make	one	CL	ball
	'Make a ball'			

GEN:	好	不	好
	hao3	*bu4*	*hao3*
	good	NEG	good
	'OK?'		

ANN:	好
	hao3
	good
	'Alright'

About one minute later

YAN:	你	也	做	星星	喔
	ni3	*ye3*	*zuo4*	*xing1-xing1*	*o5*
	you	also	make	star	SFP
	'You made a star also'				

GEN:	你	做	的	比較	好看
	ni3	*zuo4*	*de5*	*bi3jiao4*	*hao3kan4*
	you	make	modifier marker (MOD)	compare	good-looking
	'You made a good-looking star'				

ANN:	做	成	一	顆	星星	給	你
	zuo4	*cheng2*	*yi4*	*ke1*	*xing1-xing1*	*gei3*	*ni3*
	make	become	one	CL	star	give	you
	'I made a star for you'						

In this conversation, the investigator asked if Ann could make a ball and she used the classifier 顆 *ke1* in 一顆球 *yi4 ke1 qiu2* 'one CL ball'. A minute later, Ann used 顆 *ke1* with a different noun 星星 *xing1-xing1* 'star' when she talked about the star that she had made. Ann's use of 顆 *ke1* is not a direct imitation of the adult, but adult input played a role. Ann (as well as Howard) may have previously learned these classifiers, but they needed a stronger contextual support for the activation of these lexical items.

On the other hand, for the 10 language samples in the two controls, there were no similar intensive object manipulation activities and their specific classifiers were evenly distributed across all the samples. Therefore, even though the advancement in the use of classifiers observed in MSLI children could be interpreted as a case of sampling error, it is at least equally likely that Ann and Howard were weak in their lexical access during the process of production.

The last point for discussion in this section is the use of the deictic pronoun 這個 *zhe4-ge5* 'this'. In the beginning of this study, it was speculated that the two MSLI children might have problems accessing words in the lexicon and they may use 這個 *zhe4ge5* 'this' as a substitute. In fact, only Howard used 這個 *zhe4ge5* 'this' frequently, while Ann's use was similar to the MLU controls. However, Howard's high frequency of using 這個 *zhe4ge5* 'this' did not affect his overall performance in classifiers. As only two MSLI children were examined in this study, the use of 這個 *zhe4ge5* 'this' as a substitute device for nouns should be examined in future studies.

Aspect markers

Four types of aspect markers, namely perfective 了 *le5*, progressive 在 *zai4*, durative 著 *zhe5* and experiential 過 *guo4* are examined. Perfective 了 *le5*, progressive 在 *zai4* and durative 著 *zhe5* were used by all four children (see Table 3.6). Experiential 過 *guo4* was used by three subjects, Ann, GI and JC. Howard did not use 過 *guo4*, even though he had produced the highest number of utterances with predicates (1402 utterances). Howard's weakness in aspect markers was also witnessed in their frequencies of use. He used aspect markers 8%[2] (115/1402) of the time, while Ann, the other MSLI, used them 12% (101/879) of the time. Both of the typically developing controls also had higher frequency of use, 14% (97/685) for GI and 15% (68/15.2) for JC. Howard clearly displayed a weakness in aspect marking, but Ann's 2–3% below par in using aspect markers could possibly be a sampling error, as it is evident that there is a 1% difference between the two controls. Given that the understanding about MSLI children is very limited, it is not easy to determine if Ann and Howard's use of aspect markers is typical of MSLI

Table 3.6 The use of aspect markers in the two children with SLI and their controls

	Ann (SLI)	*Howard (SLI)*	*GI (TD)*	*JC (TD)*
Utterance final 了 *le5*	77	90	62	52
Nonutterance final 了 *le5*	11	6	4	2
在 *zai4*	7	9	18	7
著 *zhe5*	3	10	8	5
過 *guo4*	3	0	5	2
Total	101	115	97	68
Total utterances with a predicate (TUP)	879	1402	685	448
Aspect marker/TUP	11.5%	8.2%	14.2%	15.2%

children. This issue of individual variations in MSLI children will be left for further research.

In the original plan, four aspect markers and their distributions among six types of verb (i.e. accomplishment, achievement, activity, mixed telic-stative, semelfactive and stative[3]) were to be examined to understand the associations between lexical and grammatical aspects. However, such analyses were not performed for two reasons. First, the very limited use of progressive 在 *zai4* and durative 著 *zhe5* in both MSLI and MLU controls nullified the significance for implementing such an analysis. Secondly, more than 75% (281/304) of the 了 *le5* observed in this study are found in the final position of the utterance. As mentioned earlier, when the form 了 *le5* is found in the final position of the sentence, it can also be interpreted as a SFP marker for highlighting the 'current relevance' of the statement. When utterance final 了 *le5*s are excluded, the remaining 23 tokens of nonfinal 了 *le* do not provide enough data for the analysis on the association between lexical and grammatical aspects.

Complex sentence

Four types of sentences have been analyzed for the purpose of understanding MSLI children's capacity in deriving proper clausal structures and the role of memory loading in the process. These four types of sentences contain at least two verb phrases, but only three of them, namely, pivotal constructions, clausal subjects and clausal objects are complex sentences. This is in accordance with the definition that a complex sentence consists of one independent clause and one, two or more dependent clauses. Serial verb constructions are monoclausal and, therefore, are not complex sentences. They are examined here as a contrast with pivotal constructions. From Table 3.7, it is evident that serial verb constructions are used by all four children. Pivotal construction and clausal object are used by Ann, Howard and GI. Clausal subject is produced only by the two MSLI children. From this distribution pattern, it can be inferred that sentences with clausal subjects are the most difficult. Pivot construction and clausal object rank next in difficulty, and serial verb constructions are the least difficult.

Analyses on the use of sentence types demonstrated that the two MSLI children were somehow more advanced than the TD controls. They produced sentences with clausal subjects, which were not found in the language samples of the two controls. When the frequency of use is examined, Ann was found to be the most productive in complex sentences, with 3.5% (31/879) of use, while Howard and GI performed at the same level (Howard: 0.8% and GI: 0.9%). JC did not use any complex sentences and he only used serial verb constructions. However, if the total number of sentences with two verb phases (that is, all four sentence types are included) were compared, Howard, the boy with MSLI, had a lower percentage of use. His usage of these sentence types was around 3% of the time, which is lower than Ann's 7%. When compared with the two younger controls, Howard is the least productive

Table 3.7 Serial verb construction and complex sentences in the two children with SLI and their controls

	Ann (SLI)	*Howard (SLI)*	*GI (TD)*	*JC (TD)*
(1) Serial verb	30	30	36	23
(2) Pivotal	2	3	2	0
(3) Clausal subject	4	3	0	0
(4) Clausal object	25	5	4	0
Total number of complex sentences (percentage)	31 (3.5%)	11 (0.8%)	6 (0.9%)	0 (0%)
Total number of sentences with two verb phrases (percentage)	61 (6.9%)	41 (2.9%)	42 (5.9%)	23 (5.1%)
Total number of utterances with predicates	879	1402	685	448

(Howard: 3%; JC: 5%; GI: 6%) while Ann's performance was very close to the younger peers.

Two points can be further elaborated from these results. First, the rarity of clausal subjects in younger children's language samples can be explained in terms of memory loading. According to Baddeley's (1986) working memory model, articulations will suppress the rehearsal process that refreshes the decaying memory trace and thus will reduce the memory capacity. Therefore, it should be quite a burden for the child to hold up the matrix verb phrase that was formulated in memory while articulating the clausal subject at the same time. A sentence with a clausal object does not impose such a memory burden because the clausal object is the last unit to be produced. As the two MSLI children were four years older than the two TD controls, they might have a relatively larger memory span and be able to produce sentences that were more demanding in processing load. However, since their memory spans were not measured, the above account cannot be verified in this instance.

Secondly, although both serial and pivotal constructions are sentences with two verb phrases, they differ in the control of the subject for the second verb phrase. In a serial verb construction, the two involved verb phrases share the same subject. This sharing of subjects is relatively simple because in situations where a chain of actions performed by the same agent is expressed, children may just concatenate any two verb phrases to form a serial verb construction. They do not need to spend much effort on the sentence structure. However, in a pivotal construction, the object of the first verb phrase acts as the subject of the second verb phrase. Therefore, when producing a pivotal construction, the child has to come up with a proper structural representation so that the syntactic information specified in the first verb phrase can be properly relayed to the second one. A mere concatenation of two verb phrases does not always constitute a well-formed pivotal construction. From the results, it is evident that the use of pivotal constructions is determined by children's general grammatical development as measured by their MLU. JC, the child with the lowest mean MLU scores among the four, produced a couple of serial verb constructions, but not any pivotal constructions. On the other hand, GI, Howard and Ann have higher MLU scores and they produced both serial verb constructions and pivotal constructions.

General Discussion

Three different grammatical components have been examined in this study. The results indicated first, that the two MSLI children used fewer types of specific classifiers in free-play contexts, but managed to produce some new types when proper situational leads were provided. Their need of contextual support in using classifiers echoes the performance of children with language disorders in Hsu's (2004) learning task. In her thesis study, children with language disorders had a lower success rate for learning new classifiers and they produced the general classifier 個 *ge5* in lieu of the target. In an experimental study, an examiner is not allowed to provide prompts and other encouragement freely, so that if children with language disorders need more support from their conversational partners to produce the classifiers that are required, they will not receive any help. Yet, the language samples analyzed in the present study were collected in a spontaneous setting and the adults were free to interact with the children. The facilitative effect of adults' lead in using classifiers suggested that the MSLI children possessed the capacity for learning new classifiers, but they needed a stronger contextual support to activate these words during the production process. Secondly, the two MSLI children differed in their productivity during the use of aspect markers. Ann performed at the same level of the typically developing children, but Howard was not as capable. Howard did not use the experiential marker *guo4* and he was not as productive in the use of the three other aspect markers. Thirdly, both MSLI children produced some complex sentences that were not used by the MLU controls.

These findings provide a sketch of a grammatical profile for MSLI children. In many situations, their grammatical performance is similar to the MLU controls. They used most of the aspect markers, although the frequency was lower in one MSLI child. Without the burden of acquiring an inflectional system, clausal embedding in Mandarin appears to be easier, which is quite different from the literature with respect to English-speaking children with SLI. However, MSLI children were subject to certain limitations in their use of classifiers, which appeared to parallel English SLI children's low percentage of grammatical morpheme usage.

Jointly, the results suggest that the two MSLI children possessed linguistic knowledge that is comparable to their MLU controls. Their linguistic problems could be caused by a limited processing capacity that mostly affected their lexical access in the process of production. They might have acquired the linguistic items, but have difficulties in activating them. Therefore, they showed a lower percentage in the use of classifiers and aspect markers. The use of clausal subjects in MSLI children suggests that their memory spans allow them to produce embedded clauses, which were still beyond the capacity of the MLU controls. However, it is cautioned that there are individual differences found in the two MSLI children and between the controls, which then lead to the question about the appropriateness of matching subjects by MLU in SLI studies (Leonard, 1998). As indicated earlier, Ann and Howard differed in their use of aspect markers. Such a difference could be explained by the fact that Ann had higher MLU scores (2.22–2.55) than Howard (2.08–2.27). Nevertheless, this account cannot be extended to the two controls' performance in complex sentences. Between the two controls, GI and JC, only minimal differences in MLU scores were found (GI: 2.04–2.30; JC: 1.97–2.37). If utterance length reflects productivity in aspect markers, classifiers and complex sentences, then GI and JC would not differ in the use of all of these components. Yet, it was found that GI used three types of complex sentences, while JC used just one. The picture became more complicated when JC was compared with Howard. Howard was found to be more advanced than JC in using complex sentences, but their MLU ranges were quite similar (Howard: 2.08–2.27; JC: 1.97–2.37). From these comparisons, it is evident that MLU may not be sensitive enough to reflect the grammatical development of Howard and other children in areas such as clausal objects and subjects. If this is true, the use of MLU as a matching criterion in MSLI studies should be reconsidered. This methodological issue needs to be clarified in future research.

Acknowledgements

This study is supported by a grant from the National Science Council, Taiwan (NSC-89-2411-H-002-057). I would like to thank Genie Ou and Shu-wen Yang for data collection, and Dr Chaou Wun-Tsong and Chao Ke-Ping of Chang Hua Christian Hospital for assistance in clinical assessment.

Notes

1. Li and Thompson (1981) put these four types of sentences under the heading of serial verb constructions. Matthews (2006) argued that pivotal constructions are not truly serial verb constructions. Therefore, in this chapter we use the term serial verb constructions only for the first group of sentences listed in Table 3.2.
2. The total number of utterances with a predicate is used here as the denominator because in conversational Mandarin, many utterances contain noun phrases only. Since aspect markers are used with predicates, using the number of total utterances with a predicate can provide a better estimation.
3. Examples for the six verb types in Mandarin:
   (1) Accomplishment: 買 *mai3* 'buy' in 買衣服 *mai3 yi1fu2* 'buy clothes'.
   (2) Achievement: 掉 *diao4* 'drop' in 杯子掉了 *bei1zi5 diao4 le5* 'cup dropped'.
   (3) Activity: 跑 *pao3* 'run' in 小朋友在跑 *xiao3peng2you3 zai4 pao3* 'a boy is running'.
   (4) Mixed telic-stative: 穿 *chuan1* in 在穿衣服 *zai4 chuan1 yi1fu2* 'is putting on clothes'.
   (5) Semelfactive: 跳 *tiao4* 'jump' in 他一直跳 *ta1 yi1zhi2 tiao4* 'he is jumping'.
   (6) Stative: 坐 *zuo4* 'sit' in 坐在上面 *zuo4 zai4 shang4mian4* 'sitting on top (of something)'.

References

Baddeley, A.D. (1986) *Working Memory.* Oxford: Oxford University Press.

Bishop, D.M.V. (1997) *Uncommon Understanding: Development and Disorders of Language Comprehension in Children.* Hove: Psychology Press.

Brown, R. (1973) *A First Language: The Early Stages.* Cambridge, MA: Harvard University Press.

Chen, R-H. (1997) *Wechsler Preschool and Primary Scale of Intelligence – Revised Edition.* Taipei: Chinese Behavioral Science Corporation. (In Chinese.)

Cheung, H. (1998) The application of MLU in Chinese. *Journal of Speech-Language-Hearing Association of the Republic of China* 13, 36–48.

Cheung, H. (2000) An investigation of the language and cognitive abilities of children with specific language impairment (Project No. NSC-89-2411-H-002-057). Technical report for National Science Council, Taiwan.

Cheung, H. and Fon, J. (2002) The construction of classifier phrase in child Mandarin. In Y.E. Hsiao (ed.) *Proceedings of the First Cognitive Linguistics Conference* (pp. 42–57). National Cheng-Chi University, Taipei.

Cheung, H. and Kemper, S. (1992) Competing complexity metrics and adults' production of complex sentences. *Applied Psycholinguistics* 13, 53–76.

Erbaugh, M. (1992) The acquisition of Mandarin. In D.I. Slobin (ed.) *The Crosslinguistic Study of Language Acquisition* (Volume 3, pp. 373–456). Mahwah, NJ: Lawrence Erlbaum.

Erbaugh, M. (2006) Chinese classifiers: Their use and acquisition. In P. Li, L.H. Tan, E. Bates and O. Tzeng (eds) *The Handbook of East Asian Psycholinguistics: Volume 1 Chinese* (pp. 39–51). Cambridge: Cambridge University Press.

Fletcher, P., Leonard, L., Stokes, S.F. and Wong, A.M-Y. (2005) The expression of aspect in Cantonese-speaking children with specific language impairment. *Journal of Speech, Language, and Hearing Research* 48, 621–634.

Gathercole, S. and Baddeley, A. (1990) Phonological memory deficits in language disordered children: Is there a causal connection? *Journal of Memory and Language* 29, 336–360.

Hsu, H. (2004) The association of phonological disorders and syntactic disorders: A study of Mandarin-speaking children. Unpublished Master's Thesis, National Taiwan University, Taipei.

Hsu, J. (1986) *A Study of the Stages and Development and Acquisition of Mandarin Chinese by Children in Taiwan.* Taipei: Crane.

Hu, Q. (1993) The acquisition of Chinese classifiers by young Mandarin-speaking children. Unpublished doctoral dissertation, Boston University, Boston.

Klee, T., Stokes, S.F., Wong, A.M-Y., Fletcher, P. and Gavin, W. (2004) Utterance length and lexical diversity in Cantonese-speaking children with and without specific language impairment. *Journal of Speech, Language, and Hearing Research* 47, 1396–1410.

Lee, T.H-T. (1996) Theoretical issues in language development and Chinese child language. In C-T.J. Huang and A.Y-H. Li (eds) *New Horizons in Chinese Linguistics* (pp. 293–356). Dordrecht: Kluwer Academic.

Leonard, L.B. (1998) *Children with Specific Language Impairment.* Cambridge, MA: The MIT Press.

Leonard, L.B., Wong, A.M-Y., Deevy, P., Stokes, S.F. and Fletcher, P. (2006) The production of passives by children with specific language impairment acquiring English or Cantonese. *Applied Psycholinguistics* 27, 267–299.

Li, C.N. and Thompson, S. (1981) *Mandarin Chinese: A Functional Reference Grammar.* Berkeley, CA: University of California Press.

Li, P. and Bowerman, M. (1998) The acquisition of lexical and grammatical aspect in Chinese. *First Language* 18, 311–350.

Lin, B. and Lin, M. (1993) *Test on Preschool Language Development.* Taipei: Center for Special Education, National Taiwan Normal University. (In Chinese.)

Lin, O-H. (1986) A developmental study of the acquisition of aspect markers in Chinese children. Unpublished MA thesis, Fu Jen Catholic University, Taipei.

Lu, H. (2003) Linguistic deficits observed in the narratives of reading disabled children in Taiwan. Unpublished MA thesis, Fu Jen Catholic University, Taipei.

Lu, L. and Liu, M-X. (1998) *Peabody Picture Vocabulary Test – Revised.* Taipei: Psychological Publishing. (In Chinese.)

Matthews, S. (2006) On serial verb constructions in Cantonese. In A.Y. Aikhenvald and R.M.W. Dixon (eds) *Serial Verb Constructions* (pp. 69–87). Oxford: Oxford University Press.

Myers, J. (2000) Rules vs. analogy in Mandarin classifier selection. *Language and Linguistics* 1, 187–210.

Rice, M., Wexler, K. and Cleave, P. (1995) Specific language impairment as a period of extended optional infinitive. *Journal of Speech, Language, and Hearing Research* 38, 850–863.

Stokes, S.F. and Fletcher, P. (2000) Lexical diversity and productivity in Cantonese-speaking children with specific language impairment. *International Journal of Language & Communication Disorders* 35, 527–541.

Stokes, S.F. and Fletcher, P. (2003) Aspectual forms in Cantonese children with specific language impairment. *Linguistics* 41, 381–405.

Stokes, S.F. and So, L.K.H. (1997) Classifier use by language disordered and age matched Cantonese-speaking children. *Asia Pacific Journal of Speech, Language and Hearing* 2, 83–101.

Tallal, P. and Piercy, M. (1973) Defects of non-verbal auditory perception in children with developmental aphasia. *Nature* 241, 468–469.

Wong, A.M-Y., Leonard, L., Fletcher, P. and Stokes, S.F. (2004) Questions without movement: A study of Cantonese-speaking children with and without specific language impairment. *Journal of Speech, Language, and Hearing Research* 47, 1440–1453.

Chapter 4

A Construction Account of Question Acquisition in Cantonese-speaking Children with Specific Language Impairment

ANITA M-Y. WONG and STEPHANIE F. STOKES

Introduction

Children with specific language impairment (SLI)

A large-scale epidemiological study conducted in the USA (Tomblin *et al.*, 1997) reported that 7.4% of five-year-old children met the diagnostic criteria for SLI. The language levels of these children are significantly below their age peers in the absence of hearing, psychosocial or cognitive impairment. Using a chronological age and language age discrepancy criterion, Wong *et al.* (1992) reported a prevalence of 3% in four-year-old Cantonese-speaking children in Hong Kong. Based on this criterion, a child who scored about three standard deviations below the mean in a general test of language would be considered language impaired. Such a cutoff was much lower than the cutoffs generally adopted in the research literature (Leonard, 1998). There are no other statistics on the prevalence of SLI in Chinese-speaking children. Nevertheless, SLI does affect children learning Cantonese in Hong Kong (e.g. Stokes & Fletcher, 2003; Wong *et al.*, 2004) and children learning Mandarin in Taiwan (Chapter 3 in this volume).

Research in the last 30 years (see Leonard, 1998 for a review) has revealed that children with SLI show both a delayed and a disordered pattern of development. They learn items within a language domain in the same order and in the same way as typically developing children, only they learn them at a slower rate and hence at a later age (e.g. Johnston & Schery, 1976). Their language development, when examined across domains, shows a disordered pattern. They have special difficulties with certain forms and structures and these difficulties are not seen in typically developing children at the same level of language development. In English, these are grammatical morphemes. Their difficulties appear to be due to infrequent or restricted use rather than a lack of knowledge. Growth in these special areas of difficulties is slow and they need more frequent (Rice *et al.*, 1994) and salient input

(Ellis Weismer, 1997) to achieve the same level of competence as their typically developing peers.

Usage-based theory of language development

Reviews of research evidence generally report that intervention is effective for children with primary speech and language impairments (Gillam *et al.*, 2008; Law *et al.*, 1998; Yoder & McDuffie, 2002). Despite recent efforts to compare the efficacy of different intervention approaches (e.g. Yoder & Stone, 2006), more research is needed to examine which intervention approach works better for which population of children for which intervention goal. Before such evidence is available, the theory of language impairment, the theory of language and the theory of language development that speech-language pathologists ascribe to will continue to guide their choice of intervention approaches for each child they work with (Johnston, 1985).

Tomasello (2003) presented a usage-based theory of language development, and this theory built on work from cultural psychology, psycholinguistics, and most importantly from functional and cognitive linguistics, construction grammar and the usage-based model in particular. The thesis of the usage-based theory of language development is that linguistic knowledge is not prewired; instead it is the outcome of the child acting on the language input available in the ambient environment using his/her general cognitive mechanisms and psychological processes for the purpose of social interactions. Some of the key arguments and recent evidence are:

(1) Children learn language during social interactions with other people (Clark, 2003; Snow, 1999; Tomasello, 2003). During social interactions, linguistic expressions are used in pragmatically meaningful situations, and therefore children construct their linguistic knowledge on the basis of how forms are mapped onto meanings and functions.

(2) Children's language learning is reflective of the relative frequencies of constructions in the input. Other things being equal, children are more likely to learn constructions that occur frequently in the adult speech than those that are used infrequently (Diessel, 2004; Kidd, 2006).

(3) Children learn language gradually in a piecemeal fashion. Over time, they develop adult competence of the ambient language, which are form-meaning to function mappings known as constructions. Constructions come in different shapes, sizes and levels of abstraction. They may also vary in complexity depending on the number and the relations of the linguistic elements involved (Tomasello, 2003). The English regular plural construction is

relatively simple and the English transitive construction is more complex. Children's first constructions are simple, concrete and built around specific lexemes and are independent of one another (Tomasello, 1992). These lexically specific constructions include pivot schema, verb island and item-based constructions. Pivot schema are comprised of well-used lexical items in familiar slots or frames, e.g. eat bread, eat cake, cake gone, ball gone, milk gone, where one lexeme provides a pivot slot around which other lexemes slot in. In the earliest phases of development, pivot schemas are developed by the child mapping words to referents or events, and engaging in social activities like shared eye-gaze and joint attention. Verb island constructions are one special type of item-based constructions and they result from the instantiation of an action word with a semantic role (e.g. *eat* = to consume food) to which lexemes and syllables are attached to transmit variable meanings (e.g. eat+-ed; eat all, don't eat, I eat, you eat, eat+ing...). This phase of development is achieved through the process of schematization, where the child modifies the schema (consuming food) to communicate different communicative intentions (e.g. finished eating).

(4) More complex and abstract representations such as paradigmatic categories and construction schemas develop over repeated exposure of different exemplars of the constructions. Children learn construction schemas through inductive analyses of patterns in the input using general cognitive mechanisms including pattern-finding (Tomasello, 2003) and analogical reasoning (Diessel, 2004; Kidd, 2006; Tomasello, 2003). They compare constructions in the input, recognize their structural similarities and build their own constructions for use in social interactions. Inductive analyses also involve psychological processes such as habituation and entrenchment (Diessel, 2004; Kidd, 2006; Tomasello, 2003), and these processes are affected by frequency of use of the constructions. The more often the constructions are used, the more automatized or habituated they are, and the more highly activated they are in the child's network of linguistic knowledge (Diessel, 2004). Over time, using functionally based distributional analysis, children also begin to form categories by recognizing the possible distributional properties of words and phrases that perform the same functions in different utterances (groups or categories, such as noun phrase (NP) modifiers, verb phrase (VP) modifiers, temporal markers). They mark the verb with different morphological markers to encode perspectives for time/aspect (eat+-ing, eat+-ed, eat+-en), leading to creativity and productivity (e.g. wugs).

Constructing Cantonese

Several recent studies provided insights into how children with SLI construct Cantonese from the perspective of the usage-based theory of language development. In one study, Wong *et al.* (2004) compared children's use of 邊個 *bin1go3* 'who' subject and 邊個 *bin1go3* 'who' object questions in two elicited tasks. Children with SLI had more difficulties with 'who' object questions than younger children at the same level of language development, but the two groups were comparable in their performance on 'who' subject questions. A *post-hoc* analysis of 16 consecutive conversational samples from one of the eight children in the Hong Kong Cantonese Child Language Corpus (CANCORP; Lee *et al.*, 1996) revealed that there were much fewer 'who' object than 'who' subject questions in the adult input. These findings suggest that children with SLI are sensitive to input frequency, but they seem to require a higher frequency threshold than children at the same language level for constructing certain forms in their ambient language.

In a study that examined lexical diversity, Stokes and Fletcher (2000) reported that as a group, the 15 children with SLI used the earliest developing perfective aspect marker 咗 *zo2* with 14 different verbs. However, two thirds of these perfective aspect marker tokens were used in only three of these 14 verbs (i.e. 唔見 *m4gin3* 'disappear', 跌 *dit3* 'fall' and 食 *sik6* 'eat'). Such item-based use of the perfective aspect marker was not seen in the group of younger typically developing children at the same level of language development. These children used the perfective aspect marker across a larger set of 23 different verbs.

Similar findings were reported in a study of aspect marker development in Fletcher *et al.* (2006). Each of the eight typically developing children in the CANCORP (Lee *et al.*, 1996) was matched with a child with SLI (Stokes *et al.*, 1998) on the mean length of utterance (MLU) that was obtained from their first conversational sample. Children's use of aspect markers was examined in this and two subsequent language samples. In all three data points, the two groups of children did not differ in the tokens of aspect markers produced. An aspect marker was considered productive if the verb types to which it was attached were larger than the verb tokens, and if the number of verb tokens was more than six. Children with SLI showed productive use of fewer aspect markers than their language-matched peers in two data points. In the first data point, while children with SLI were not productive with any aspect markers, the language-matched controls were already productive with the perfective aspect marker 咗 *zo2*. In the third data point, the language-matched controls were once again more advanced than the children with SLI, as they were productive with three more aspect markers, the delimitative 吓 *haa2*, the continuous 住 *zyu6* and the habitual

過 *gwo3*. Children with SLI were only productive with one additional aspect marker 吓 *haa2*. Compared with children at the same language level, item-based use of aspect markers seemed to be extended in children with SLI.

Aspect markers are not syntactically obligatory in Cantonese and their use is pragmatically controlled. The speaker can use one of the six aspect markers to restrict the hearer's interpretation of the temporal contour of the event denoted by the verb. For example, the use of the perfective aspect marker 咗 *zo2* with the accomplishment verb 食 *sik6* 'eat' will draw the hearer's attention to the end-point of the eating event, whereas the use of the progressive 嚟 *gan2* focuses on its process. The speaker can alternatively use the verb without an aspect marker, thereby taking a neutral temporal perspective on the event. Such a variable use and nonuse of aspect markers will result in structural inconsistencies in the constructions involved. There are other constructions in Cantonese that are structurally more consistent. One example is A-not-A questions. A-not-A questions involve the juxtaposition of the positive and the negative counterpart of the lexeme A, and they do not allow omissions of any of these components. They are posed as yes/no questions when one wants to find out 'Is A the case or not?' The lexeme can either be an adjective, a lexical or a modal verb. An example is 你 食-唔-食 呀? *nei5 sik6-m4-sik6 aa3?* 'you eat-not-eat + SFP?' The syllabic nasal 唔 *m4* is the negative marker, SFP stands for sentence-final particles, and the question means 'Are you eating or not?'. The first part of the question is always monosyllabic even if the lexeme A is disyllabic (e.g. 記得 *gei3dak1* 'remember'), and in such cases only the first syllable is included (e.g. 記-唔-記得 佢 呀? *gei3-m4-gei3dak1 keoi5 aa3?* meaning 'remember him/her or not?'). Do children with SLI show an extended item-based lexically specific phase in the learning of structurally more consistent constructions such as A-not-A questions? And can item-based lexically driven learning be tracked through longitudinal language sampling? These were the questions that motivated this study.

The first task was to establish the pattern of construction of questions in typically developing children at a language level similar to a sample of children with SLI. Stokes and Wong (2006) examined the emergence of A-not-A questions in the eight typically developing children reported in the CANCORP (Lee *et al.*, 1996). Sixteen consecutive conversational samples from each child were included in this analysis and the children were aged between 1;10 (year;month) and 2;08 for their first sample. These samples were collected once or twice each month for a period between 8 and 12 months. In these conversational samples, the child engaged in play with a research assistant, his/her caretaker(s) and other family members who were present at the time of the recording. Each sample was approximately one hour long and included between

45 to 1201 utterances. One of the oldest and developmentally more advanced children in the group, LLY, demonstrated the transition from the lexical-grammaticalization to the construction phase in his acquisition of A-not-A questions. The other children in this study were either at the earlier social imitation and chunking or the lexical-grammaticalization phase. Together the eight children presented evidence of the three phases in children's learning of new constructions, as discussed in Tomasello's (2003) usage-based theory of language development.

Stokes and Wong (2006) described the three phases of development of A-not-A questions as follows. Initially, children's use of A-not-A questions was a result of chunking from the input. Children imitated utterances from the input in an attempt to obtain the same social consequence as the adults with whom they were interacting. In the next phase, children began to produce A-not-A questions with specific lexemes. These lexemes were ones they had used and heard frequently in their conversations with the adult speakers, and ones they had negated with the syllabic nasal. For example, a child would have used 食 呀 *sik6 aa3* 'eat' many times in prior exchanges, and then used 唔 食 呀 *m4 sik6 aa3* 'not eat SFP', before producing 食-唔-食 呀? *sik6-m4-sik6 aa3*? 'you eat-not-eat SFP?'. Production of the 唔 *m4* + A frame appeared to be a prerequisite in the construction of children's first A-not-A questions. In this lexical-grammaticalization phase, children used the 'cut-and-paste' operations to merge two utterances A (+ SFP) and 唔 *m4* + A (+ SFP) with the same lexeme to form A-not-A questions. With three lexically specific A-not-A questions in her inventory of constructions, LLY moved on to the construction phase. Using analogy and distributional analysis, she began to pose A-not-A questions productively with no prior use of the 唔 *m4* + A frame. Children at this point were developing a more abstract construction schema for A-not-A questions, and therefore began to use them more often and with more different new lexemes.

Research questions

Building on our earlier work with typically developing children (Stokes & Wong, 2006), this study aimed to examine the development of A-not-A questions in eight children with SLI on a case-by-case basis to see if children with SLI followed the same routes of A-not-A question development as reported for typically developing children. Specifically, our two research questions were:

(1) Do children with SLI produce lexeme-specific A-not-A questions that require prior use of the not-A component with that specific lexeme? This requires schematization and cut-and-paste operations.
(2) Do children with SLI generate A-not-A questions from an abstract schema without prior use of the not-A component after they have

produced several lexeme-specific questions? This requires analogical learning and distributional analysis.

On the basis of their pattern of aspect marker use, we predicted that Cantonese-speaking children with SLI do not have problems with schematization and cut-and-paste operations, and the learning of lexeme-specific A-not-A questions. If their difficulties with aspect markers were related to these markers' variable pattern use and nonuse, the consistent structure of A-not-A questions should pose no special difficulties for these children's analogical learning and distributional analysis. We therefore predicted that Cantonese-speaking children have no problems constructing an abstract schema for generating new A-not-A questions.

Method

Data and participants

Data for this study came from the eight children with SLI who were previously reported in Fletcher *et al.* (2006) and Klee *et al.* (2004). These children all received a score that was more than 1.5 standard deviations below the mean on the Cantonese version of the Reynell Developmental Language Scale (RDLS; Reynell & Huntley, 1987) expressive subscale. The score on the RDLS receptive subscale was also more than 1.5 standard deviations below the mean for six of the eight children. All children received a score that was no less than 1 standard deviation below the mean on the Columbia Mental Maturity Scale (Burgemeister *et al.*, 1972), a test of non-verbal cognitive abilities. They all passed a hearing and oral motor screening, and showed no signs of psychosocial impairment. They were between age 3;10 and 5;0 when they were first seen, with a mean age of 4;07. These children were participants in a longitudinal study of SLI (Stokes *et al.*, 1998). Language samples were collected for each of the children in their own home once a month in the first six or seven months, and subsequently twice every three months or once after a year for some of the children. In these samples, the children engaged in a conversation with the same investigator, a trained speech therapist, around toy sets they were playing with at the time. In the first sample for all, and also the fourth sample for some children, the children played with the same birthday party set and talked about things related to this event. Each sample included 150 child utterances. To compare results from the typically developing children, only the first six or seven consecutive monthly samples were used in this study. These eight children with SLI were at roughly comparable language levels, as measured by their MLU, as the eight typically developing children reported in Stokes and Wong (2006). Table 4.1 gives the age range of the children with SLI in this study, and that of the younger typically

Table 4.1 Age, total number of questions, and number of A-not-A questions produced by the children with SLI and the children reported in Stokes and Wong (2006)

	Age range (months)	*No. of samples*	*No. of questions*	*No. of A-not-A questions*
Children with SLI				
R05	54–60	7	31	9
R07	55–62	7	44	6
R08	57–63	7	56	8
R09	49–55	7	58	11
R10	46–52	6	66	13
R11	56–60	6	16	1
R13	60–63	4	1	0
R16	54–62	6	48	1
Typically developing children				
CGK	23–32	12	130	0
CKT	22–31	12	286	1
LTF	26–38	12	1037	12
LLY	32–40	12	563	12
MHZ	24–32	12	67	1
CCC	23–33	12	510	1
WBH	28–38	12	166	0
HHC	28–40	12	396	1

developing children reported in Stokes and Wong. Table 4.2 shows how each child with SLI was matched with one of the younger typically developing children on the MLU of their first and last samples.

Procedures

All questions produced by the child were first identified using the CLAN command kwal + s"?" + w2–w5 + t*CHI (child). The first author extracted all of the A-not-A questions from the list. If the A-not-A piece of the question appeared in the last three adult turns, that question was

Table 4.2 The developmental phase of the seven children with SLI in this study and the eight typically developing children reported in Stokes and Wong (2006), starting from the children with the lowest initial MLU

Child	*MLU range*	*Developmental phase*	*Child*	*MLU range*	*Developmental phase*
CKT	1.5–2.5	Lexical-grammaticalization	R07	1.3–2.6	Lexical-grammaticalization
MHZ	1.6–2.8	Social imitation and chunking	R10	1.8–2.5	Construction
HHC	1.7–3.8	Social imitation and chunking			
WBH	1.8–3.1	NA	R16	1.9–3.1	Lexical-grammaticalization
CGK	2.1–3.7	NA	R05	2.0–3.7	Lexical-grammaticalization
CCC	1.7–3.1	Social imitation and chunking	R11	2.1–3.0	NA
LLY	2.2–4.1	Construction	R09	2.1–3.8	Construction
LTF	1.9–3.7	Construction	R08	2.3–3.6	Construction

marked as an imitation. Another clan command kwal + s"A" + t*CHI (or + t*INV (adult investigator)) was used to search for all instances of the lexeme A (e.g. 食 *sik6* 'eat') and its negative counterpart 唔 *m4*-A in the child and INV's utterances in all of the language samples up to the child's production of the A-not-A question with that specific lexeme. The INV's uses of A-not-A questions with these same lexemes were also identified from the samples. With these data, we traced the emergence of A-not-A questions in each of the children, and determined the developmental phase they were in. The three developmental phases are defined as follows:

(1) Social imitation and chunking phase: the child's A-not-A questions are imitative productions of an adult utterance.
(2) Lexical-grammaticalization phase: the child's spontaneous A-not-A questions are preceded by the prerequisite 唔 *m4*-A component involving the specific lexemes.
(3) Construction phase: the child successfully constructs his/her A-not-A questions on the basis of an abstract schema without prior use of the 唔 *m4*-A component.

Results

Table 4.1 shows the total number of questions and number of A-not-A questions produced by the children with SLI. The same information for the younger typically developing children is also included for reference. We now discuss each of the children with SLI in turn. Only four monthly samples were collected for R13, with an MLU of 1.3 for the first and 1.6 for the last sample. He was at a much lower level of language development than the rest of his group, and a language-matched typically developing child could not be identified for him. R13 produced one 咩 *me1* 'what' question during this period, no A-not-A question was observed. He was therefore excluded from further discussion. R11 produced 16 questions, and there were no A-not-A questions except for the one 係-咪 *hai6-mai6* question. 係-咪 *hai6-mai6* was a reduced version of 係-唔-係 *hai6-m4-hai6* 'is-not-is' where 唔-係 *m4-hai6* 'not is' was produced together as 咪 *mai6*, which is common in conversational speech. Except for R11 who was low in question production, the other six children produced between 31 and 66 questions, and of these, between 1 and 13 were A-not-A questions. Next, we describe the pattern of emerging question use for each SLI child.

R05

R05 attempted a total of nine A-not-A questions. The first four were produced in the first sample at 4;06, and resulted in an error pattern also used by typically developing children; the verbs were 去 *heoi3* 'go', 食 *sik6* 'eat' and 鍾意 *zung1ji3* 'like'. These questions were all in error as none of them included the required negative marker 唔 *m4*, e.g. 食-食 呀 *sik6-sik6 aa3* 'eat-eat SFP'. Prior to these error questions, the prerequisite 唔-去 *m4-heoi3*, 唔-食 *m4-sik6* and 唔-鍾意 *m4-zung1ji3* frames were not observed in R05's productions. At 4;07, R05 produced her first spontaneous A-not-A question with the lexeme 啱 *ngaam1* 'correct'. Prior to this question, R05 used the lexeme 啱 *ngaam1* 'correct' four times, and the prerequisite 唔-啱 *m4-ngaam1* four times. Correct use (as the model predicts) seems dependent on using the cut-and-paste operation correctly, with prior use of the component forms.

R05's next four A-not-A questions involving the lexeme 嚟 *lei4* 'come' were observed at 4;09. The first two were produced appropriately without prior use of the prerequisite 唔-嚟 *m4-lei4*. This seemed to suggest that R05 was already constructing an abstract representation for A-not-A questions. However, her next two 嚟-唔-嚟 *lei4-m4-lei4* questions were produced without the syllabic negative marker (i.e. 嚟-嚟-呀 *lei4-lei4 aa3*). The attempt to skip the lexical-grammatical phase might have been premature. Given that she had only successfully produced A-not-A questions with two different lexemes, her abstract representation was not complete or stable enough for consistent production. R05 did not produce other A-not-A questions in the next three monthly sessions, and hence no further observation of her developmental path could be made.

R07

R07 produced all six of his A-not-A questions in the sixth of his seven monthly samples. These A-not-A questions involved three different lexemes. R07's first two A-not-A questions involved the lexeme 得 *dak1* 'okay' and 識 *sik1* 'know' and both were exact imitations of the adult input. Before these productions, R07 did not produce the prerequisites 唔-得 *m4-dak1* or 唔-識 *m4-sik1*. R07's second 識-唔-識 *sik1-m4-sik1* question was a spontaneous production, and prior to this question, the child used the prerequisite 唔-識 *m4-sik1*. R07's next two A-not-A questions involved the same lexeme 睇 *tai2* 'watch'. The first 睇-唔-睇 *tai2-m4-tai2* question was an imitative one. Although R07 used the 唔 *m4*+A frame with seven different lexemes before his second spontaneous production of 睇-唔-睇 *tai2-m4-tai2* question, none of them included the verb 睇 *tai2*. At this point, R07 had only spontaneously produced one lexeme-specific A-not-A question, and it was possible that he had not formed an abstract construction schema for A-not-A questions. R07's second 睇-唔-睇 *tai2-m4-tai2* question was produced only after a failed attempt, and a request for clarification question 吓 *haa2?* from the adult. R07's last A-not-A question was a spontaneous production involving the same lexeme 識 *sik1* 'know'.

R08

R08 produced eight A-not-A questions, and the first three, which involved the same lexeme 係 *hai6* 'is', were produced in the second sample at 4;10. The first of these questions was the full form 係-唔-係 *hai6-m4-hai6*. R08 used the word 係 *hai6* 'is' six times and three tokens of 係-唔-係 *hai6-m4-hai6* question were observed in the input. Although the prerequisite 唔-係 *m4-hai6* did not appear before the child's first production of these questions, the child did use it once in the first sample. R08's next two 係-唔-係 *hai6-m4-hai6* questions were given in the reduced form 係-咪 *hai6-mai6*, and they were preceded by two productions of the prerequisite. In the fourth sample, R08 produced one A-not-A question with the lexeme 識 *sik1* 'know'. The prerequisite 唔-識 *m4-sik1* was observed in R08's third sample.

R08 produced two A-not-A questions using the lexemes 係 *hai6* 'is' and 靚 *leng3* 'pretty' in the fifth sample at 5;00. The prerequisite 唔-靚 *m4-leng3* did not appear in R08's utterances prior to his first 靚-唔-靚 *leng3-m4-leng3* question, nor was it used in the adult input in this sample. R08, however, was prepared to produce this question in two ways. In the previous sample at 4;11, R08 used the 唔 *m4*-A frame 19 times with 11 different lexemes, showing solid knowledge of the construction schema for generating the 唔-靚 *m4-leng3* prerequisite when situations required its production. This question was also produced in the context of two earlier 係-唔-係 *hai6-m4-hai6* questions, which could have provided the data for analogical reasoning and construction of new A-not-A questions. In the sixth sample at 5;02, R08 produced one more 靚-唔-靚 *leng3-m4-leng3* question, and a new A-not-A question with the lexeme 啱 *ngaam1* 'correct'. The prerequisite 唔-啱 *m4-ngaam1* was produced in the sample collected three months previously at 4;11.

R09

R09 produced a total of 11 A-not-A questions. Her first A-not-A question involving the lexeme 嚟 *lei4* 'come' was an immediate repetition of the adult input. Prior to this question in the first sample at 4;00, there was no use of its prerequisite 唔-嚟 *m4-lei4* in R09's utterances. R09 did not seem prepared for a spontaneous production. However, there were six 嚟-唔-嚟 *lei4-m4-lei4* questions in the input, and R09 was certainly socially motivated to learn this question as could be seen by her two inaccurate attempts to repeat after the adult model, which eventually led to the successful imitation.

R09 produced four A-not-A questions at 4;01. R09's first spontaneous 要-唔-要 *jiu3-m4-jiu3* 'want-not-want' question was produced in the middle of the sample. Although the prerequisite 唔-要 *m4-jiu4* was not observed, R09 did use it twice in the sample collected a month earlier. Her next spontaneous production of 好-唔-好 *hou2-m4-hou2* 'good-not-good' question was preceded by its prerequisite in the form of a question 唔-好 呀? *m4-hou2 aa4?* R09's production of 識-唔-識 *sik1-m4-sik1* 'know-not-know' question was also preceded by her use of its prerequisite 唔-識 *m4-sik1*, as well as an immediate adult model. After three A-not-A questions with three different lexemes, R09 produced her first A-not-A question involving the lexeme 得 *dak1* 'okay' without going through the lexical-grammaticalization phase. At this point, R09 began to develop an abstract representation of A-not-A questions, and generate the use of this question construction to other lexemes.

At age 4;03, R09 produced five A-not-A questions, of which four were imitations of the adult input. Would this regression to the earlier imitative learning or chunking phase invalidate the conclusion we have just drawn on R09? The answer was no, for two reasons. The first reason was that all of these imitations involved the same lexeme 會 *wui5* 'would' and these questions were requested of the child by the adult to find out if the different stuffed animals would come to the pretend birthday party. The child needed a lot of prompting and scaffolding in order to fulfill the adult's request, and in the sample the transcriber also noted that 'the child seemed a bit confused'.

INV: 你 問 佢 會 唔 會 嚟 啦.
nei5 man6 keoi5 wui5 m4 wui5 lei4 laa1.
You ask s/he would not would come SFP
'You ask him/her if s/he will come or not'

CHI: 佢 問 你 會 + . . . ?
keoi5 man6 nei5 wui5 + . . . ?
S/he asks you would + . . . ?
'S/he asks if you would + . . . ?'

R09's difficulty was not with the structure of this question *per se* but posing a question that was not out of an intention of her own. This difficulty was also observed in young typically developing children. The second reason was that R09 successfully produced another A-not-A question with the lexeme 返 *faan1* 'return' without earlier production of the prerequisite 唔-返 *m4-faan1* in any of her previous samples. This child was in the construction phase at this point. At 4;05, R09 produced her first spontaneous 會-唔-會 *wui5-m4-wui5* question.

R10

R10 used a total of 14 A-not-A questions, and two of them were produced in the first session when he was 3;10. They involved the lexemes 啱 *ngaam1* 'correct' and 嚟 *lei4* 'come'. Prior to the 啱-唔-啱 *ngaam1-m4-ngaam1* question, the prerequisite 唔-啱 *m4-ngaam1* was not observed in R10's utterances. The 嚟-唔-嚟 *lei4-m4-lei4* question was an imitation of the adult input.

In the next monthly session, R10 produced five A-not-A questions, using the lexemes 食 *sik6* 'eat' and 好 *hou2* 'good'. The first 食-唔-食 *sik6-m4 sik6* question was an imitation of the adult production, and the second 食-唔-食 *sik6-m4-sik6* question followed shortly after the first one. R10 did not use the prerequisite 唔-食 *m4-sik6* before either one of these questions. R10's next A-not-A question involved the lexeme 見 *gin3* 'see', and it was again an imitative production. His third 食-唔-食 *sik6-m4-sik6* question was an exact repetition of the adult input, although prior to this question, there were three spontaneous uses of the prerequisite 唔-食 *m4-sik6*. R10's last A-not-A question in this sample was a spontaneous production and it involved the lexeme 好 *hou2* 'good'. There was no use of the prerequisite 唔-好 *m4-hou2* frame in R10's utterances. In the adult input, however, half of all A-not-A questions involved the lexeme 好 *hou2*.

In the third session at 4;00, R10 produced four A-not-A questions involving the two lexemes 啱 *ngaam1* 'correct' and 好 *hou2* 'good' which he had used before. As with his previous production, none of R10's three 啱-唔-啱 *ngaam1-m4-ngaam1* questions were preceded by the prerequisite 唔-啱 *m4-ngaam1*. The 好-唔-好 *hou2-m4-hou2* question was the second one produced in this sample, and it was an exact repetition of the adult input. In this session, as in the first, the adult produced a substantial number of 63 A-not-A questions involving 14 different lexemes.

In the fifth sample, R10 produced one A-not-A question using the lexeme 相同 *soeng1tung4* 'same'. There was no use of the prerequisite 唔-相同 *m4-soeng1tung4* in this or earlier samples in the child's production or the adult input. In the sixth sample, R10 produced one A-not-A question using the familiar lexeme 食 *sik6* 'eat'. In the last sample at 4;03, R10 produced a spontaneous 係-唔-係 *hai6-m4-hai6* question and he produced the prerequisite 唔-係 *m4-hai6* once in his sample two months previously.

R16

R16 produced his only A-not-A-question with the lexeme 知 *zi1* 'know' in his fifth sample at 4;11. It was a spontaneous production. Although there was no occurrence of the prerequisite 唔-知 *m4-zi1* in this sample, R16 produced it four times in three of his previous monthly samples. The child also produced seven 唔 *m4*-A frames with six different lexemes prior to the production of this A-not-A question in this sample. There were no other instances of A-not-A question to ascertain what phase R16 was at, but he was likely to be at least at the lexical-grammaticalization phase.

Summary

Based on descriptions of their A-not-A question use, we identified the developmental phase for the seven children with SLI. We also did the same for the typically developing children reported in Stokes and Wong (2006). Table 4.2 summarizes the developmental phase of each of the children and Table 4.3 lists the lexemes used in the A-not-A questions produced by each child with SLI. It was quite straightforward for all children except R10. R10's development of A-not-A questions did not seem to go through the lexical-grammaticalization phase. He was in the chunking-social imitation phase in the first two months. In the subsequent months, he produced three spontaneous A-not-A questions but none of them was preceded by their prerequisites except for the last one involving the lexeme 係 *hai6* 'is'. Given the presence of frequent and diverse exemplars in the input, it was very plausible that R10 had successfully learned the construction schema for A-not-A questions

Table 4.3 Lexemes used in the A-not-A questions produced by the children with SLI

Child	*Lexemes used in A-not-A questions*
R07	得 *dak1* 'okay', 識 *sik1* 'know', 睇 *tai2* 'watch'
R10	啱 *ngaam1* 'correct', 嚟 *lei4* 'come', 食 *sik6* 'eat', 好 *hou2* 'good', 見 *gin3* 'see', 相同 *soeng1tung4* 'same', 係 *hai6* 'is'
R16	知 *zi1* 'know'
R05	去 *heoi3* 'go', 食 *sik6* 'eat', 鍾意 *zung1ji3* 'like', 啱 *ngaam1* 'correct', 嚟 *lei4* 'come'
R09	嚟 *lei4* 'come', 要 *jiu3* 'want', 好 *hou2* 'good', 識 *sik1* 'know', 得 *dak1* 'okay', 會 *wui5* 'would', 返 *faan1* 'return'
R08	係 *hai6* 'is', 識 *sik1* 'know', 靚 *leng3* 'pretty', 啱 *ngaam1* 'correct'

through inductive analysis, although the prerequisites were not observed in the samples.

These seven case studies together showed that children with SLI generally followed the same three phases of A-not-A question development: chunking and social imitation phase, then lexical-grammaticalization phase and eventually construction phase. Both of our predictions were confirmed. As for typically developing children, the questions these children produced at the lexical-grammaticalization phase also required prior use of the 唔 *m4*-A frame with the specific lexemes. Again like typically developing children, children with SLI in this cohort were able to abstract a schema construction for A-not-A questions after they produced several lexeme-specific questions.

In the SLI group as in the typically developing group, there were two children in the construction phase (R09, R08, LLY, LTF). They were the children with a maximum MLU of 3.6 morphemes or above, and the ones who produced more A-not-A questions than most children in their respective groups. As their A-not-A questions were no longer lexically bound, they began to generate questions with new lexemes, resulting in higher frequencies of use. Individual variability was also noted in both groups. At a maximum MLU between 3.0 and 3.8, two children in the SLI group (R05, R16) were still at the lexical-grammaticalization phase, and one (R11) did not produce any A-not-A questions. At the same MLU range in the typically developing group, two children (CGK, WBH) did not produce any A-not-A questions, and two (CCC, HHC) were in the social imitation and chunking phase. At a maximum MLU level between 2.5 to 2.9, two children, one from each group (R07, CKT), were in the lexical-grammaticalization phase. One child in the SLI group (R10) was in the construction phase while one child in the typically developing group (MHZ) was in the social imitation and chunking phase.

As revealed in Table 4.2, seven children in the SLI group showed a comparable range of MLUs with a child in the typically developing group reported in Stokes and Wong (2006). Children in the SLI group seemed to be at a more advanced phase of development than the children in the typically developing group. In the SLI group, no children were in the earliest social imitation and chunking phase, whereas there were three in the typically developing group. There were more children in the SLI group who were in the two later lexical-grammaticalization and construction phases than in the typically developing group. The second piece of evidence came from the fact that the typically developing children produced fewer A-not-A questions than the children with SLI. The SLI group's maximum number of A-not-A questions was 13 compared to 12 produced in the typically developing group. Note, however, that 16 samples were examined for A-not-A questions for each child in the typically developing group and most of the samples were longer than the 150 utterances included for children in the SLI group. Unlike the SLI group where only three of the eight children produced only one or fewer questions of this type, six children in the typically developing group had this low (or nil) frequency pattern.

It is possible that some children with SLI had special difficulty with the abstraction of the construction schema for A-not-A questions. They were caught at the lexical-grammaticalization phase when other children at the same MLU level had moved on to the construction phase (e.g. R05 vs R08). But then the same was observed for children in the typically developing group (HHC vs LTF). Findings from this study suggest that the construction of A-not-A questions did not appear to be an area of special difficulty for children with SLI. Evidence from an earlier study (Leonard *et al.*, 2007) supports this conclusion. The study examined Cantonese-speaking children's use of the modal auxiliary 可以 *ho2ji3* 'can' in the form of A-not-A questions. The performance of the children with SLI was comparable to that of the younger language-matched typically developing controls, although they did more poorly than their typically developing age peers.

Given that the children with SLI in this study were on average two years older, increased social and world experience might have given them a stronger motivation to seek out others' opinions through the use of A-not-A questions. This motivation would be matched with a greater understanding of the role of this question form in social interaction. This conclusion needs to be further confirmed with longitudinal language samples of the sort reported in Rice (2004), or preferably with more intensive samples collected between children and their primary caregiver(s), as suggested by Tomasello and Stahl (2004). Another alternative will be the use of experimental data (Riches *et al.*, 2006). Experimental data will also allow us to examine children's use of A-not-A questions where the lexeme A is disyllabic. These questions are not as common as those with a monosyllabic lexeme, but they are formulated slightly differently and therefore potentially might create difficulties for children with SLI.

Discussion

Implications for intervention

(1) The usage-based theory of language development places an emphasis on the exposure to relevant adult input; however, the contribution of input is not absolute, but seems to require intentional knowledge and the emergence of structural prerequisites (唔 *m4* + A + SFP and A + SFP) in the child. The most frequently occurring A-not-A questions in the adult input were ones that involved the lexemes 係 *hai6* 'is' and 好 *hou2* 'good'. However 係-唔-係 *hai6-m4-hai6* and 好-唔-好 *hou2-m4-hou2* questions were not one of the first A-not-A questions produced by any of the children, except one (R10). In addition to input, the intervention literature on children with language impairment reported that children were more successful in learning what they were ready to learn (Bain & Olswang, 1995; Olswang *et al.*, 1992). When the child is ready, that is when s/he has the structural prerequisites for the construction, learning is likely to take place with increased and focused input.

(2) Children with SLI and typically developing children reported in Stokes and Wong (2006) generally went through the lexical-grammaticalization phase before they developed an abstract schema for A-not-A questions. Intentional knowledge is not enough to support learning, and social imitation and chunking does not lead directly to the construction phase. It only allows children to experience the communicative function of A-not-A questions, and provides the motivation needed for its learning and use. Opportunities should therefore be given to children at the social imitation and chunking phase to use the prerequisite 唔 *m4*-A with a few lexemes to prepare them for their first spontaneous production of A-not-A questions.

(3) As reported for English-speaking children with SLI, Cantonese-speaking children with SLI made the same developmental errors as their typically developing peers (Wong *et al.*, 2004). This study provided further evidence for this. R05's early attempts of A-not-A questions without the prerequisite 唔 *m4*-A resulted in the omission of the syllabic nasal negative marker. Stokes and Wong (2006)

reported the same error in a typically developing child (LLY). Similarities such as this provide the justification for our application of theories of normal language learning to language-impaired populations.

(4) Despite the fact that there were fewer utterances in her samples, the child with SLI (R09) was observed to successfully transition to the construction phase after she produced three lexeme-specific A-not-A questions, just like the typically developing child, LLY. The two children with SLI who attempted but failed to do so produced only one (R07) or two (R05) of these questions. Having said that, one child with SLI (R08) who was in the construction phase only produced two lexeme-specific questions before he generated a new A-not-A question without use of the prerequisite. This child, however, produced the 唔 *m4*-A frame with many different lexemes prior to this production. Given sampling limitations, it is very likely that children in this study produced the prerequisite 唔 *m4*-A frames and other lexeme-specific questions when not being recorded. This might be the case for the third child (R10) who appeared to have reached the construction phase without going through the lexical-grammaticalization phase.

As for the children who were reported in Stokes and Wong (2006), we were only able to examine children's learning in relation to the immediate input at the time of the recording, and we had no information of input from the children's caregivers (interaction was only with the research assistant). We therefore could not conclude on the specific effect of caregiver input or the number of lexeme-specific questions a child with SLI had to produce before s/he was able to abstract the construction schema or how that number compared with typically developing children or related to the severity of the children's language impairment. Again, more intensive and longitudinal language samples (between children and their primary caregiver) must be collected and analyzed to provide a microgenetic database (Siegler & Crowley, 1991) for analysis of emergence patterns. This study does provide a rough benchmark, however, for the speech-language pathologist who is not the primary provider of language input for children with SLI and who will not be able to observe the child's use of A-not-A questions all the time.

Accounting for SLI

General information processing deficit accounts of SLI (see Leonard, 1998 for a review) and the usage-based theory of language development share the assumption that children learn language using general cognitive mechanisms and psychological processes. From cross-linguistic studies of SLI, we learn that the pattern of impairment is the outcome of an inadequate general information processing system failing to meet the online processing demands of forms and constructions. Among the several general processing deficit accounts proposed, the morphological sparseness account (Bortolini *et al.*, 1997) offered some explanations for Cantonese-speaking children with SLI's difficulties with aspect markers, but was inadequate for the difficulties in who-object questions that Wong *et al.* (2004) observed in these children. The usage-based theory of language development, which specifies the cognitive mechanisms and psychological processes involved in language learning, might provide an insight for further studies on Cantonese-speaking children with SLI.

Cantonese-speaking children with SLI showed exceptional difficulties with aspect markers (Fletcher *et al.*, 2005), and it was suggested that they were in a prolonged lexical-grammaticalization phase when compared to their language-matched peers (Fletcher *et al.*, 2006). Evidence from this study suggested that these children did not have particular difficulties with A-not-A questions, and they were able to move away from lexeme-specific learning to the abstraction of construction schema in the same way as typically developing children at comparable language levels.

According to the usage-based theory, the cognitive mechanisms that are involved in the abstraction of construction schema are analogical reasoning and pattern-finding. Given a very consistent pattern like A-not-A questions, Cantonese-speaking children with SLI did not seem to have problems with these cognitive mechanisms. However, as mentioned earlier, using a cross-sectional methodology, Stokes and Fletcher (2000) found that children with SLI restricted their use of aspect markers to a few verbs. How do we explain their problems in building a construction schema that allows them to use aspect markers with a wider set of verbs of different semantic types?

We have two plausible answers for this question. Faulty learning of aspect marker forms in children with SLI could be due to either their input characteristics or the conceptual underpinnings of aspect marker deployment in discourse. When constructions are inconsistent (as in aspect marker use) and do not allow comparisons of structural similarities across instances of use, children with SLI may have more difficulty in recognizing analogous forms. That is, variations in forms in the input (飲 水 *jaam2 seoi2* = 'drink water' *or* 'drinking water; and 飲 嚟 水 *jaam2 gan2 seoi2* = 'drinking water') may pose particular difficulties for learners who are not as proficient at pattern recognition when the input is inconsistent. Alternatively, or even additionally, children with SLI have difficulties appreciating the speaker's perspective on the event when there is no aspectual marking on the verb, and recognizing the difference in perspectives when the verb is followed by an aspect marker. Children with SLI's difficulties with aspect markers can be due to their underdeveloped cognitive perspective-taking abilities, as discussed in

MacWhinney (1999), to appreciate the subtle perspective-driven nature of aspect marker use and nonuse (Stokes *et al.*, 2002). Here then, children with SLI's use of an aspect marker with some, but not other verbs, may become more a function of the frequency in which these combinations appear in the input. Future research is needed to test this hypothesis.

Conclusion

Over time we have tested the ability of Cantonese-speaking children with SLI to encode morphological markers and question formation using cross-sectional and longitudinal methods, psycholinguistic experiments and language sample analysis, and systematically explored accounts of language development and disorders. These studies as a whole lead us to the hypothesis that the roots of SLI may not lie in faulty cognitive mechanisms that underlie language learning (intention-reading and cultural learning; schematization; entrenchment and competition; analogy and functionally based distributional analysis), but may lie in the specific nature of the input and concomitant cognitive development. From studying a Sinitic language, we propose that factors in addition to frequency in the input are important in language learning. The two factors we have identified thus far that are in need of further empirical testing are consistency in input and the development of discourse-based perspective-taking abilities throughout childhood.

Acknowledgements

We acknowledge funding support from the Hong Kong Research Grants Council, Hong Kong-SAR-China to the first author (No. 7264/04H) and the second author (No. 7192/97H) for the research reported in this chapter.

References

Bain, B.A. and Olswang, L.B. (1995) Examining readiness for learning two-word utterances by children with specific expressive language impairment: Dynamic assessment validation. *American Journal of Speech-Language Pathology* 4, 81–91.

Bortolini, U., Caselli, M.C. and Leonard, L.B. (1997) Grammatical deficits in Italian-speaking children with specific language impairment. *Journal of Speech, Language, and Hearing Research* 40, 809–820.

Burgemeister, B., Blum, L. and Lorge, I. (1972) *The Columbia Mental Maturity Scale*. New York: Harcourt Brace Jovanovich.

Clark, E.V. (2003) *First Language Acquisition*. Cambridge: Cambridge University Press.

Diessel, H. (2004) *The Acquisition of Complex Sentences*. Cambridge: Cambridge University Press.

Ellis Weismer, S. (1997) The role of stress in language processing and intervention. *Topics in Language Disorders* 17, 41–52.

Fletcher, P., Stokes, S.F., Leonard, L.B. and Wong, A.M-Y. (2005) The expression of aspect in Cantonese-speaking children with specific language impairment. *Journal of Speech, Language, and Hearing Research* 48, 621–634.

Fletcher, P., Stokes, S.F. and Wong, A.M-Y. (2006) Specific language impairment in Chinese. In P. Li, L.H. Tan, E. Bates and O.J.L. Tzeng (eds) *Handbook of Asian Psycholinguistics* (Vol. 1, pp. 296–307). Cambridge: Cambridge University Press.

Gillam, R.B., Loeb, D.F., Hoffman, L. Bohman, T., Champlin, C.A., Thibodeau *et al.* (2008) The efficacy of Fast ForWord language intervention in school-aged children with language impairment: A randomized controlled trial. *Journal of Speech, Language, and Hearing Research* 51, 97–119.

Hong Kong Society for Child Health and Development (1985) *Reynell Developmental Language Scales: Revised*. Windsor: NFER-Nelson.

Johnston, J. and Schery, T. (1976) The use of grammatical morphemes by children with communication disorders. In D. Morehead and A. Morehead (eds) *Normal and Deficient Child Language* (pp. 239–258). Baltimore, MD: University Park Press.

Johnston, J.R. (1985) Fit, focus and functionality. *Child Language Teaching and Therapy* 1, 125–134.

Kidd, E. (2006) The acquisition of complement clause constructions. In E.V. Clark and B.F. Kelly (eds) *Constructions in Acquisition* (pp. 311–332). Stanford, CA: Center for the Study of Language and Information.

Klee, T., Stokes, S.F., Wong, A.M-Y., Fletcher, P. and Gavin, W. (2004) Utterance length and lexical diversity in Cantonese-speaking children with and without specific language impairment. *Journal of Speech, Language, and Hearing Research* 47, 1396–1410.

Law, J., Boyle, J., Harris, F., Harkness, A. and Nye, C. (1998) Screening for speech and language delay: A systematic review of the literature. *Health Technology Assessment* 2, 1–184.

Lee, T.H-T., Wong, C.H., Leung, S., Man, P., Cheung, A., Szeto, K. *et al.* (1996) *The Development of Grammatical Competence in Cantonese-speaking Children*. Report of a project funded by Hong Kong Research Grants Committee 2/91 (1991–1994).

Leonard, L. (1998) *Children with Specific Language Impairment*. Cambridge, MA: The MIT Press.

Leonard, L.B., Deevy, P., Wong, A.M-Y., Stokes, S.F. and Fletcher, P. (2007) Modal verbs with and without tense: A study of English- and Cantonese-speaking children with specific language impairment. *International Journal of Language & Communication Disorders* 42, 209–228.

Linguistic Society of Hong Kong (1994) *The LSHK Cantonese Romanization Scheme*. Hong Kong: Linguistic Society of Hong Kong.

MacWhinney, B. (1999) The emergence of language from embodiment. In B. MacWhinney (ed.) *The Emergence of Language* (pp. 213–256). Mahwah, NJ: Lawrence Erlbaum.

Olswang, L.B., Bain, B.A. and Johnson, G.A. (1992) Using dynamic assessment with children with language disorders. In S.F. Warren and J. Reichle (eds) *Causes and Effects in Communication and Language Intervention* (pp. 187–216). Baltimore, MD: Paul H. Brookes.

Reynell, J. and Huntley, M. (1987) Reynell Developmental Scales: Revised Version. Windsor: NFER-Nelson.

Rice, M., Oetting, J., Marquis, J., Bode, J. and Pae, S. (1994) Frequency of input effects on word comprehension of children with specific language impairment. *Journal of Speech and Hearing Research* 37, 106–122.

Rice, M.L. (2004) Growth models of developmental language disorders. In M.L. Rice and S.F. Warren (eds) *Developmental Language Disorders: From Phenotypes to Etiologies* (pp. 207–240). Mahwah, NJ: Lawrence Erlbaum.

Riches, N.G., Faragher, B. and Conti-Ramsden, G. (2006) Verb schema use and input dependence in 5-year-old children with specific language impairment (SLI). *International Journal of Language & Communication Disorders* 41, 117–135.

Siegler, R.S. and Crowley, K. (1991) The microgenetic method: A direct means for studying cognitive development. *American Psychologist* 46, 606–620.

Snow, C.E. (1999) Social perspectives on the emergence of language. In B. MacWhinney (ed.) *The Emergence of Language* (pp. 257–276). Mahwah, NJ: Lawrence Erlbaum.

Stokes, S.F. and Fletcher, P. (2000) Lexical diversity and productivity in Cantonese-speaking children with specific language impairment. *International Journal of Language & Communication Disorders* 35, 527–541.

Stokes, S.F. and Fletcher, P. (2003) Aspectual forms in Cantonese children with specific language impairment. *Linguistics* 41, 381–406.

Stokes, S.F., Fletcher, P. and Leung, S.C-S. (1998) *Language Growth in Cantonese-speaking Children with SLI* (RGC project No. 7192/97H). Hong Kong: Hong Kong Research Grants Council.

Stokes, S.F., Fletcher, P., Leung, S.C-S. and Kong, A. (2002) Lexical and morphological diversity in children with SLI: Evidence in support of an optionality constraint. Paper presented at the joint meeting of the IX Congress of the International Association for the Study of Child Language and the Symposium for Research on Child Language Disorders, Madison, July.

Stokes, S.F. and Wong, A.M-Y. (2006) Building questions in Cantonese. In E.V. Clark and B.F. Kelly (eds) *Constructions in Acquisition* (pp. 283–310). Stanford, CA: Center for the Study of Language and Information.

Tomasello, M. (1992) *First Verbs: A Case Study of Early Grammatical Development*. Cambridge: Cambridge University Press.

Tomasello, M. (2003) *Constructing a Language: A Usage-based Theory of Language Acquisition*. Cambridge, MA: Harvard University Press.

Tomasello, M. and Stahl, A. (2004) Sampling children's speech: How much is enough? *Journal of Child Language* 31, 101–121.

Tomblin, J.B., Records, N.L., Buckwalter, P., Zhang, X., Smith, E. and O'Brien, M. (1997) Prevalence of specific language impairment in kindergarten children. *Journal of Speech, Language, and Hearing Research* 40, 1245–1260.

Wong, A.M-Y., Leonard, L.B., Fletcher, P. and Stokes, S.F. (2004) Questions without movement: A study of Cantonese-speaking children with and without specific language impairment. *Journal of Speech, Language and Hearing Research* 47, 1440–1453.

Wong, V., Lee, P.W.H., Lieh-Mak, F., Yeung, C.Y., Leung, P.W.L., Luk, S.L., *et al.* (1992) Language screening in preschool Chinese children. *European Journal of Disorders of Communication* 27, 247–264.

Yoder, P.J. and McDuffie, A. (2002) Treatment of primary language disorders in early childhood: Evidence of efficacy. In P. Accardo, B. Rogers and A. Capute (eds) *Disorders of Language Development* (pp. 151–177). Baltimore, MD: York Press.

Yoder, P.J. and Stone, W.L. (2006) A randomized comparison of two prelinguistic communication interventions on the acquisition of spoken communication in preschoolers in ASD. *Journal of Speech, Language and Hearing Research* 49, 698–711.

Chapter 5

Morphosyntactic Deficits in Cantonese-speaking Children with Specific Language Impairment

PAUL FLETCHER, LAURENCE B. LEONARD, STEPHANIE F. STOKES and ANITA M-Y. WONG

Investigating Specific Language Impairment (SLI)

In a series of studies over two decades, Leonard and colleagues have taken advantage of typological differences between English and other languages to explore and endeavor to explain morphosyntactic deficits in children with SLI (see e.g. Bedore & Leonard, 2001 on Spanish; Dromi *et al.*, 1993 on Hebrew; Hansson & Leonard, 2003 on Swedish; Leonard *et al.*, 1987 on Italian). In these studies, the performance of children with SLI at around the age of five years is compared with that of their typically developing age peers (TD-AM) and a group of younger typical developers (TD-Y) close to three years of age, on a morphological or syntactic feature whose realization differs from English. As we know that children with SLI have delayed language development, we expect their performance on a grammatical variable of interest to be poorer than that of the TD-AM group. But their overall language ability should see them operating at the same level as the TD-Y group, who are younger than them by two years. If this is not the case – if the children with SLI do not control a morphosyntactic element or system as well as the TD-Y group – the inference is made that this constitutes a specific morphosyntactic deficit, relative to the overall grammatical system. The comparison of deficits that occur in English with either comparable deficits, or the lack of them, in other languages, allows us to go beyond description to test hypotheses about the basis for the grammatical symptoms that have been isolated.

Here we report on three areas of Cantonese grammar that have the potential to inform our perspective on SLI via comparisons between the performance of Cantonese-speaking children with SLI and their English-speaking counterparts. (For a discussion of SLI in Mandarin-speaking children, see Chapter 3 of this volume.) The design of the studies of each area adhered to the blueprint outlined earlier. There were three groups of Cantonese-speaking children from Hong Kong involved. The children with SLI, with an average age close to 60 months, were identified using comparable exclusion and inclusion criteria to those used in previous studies of English-speaking children. Their non-verbal intelligence was assessed as within normal limits using the Columbia Mental Maturity Scale (Burgemeister *et al.*, 1972). They all passed an oro-motor and hearing screenings and none of them had a history of seizures or showed any evidence of neurological or psychosocial impairment. Their language status was established via the Receptive scale of the Cantonese adaptation of the Reynell Developmental Language Scales (RDLS; Reynell & Huntley, 1987), with a criterion of more than 1.25 SD below the mean required for children to be included in the SLI group. The comparison groups of typically developing children were also tested on the Receptive scale of the RDLS. The TD-Y group mean score was not distinct from that of the SLI group, while the mean score for the TD-AM group was significantly higher. Mean length of utterance in words (MLU) was calculated for all three groups, and again the SLI and TD-Y groups were comparable on this measure, while the MLU for the TD-AM group was significantly higher than that of the other two groups.

SLI in Cantonese

The grammatical areas in Cantonese that were chosen for scrutiny were *wh*-questions, passive and aspect. These areas, while common to the two languages, present potentially informative structural differences from English or relate to current theoretical discussion of language impairment or both:

(1) *Wh*-questions in Cantonese differ from English in that the *wh*-word remains in all cases *in situ* – that is, it holds the same structural position as its analogous constituent in a declarative structure. In English, *wh*-object questions, in common with other *wh*-constituents, are located at the beginning of the sentence, and so the *wh*-constituent is some distance away from the postverbal slot in which an object noun phrase (NP) would normally be found and interpreted, which seems to cause problems for English-speaking children with SLI (van der Lely & Battell, 2003). The parallel structures for declarative and interrogative in Cantonese might be expected to facilitate the construction of *wh*-forms for children with SLI learning this language.
(2) Passives in English and Cantonese also involve constituent order differences from their active analogues, and in Cantonese the NP identifying the agent of the action is preceded by a form that corresponds to *by* in English. Cantonese does not, however, require the changes in verb modification that English displays.
(3) There is ample evidence from English that the mastery of tense and agreement is problematic for children with SLI, to the extent that these forms have been suggested as reliable markers of SLI in English (Tager-Flusberg & Cooper, 1999). They have also served as fertile

ground for theoretical discussion of SLI, specifically in relation to the agreement/tense omission model (ATOM; see Pine *et al.* 2005; Wexler, 1998). Other areas of verb modification, such as aspect, have been relatively ignored. The absence of formal tense in Cantonese allows us to look directly at the control of aspect by Cantonese-speaking children with SLI without the confounding potential that the obligatory tense entails in the study of SLI in English.

Full details of the subject groups involved, the procedures followed to explore the children's production of all of these forms, and statistical analyses of the results can be found in a series of recent articles. For *wh*-questions, see Wong *et al.* (2004); for passives, Leonard *et al.* (2006); and for aspect, Fletcher *et al.* (2005). Here we will outline the findings from each of the areas in turn and discuss their implications for our understanding of SLI.

Wh-questions

Previous work on English has identified deficits in performance by children with SLI on *wh*-subject and *wh*-object questions (e.g. van der Lely & Battell, 2003), with *wh*-object questions posing greater problems. More precisely, this pattern has been identified in a subgroup of children with SLI, referred to as G-SLI, who 'exhibit a relatively pure, domain-specific grammatical impairment' (van der Lely & Battell, 2003: 153). Their explanation of why object questions may present more difficulty comes from an account of *wh*-question formation that invokes movement. For object questions, the *wh*-operator is moved to specifier position of the complementizer phrase (CP), leaving behind a trace in the internal verb argument position. The trace is bound by the *wh*-operator. A typical structure (van der Lely & Battell, 2003: 157) appears in (1):

(1) $[_{CP}$ Who$_i$ $[_{C}$ did$_j$ $[_{IP}$ Ralph $[_{I}$ e$_j$ $[_{VP}$ $[_{V}$ see $[_{NP}$ t$_i$ $]]]]]]]$

Object questions also involve *do*-support – characterized here as I to C movement.

In subject questions, on the other hand, we find the *wh*-operator in the appropriate external argument position and no *do*-support is required, as in (2):

(2) $[_{CP}$ $[_{C}$ $[_{IP}$ Who $[_{I}$ $[_{VP}$ $[_{V}$ saw $[_{NP}$ Ralph $]]]]]]]$

The representational deficit for dependent relations (RDDR) account of G-SLI asserts that the core deficit for G-SLI children is that they treat obligatory movement as optional. The prediction then for these children's treatment of *wh*-questions is that they will perform less well on the questions that involve movement, the object questions, than on subject questions. And in treating movement as optional in *wh*-object questions, they will sometimes produce utterances such as *Ralph saw what?* or *What did Ralph see something?* The data reported in van der Lely and Battell (2003) support these predictions.

Cantonese offers an important perspective from which to study *wh*-questions used by children with SLI. As Examples (3) to (6) show, *wh*-subject and *wh*-object questions preserve the same subject-verb-object order as declaratives. So unlike English, a *wh*-word or phrase that is the object of the verb occupies the internal argument position, as in (6):

(3)	熊仔	錫	豬豬
	hung4zai2	*sek3*	*zyu1zyu1*
	TeddyBear	kiss	Piglet
	'TeddyBear kissed Piglet'		

(4)	邊個	錫	豬豬	呀?
	bin1go3	*sek3*	*zyu1zyu1*	*aa3?*
	Who	kiss	Piglet	SFP?
	'Who kissed Piglet?'			

(5)	豬豬	錫	熊仔
	zyu1zyu1	*sek3*	*hung4zai2*
	Piglet	kiss	TeddyBear
	'Piglet kissed TeddyBear'		

(6)	豬豬	錫	邊個	呀?
	zyu1zyu1	*sek3*	*bin1go3*	*aa3?*
	Piglet	kiss	who	SFP?
	'Who did Piglet kiss?'			

(In these examples, SFP indicates sentence-final particle.)

It would follow that if the structure of Cantonese object questions does not involve movement, then the performance of Cantonese children with SLI on *wh*-subject and *wh*-object questions should not differ, and the discrepancy seen in English and attributed to movement should disappear. However, the outcome of the elicitation procedures reported in Wong *et al.* (2004) confounds this prediction. The results indicated that the children with SLI were less accurate in using *wh*-questions than either same-age peers or younger, typically developing children. This difference was attributable to the difficulty that the children with SLI had with *wh*-object questions. Both the younger, typically developing children and the children with SLI were less accurate with *wh*-object questions than the typically developing children serving as age matches. However, the children with SLI were even less skilled than the younger typically developing group in using questions of this type. The three groups of children did not differ in their use of *wh*-subject questions. If the poorer performance on object questions in Cantonese is not attributable to movement, why would the discrepancy between the two types of interrogative occur?

An alternative explanation relates to animacy and input frequency. For Cantonese-speaking children with SLI, a rationale for hypothesizing both animacy effects and input-frequency effects can be formulated. A recent study by Wong and Ingram (2003) examined whether the *wh*-subject/*wh*-object asymmetry seen in English would also be evident in the speech of young typically developing Cantonese-speaking children. These investigators inspected the spontaneous speech samples of eight children between the ages of 1;5 (year;month) and 3;8. They hypothesized that no asymmetry would be found because the *wh*-word remains *in situ* in Cantonese. Wong and Ingram did not report overall accuracy levels. However, they found that the children were more likely to use 乜嘢 *mat1je5* 'what' in *wh*-object questions and 邊個 *bin1go3* 'who' in *wh*-subject questions. This finding raises the possibility that even when *wh*-object questions require no movement, the animacy of the referent will continue to play a significant role in the children's success with *wh*-subject questions.

An inspection of adults' speech to young Cantonese-speaking children provides evidence consistent with the possibility that frequency effects could influence the relative difficulty of different types of *wh*-questions. An examination of adult speech to 70 typically developing preschoolers collected by Fletcher *et al.* (2000) revealed that 87% of *wh*-questions with 邊個 *bin1go3* 'who' were *wh*-subject questions; only 13% were *wh*-object questions. This clear difference raises the possibility that *who*-object questions are less familiar to these children, and hence likely to be more difficult than *who*-subject questions, independent of movement. If input-frequency effects are operative in children's acquisition of *wh*-questions in Cantonese, they might constitute an especially strong influence in the case of children with SLI. Leonard and colleagues (e.g. Dromi *et al.*, 1993; Leonard *et al.*, 1987) have proposed that children with SLI may have processing limitations that compel them to rely heavily on the dominant grammatical characteristics of the ambient language at the expense of other grammatical details. As a result, the typical grammatical profile seen in normally developing children in any given language will be exaggerated in the case of children with SLI learning the same language. Cantonese is a hallmark case of an isolating language with no grammatical inflections for person, number or gender, and no distinctions according to case, even within the pronoun system. Given the absence of morphological cues to distinguish subjects from objects, it would not be surprising if the higher frequency of 邊個 *bin1go3* 'who' in the sentence-initial position leads children with SLI to associate this *wh*-word with subjects. This, in turn, would render *who*-object questions especially difficult for children with SLI relative to typically developing children and relative to their own use of *who*-subject questions.

Passive

As in English, passive sentences in Cantonese differ from active sentences in word order and the agent is identified by a specific marker, 畀 *bei2*. Unlike English, the Cantonese passive form has the order patient-agent-verb. Because Cantonese does not employ tense (or agreement), the same verb form is used for both active and passive sentences. Examples of active and passive sentences are provided in (7) and (8):

(7) 狗 追 貓
gau2 zeoi1 maau1
dog chase cat
'the dog chases the cat'

(8) 貓 畀 狗 追
maau1 bei2 gau2 zeoi1
cat by dog chase
'the cat is chased by the dog'

The passive in Cantonese is most likely to be used when the subject (the patient) is affected by the action, often in an adverse manner. According to Matthews and Yip (1994), passives are used less often in Cantonese than in English. They are used only infrequently by adults when speaking to their preschool-aged children (McBride *et al.*, 2004). Based on input frequency, then, Cantonese passives should hold no advantage over passives in English. A structural description of the Cantonese passive based on Li (1990), invoking movement, is shown in (9):

(9) $[_{\text{TP}}$ 貓 1_i $[_{\text{T}'}$ $[_{\text{VP}}$ $[_{\text{V}'}$ $[_{\text{PP}}$ 畀狗] $[_{\text{V}'}$ $[_{\text{V}}$ 追] $[_{\text{NP}}$ t_i]]]]]]
$[_{\text{TP}}$ *maau1*$_i$ $[_{\text{T}'}$ $[_{\text{VP}}$ $[_{\text{V}'}$ $[_{\text{PP}}$ *bei2 gau2*] $[_{\text{V}'}$ $[_{\text{V}}$ *zeoi1*] $[_{\text{NP}}$ t_i]]]]]]

As in English verbal *be* passives, the NP (貓 *maau1*) serving as the complement of the verb moves to the Spec position of TP (tense phrase), leaving a co-indexed *t*. The agent role is expressed through a prepositional phrase (PP) (畀 狗 *bei2 gau2*) that appears within VP (verb phrase). However, unlike English, the PP appears before rather than after the verb. An important difference between English and Cantonese is that the latter does not have an overt form in T representing tense (or agreement). The structure of Cantonese passives has implications for the RDDR account, at least within the movement analysis approach outlined earlier. Because they are assumed to apply movement optionally, Cantonese-speaking children with SLI should be inconsistent in placing the NP complement (貓 *maau1*, in our example) in the Spec position of TP. This should result in ill-constructed passives, e.g. productions such as 畀 狗 追 貓 *bei2 gau2 zeoi1 maau1* or even 貓 畀 狗 追 貓 *maau1 bei2 gau2 zeoi1 maau1* in place of 貓 畀 狗 追 *maau1 bei2 gau2 zeoi1*, or an over-reliance on active sentences. The RDDR account has support in relation to English passives: van der Lely (1996) found that a group of children with SLI made significantly more reversal errors in the comprehension of passives than their TD-Y counterparts. In response to the sentence *the man is eaten by the fish*, they were prone to select a picture of a man eating a fish.

The RDDR prediction based on optionality of movement is not the only explanatory account of the grammatical performance of children with SLI. In keeping with the sparse morphology hypothesis (Leonard, 1998), the noncanonical word order of passives coupled with the extremely sparse grammatical morphology of Cantonese could lead children with SLI to impose a more typical subject-verb-object order on these utterances. The RDDR and the sparse morphology hypothesis thus concur on likely outcomes but from different premises. However, the results of two passive production tasks (for details see Leonard *et al.*, 2006) provide little support for the predictions of either account. In both tasks, the children with SLI were as successful as the TD-Y children, and numerical differences between the SLI and TD-AM groups failed to reach statistical significance. The similarity in the performance of the SLI and TD-Y groups could not be attributed to the number of passive sentences attempted because the children with SLI were no more likely than the TD-Y children to produce active sentences during the two tasks. Furthermore, when the children attempted passive sentences, they neither produced many examples of ill-constructed passives nor did they confuse agent and patient, as happens in English. The following list of examples is exhaustive of productions regarded as passive attempts in the data:

(10) a. 貓 畀 狗 追 *maau1 bei2 gau2 zeoi1*
b. 畀 狗 追 *bei2 gau2 zeoi1*
c. 貓 狗 追 *maau1 gau2 zeoi1*
d. 貓 畀 追 *maau1 bei2 zeoi1*
e. 貓 追 *maau1 zeoi1*
f. 貓 畀 狗 追 佢 *maau1 bei2 gau2 zeoi1 keoi5*
g. 貓 畀 狗 追 人 *maau1 bei2 gau2 zeoi1 jan4*
h. 畀 貓 追 *bei2 maau1 zeoi1*

Here (10a) is the target utterance, and (10b) and (10f) are acceptable passives, while the remainder of the examples are errors. Examples (10f) and (10g) are interesting in relation to the RDDR account, as both could be interpreted as involving problems with movement. This would be the case both in the structural description of passives based on Li (1990), outlined earlier, and in an alternative account (Tang, 2001). In this account, 貓 *maau1* is base-generated in subject position, and a null operator undergoes movement from its position as the object of the verb and adjoins to the right of 畀 *bei2*, leaving a trace (*t*) in object position.

Examples such as (10f) and (10g), which appear to strand pronominal forms in the trace (object) position, could thus be seen as problems with movement under either account. However, examples like (10f) and (10g) are rare in the data.

Aside from failing to support movement accounts of passive in Cantonese, our findings also suggest that the sparse morphology account requires modification. It seems that if children with SLI direct the limited resources they have available to the signalling of grammatical relations by word order in languages such as Cantonese, they do not focus exclusively on the canonical word order of the language, and in cases where the word order deviates, rely on a default subject-verb-object interpretation. Rather they become sensitive to word order cues in general. Passive word order in Cantonese, in which both nouns precede the verb, provides clear evidence that the sentence deviates from the canonical order; this difference would be clear even if children did not attend to the morpheme 畀 *bei2*.

Aspect

Tense is not grammaticalized in Cantonese, and this allows us to look directly at its complex aspectual system without the confound that obligatory tense adds to any verb modification in English. An account of Cantonese grammar identifies six morphemes which have aspectual meanings (Matthews & Yip, 1994: 198). Two of these forms are perfective and two imperfective, while the set is completed by a morpheme that denotes repeated or habitual activity, and another which is described as 'delimitative'. We will not consider further the habitual or delimitative forms, and will confine further discussion to perfective and imperfective forms. The two imperfective forms, 緊 *gan2* and 住 *zyu6*, are described as 'progressive' and 'continuous', respectively (Matthews & Yip, 1994: 202). The 緊 *gan2* form applies to dynamic, ongoing activity, while 住 *zyu6* indicates a continuous activity or state. The contrast between the two perfective forms, 咗 *zo2* and 過 *gwo3*, hinges on whether the event on which they provide a viewpoint of completion or termination still applies (咗 *zo2*) or has been experienced but does not now hold (過 *gwo3*).

All aspect markers are bound morphemes, which behave in the same way distributionally. They occur immediately after the verb to which they apply (or between words in verb compounds), though they are not inflections and do not undergo any morphophonemic processes. They are grammatically optional: 'for every context in which one occurs it is possible to have the same sentence without the aspect marker' (Matthews & Yip, 1994: 200). There are, however, syntactic contexts in which an aspect marker is at least strongly preferred, if not obligatory. For example 咗 *zo2*, a perfective marker, seems to be required when a transitive verb is accompanied by a past time referring adverbial, and the object of that verb is quantified. And there are pragmatic conditions in which the omission of an aspect marker would seem inappropriate.

The segmentability of Cantonese syllables, the requirement for a full tone on each syllable and the lack of any morphophonemic modification when an aspect marker is added to a verb, are all factors which would seem to conspire to ensure that the aspect morpheme is salient in perception for the Cantonese learner. The available acoustic evidence tends to support that view. For example, durations for the aspect forms of Cantonese range from a mean of 140 ms for perfective 過 *gwo3* to 380 ms for imperfective 緊 *gan2* (Ansaldo & Lim, 2004). By comparison, function words in English appear to be much shorter. Vowel durations in monosyllabic English function words – even in child-directed speech – are usually 50 ms or shorter (Swanson *et al.*, 1992), and whole word durations of monosyllabic function words are usually under 100 ms (e.g. Cooper & Paccia-Cooper, 1980). The facts of the language would seem to rule out the possibility that aspect morphemes in Cantonese could cause perception problems. The same set of observations, together with the similar token frequencies observed in children with SLI and their younger MLU-matched counterparts (Stokes & Fletcher, 2003), suggest that these forms will not lead to production problems. If aspect morphemes do cause particular difficulty for Cantonese children with SLI, relative to younger typically developing children, it will not be plausible to attribute this to the phonological nature of these forms.

Aspect markers in Cantonese should not be especially problematic according to surface accounts of morphosyntactic deficit. But the morphological sparseness of Cantonese, the optional nature of the forms and their dependence on specific pragmatic conditions, predicts difficulties for impaired learners in mastering these forms. In addressing the abilities with aspect markers of children with SLI, we created communication contexts which would require the adult speaker to express viewpoint aspect. Carefully constructed tasks were employed to examine the use of aspect markers, focusing on one of the perfective markers, 咗 *zo2*, and one of the imperfective forms, 緊 *gan2*. The latter was tested in both ongoing and past time contexts. We selected 咗 *zo2* because previous studies indicate it is the first form to appear in typically developing children (Stokes & Fletcher, 2003). The 緊 *gan2* form, while acquired later than the other imperfective form, 住 *zyu6*, is still relatively early to appear, and is less restricted than 住 *zyu6* in the verbs it can co-occur with (Matthews & Yip, 1994: 203). To gain insight into the possible sources of any differences observed among the three groups of children, we also assessed the children's use of temporal meaning as expressed through a nonaspectual form, the temporal adverb 琴日 *kam4jat6* 'yesterday'. Difficulties with temporal adverbs as well as aspect markers could suggest that the problem rests in the expression of temporal notions more generally rather than in the grammatical expression of aspect in particular, and it was important to rule this possibility out.

Our findings indicate that in Cantonese, the first Sinitic language to be thus studied, children with language impairment appear to be disadvantaged with regard to verb morphosyntax, as they have been demonstrated to be in English (Leonard, 2000). As in English however, the difference between children with SLI and their typically developing counterparts is in degree of use: the SLI group can use aspect morphemes in Cantonese, but they use them on significantly fewer occasions than younger typically developing children. When they do select the forms however, they use them appropriately in terms of syntactic distribution and pragmatic context. Cantonese-speaking children with SLI do not seem to differ significantly from TD-Y children in the lexical expression of a temporal concept, as measured by temporal adverbials. And their morphosyntactic deficit also has to be set against a sentence length equivalence to the TD-Y group: they are as capable as their younger counterparts at producing sentences long enough to accommodate the expression of aspect.

Not all languages provoke verb morphology deficits in children with SLI. While English present tense agreement morphemes seem to cause special problems, this is not the case in Spanish and Italian, where children with SLI match their typically developing peers' performance with singular present tense forms. Leonard and colleagues have attributed the relative success of the Spanish and Italian children to the phonetic salience of these forms, by comparison with English, and to the rich inflectional systems within which they cohere (e.g. Bedore & Leonard, 2001; Bortolini *et al.*, 1997). As we have seen, because of the phonological system of Cantonese, lexical and grammatical forms are equally salient, and it is not possible to attribute the deficits in the SLI group to differential phonetic realizations. It seems that reasons for the deficit in the children with SLI have to be sought in other dimensions of the language that the child hears. There are features of the language which separately or in combination could make it problematic for a vulnerable system to analyze the conditions under which aspect markers apply. They are its morphological sparseness and the optionality of aspectual forms.

The aspectual system of Cantonese, as of other Chinese languages, is in one sense 'rich', compared to English. It has six aspectual morphemes, and of these, two are perfective and two imperfective. English has one imperfective form (progressive) and another form which is referred to as perfect, but which some commentators do not consider to be an aspectual category (Huddleston & Pullum, 2002: 116). Cantonese is morphologically sparse in the sense that each of its aspectual categories is represented by a phonologically unvarying form. Unlike tense and agreement forms in, say, Spanish, aspect forms in Cantonese do not contrast person and number forms within a paradigm with a single temporal meaning such as future. Presumably in Spanish, the commonalities between the various forms within a paradigm (e.g. the consistent appearance of the stem, *hablar*, in every future form), plus the existence of identical morphemes with the same meanings across paradigms (e.g. the *-an* ending for third person plural in Spanish present tense *hablan* and future tense *hablaran*), should facilitate the identification of these forms and their semantic interpretation. No such formal support is provided for the interpretation of aspect forms by the Cantonese learner.

In English, children with SLI are said to show optional use of tense morphemes (Rice & Wexler, 1996). In an important sense, this optionality differs from the kind of variable use observed in the present study. We suspect that the optional nature of aspect in input in Cantonese poses problems for the learner that are simply not the same as those seen in English. Verbs appearing without aspect morphemes do not render sentences ungrammatical or unacceptable. It follows that the child will hear many instances of any individual verb without aspect markers, as well as hearing instances with these forms. It is this variability that can serve as a cue as to which contexts are especially appropriate to convey the completion or continuation of an action. Given our findings, working out when to apply this viewpoint aspect may take the child with SLI longer than typically developing peers.

In summary, it would appear that we can identify this area of Cantonese verb morphosyntax as problematic for the child with SLI. In the absence of grammatical tense, we have a clear window on the vulnerability of aspect in this language, as it interacts with a less than adequate acquisition system. In other languages, it has been demonstrated that the phonetic salience of grammatical morphemes is an advantage for children with SLI, especially in the context of a rich inflectional system. In Cantonese however, it would appear that this potential advantage is neutralized by a system of aspectual morphemes that does not cohere within a rich inflectional system, and by the optionality of these forms.

Conclusion

The structure of Cantonese offers the opportunity to shed new light on the vulnerabilities of children with SLI in their attempts to learn grammar. Its tonal character eliminates any realizational difference between members of lexical and grammatical categories. The presence of a tone on each syllable renders all forms equally salient, and rules out the possibility that stress reduction, for example, makes some grammatical categories difficult for children with SLI. As varying surface realizations are unlikely to explain any deficits that we do find in Cantonese-speaking children with SLI, we turn to accounts derived from linguistic theory, such as the RDDR, or to explanations which emphasize the tendency of the child with SLI, with limited processing resources available, to concentrate on the dominant characteristics of the ambient language in learning how to use it. It is these latter accounts which seem to come out best, in relation to the series of studies reported here. Under the RDDR, the *in situ* location of the *wh*-word in Cantonese should give children with SLI no advantage in the use of *who*-subject questions over *who*-object questions. This is not the case – *who*-object questions cause problems for these children. An alternative account suggests that input-frequency effects which, allied to an expectation that animate agents appear in subject rather than object position, reduces accuracy with *who*-object questions.

The RDDR predictions again appear confounded by the results from passive in Cantonese. If the alternative word order for passive is interpreted in terms of movement, with the passive derived from an active form, then children with SLI learning this language should find difficulties with passive forms. They do not, and it might be supposed that the attention they have to pay to the dominant characteristic of the language in determining structural relations, namely word order, is of service in working out agent and patient roles. In this, they are presumably aided by the salient 畀 *bei2* morpheme, and a constituent order which in Cantonese cannot be interpreted as subject verb object (SVO) with S as agent. Finally, the problems Cantonese-speaking children with SLI evince with aspect morphemes echo the difficulties with verb-forms long identified in their English-speaking counterparts. Again, it seems unlikely the phonological realizations of these forms are responsible for their relative difficulty. However, their lack of what might be referred to as paradigm status seems to render them, by comparison to constituent order, less salient in a grammatical sense. While extensive in the meaning range they cover, aspect morphemes do not cohere in a paradigm that rings inflectional changes around a consistent stem form, which seems to be the factor that assists children with SLI learning Spanish, for example.

Cantonese can be added to the list of languages scrutinized in relation to SLI. The series of studies summarized here underline once again the utility of cross-linguistic comparisons, in refining our understanding of the problems posed for children with SLI by their ambient language. The studies also take us a little further in isolating what it is about the interaction between an impaired mechanism and the structure of a language which leads to the deficits these children demonstrate.

Acknowledgements

The research reported in this article was supported by research grant R01 00-458 from the National Institute on Deafness and Other Communication Disorders of the National Institutes of Health (USA), and by the Hong Kong Christian Service Choi Wan and Yuen Long Early Education and Training Centers, the Spastics Association of Hong Kong Wang Tau Hom and Tak Tin Early Education and Training Centers, the Speech and Language Clinic at the Division of Speech and Hearing Sciences, University of Hong Kong, Pamela Youde Child Assessment Center, Yan Chai Hospital and other speech therapy service providers in Hong Kong. We thank the children and families who participated. We gratefully acknowledge the assistance of Anna Lee, Eva Chau, Serena Chan, Patricia Deevy, Alice Lee, Cora Lee, Lina Wong and Richard Wong.

References

Ansaldo, U. and Lim, L. (2004) Phonetic absence as syntactic prominence: Grammaticalization in isolating tonal languages. In O. Fischer, M. Norde and H. Perridon (eds) *Up and Down the Cline – the Nature of Grammaticalization* (pp. 345–362). Amsterdam: John Benjamins.

Bedore, L. and Leonard, L. (2001) Grammatical morphology deficits in Spanish-speaking children with specific language impairment. *Journal of Speech, Language, and Hearing Research* 44, 905–924.

Bortolini, U., Caselli, M. and Leonard, L. (1997) Grammatical deficits in Italian-speaking children with specific language impairment. *Journal of Speech, Language, and Hearing Research* 40, 809–820.

Burgemeister, B., Blum, L. and Lorge, L. (1972) *The Columbia Mental Maturity Scale*. New York: Harcourt Brace Jovanovich.

Cooper, W.E. and Paccia-Cooper, J. (1980) *Syntax and Speech*. Cambridge, MA: Harvard University Press.

Dromi, E., Leonard, L. and Shteiman, M. (1993) The grammatical morphology of Hebrew-speaking children with specific language impairment: Some competing hypotheses. *Journal of Speech and Hearing Research* 36, 760–771.

Fletcher, P., Leonard, L., Stokes, S. and Wong, A.M-Y. (2005) The expression of aspect in Cantonese-speaking children with specific language impairment. *Journal of Speech, Language, and Hearing Research* 48, 621–634.

Fletcher, P., Leung, C-S., Stokes, S. and Weizman, Z. (2000) *Cantonese Pre-school Language Development: A Guide*. Hong Kong: University of Hong Kong, Department of Speech and Hearing Sciences.

Hansson, K. and Leonard, L. (2003) The use and productivity of verb morphology in specific language impairment: An examination of Swedish. *Linguistics* 41, 351–379.

Huddleston, R. and Pullum, G. (2002) *The Cambridge Grammar of the English Language*. Cambridge: Cambridge University Press.

Leonard, L. (1998) *Children with Specific Language Impairment*. Cambridge, MA: The MIT Press.

Leonard, L. (2000) Specific language impairment across languages. In D.V.M. Bishop and L. Leonard (eds) *Speech and Language Impairments in Children: Causes, Characteristics, Intervention and Outcome* (pp. 115–129). Hove: Psychology Press.

Leonard, L., Sabbadini, L., Leonard, J. and Volterra, V. (1987) Specific language impairment in children: A crosslinguistic study. *Brain and Language* 32, 233–252.

Leonard, L., Wong, A.M-Y., Deevy, P., Stokes, S. and Fletcher, P. (2006) The production of passives by children with specific language impairment. *Applied Psycholinguistics* 27, 267–299.

Li, Y-H.A. (1990) *Order and Constituency in Mandarin Chinese.* Dordrecht: Kluwer Academic.

Linguistic Society of Hong Kong (1994) *The LSHK Cantonese Romanization Scheme.* Hong Kong: Linguistic Society of Hong Kong.

Matthews, S. and Yip, V. (1994) *Cantonese: A Comprehensive Grammar.* London: Routledge.

McBride, C., Tardif, T., Fletcher, F., Shu, H. and Wong, A.M-Y. (2004) *Developmental Precursors to Early Literacy in Chinese Children.* Hong Kong: Hong Kong Research Grants Council.

Pine, J., Rowland, C., Lieven, E. and Theakston, A. (2005) Testing the agreement/tense omission model: Why the data on children's use of nominative 3psg singular subjects counts against the ATOM. *Journal of Child Language* 32, 269–289.

Reynell, J. and Huntley, M. (1987) *Reynell Developmental Language Scales: Cantonese Version.* Windsor: NFER-Nelson.

Rice, M. and Wexler, K. (1996) Toward tense as a clinical marker of specific language impairment. *Journal of Speech, Language, and Hearing Research* 39, 1236–1257.

Stokes, S.F. and Fletcher, P. (2003) Aspectual forms in Cantonese children with specific language impairment. *Linguistics* 41, 381–406.

Swanson, L., Leonard, L. and Gandour, J. (1992) Vowel duration in mothers' speech to young children. *Journal of Speech and Hearing Research* 35, 617–625.

Tager-Flusberg, H. and Cooper, J. (1999) Present and future possibilities for defining a phenotype for specific language impairment. *Journal of Speech, Language, and Hearing Research* 42, 1261–1274.

Tang, S-W. (2001) A complementation approach to Chinese passives and its consequences. *Linguistics* 39, 257–295.

van der Lely, H. (1996) Specifically language impaired and normally developing children: Verbal passive vs. adjectival passive interpretation. *Lingua* 98, 243–272.

van der Lely, H. and Battell, J. (2003) Wh-movement in children with grammatical SLI: A test of the RDDR hypothesis. *Language* 79, 153–181.

Wexler, K. (1998) Very early parameter setting and the unique checking constraint: A new explanation of the optional infinitive stage. *Lingua* 106, 23–79.

Wong, A.M-Y., Leonard, L., Fletcher, P. and Stokes, S. (2004) Questions without movement: A study of Cantonese-speaking children with and without specific language impairment. *Journal of Speech, Language, and Hearing Research* 47, 1440–1453.

Wong, W. and Ingram, D. (2003) Question acquisition by Cantonese-speaking children. *Journal of Multilingual Communication Disorders* 1, 148–157.

Chapter 6

Assessing Cantonese-speaking Children with Language Difficulties from the Perspective of Evidence-based Practice: Current Practice and Future Directions

THOMAS KLEE, ANITA M-Y. WONG, STEPHANIE F. STOKES, PAUL FLETCHER and LAURENCE B. LEONARD

In this chapter, we review the current state of the art with regard to speech and language assessment of Cantonese-speaking children suspected of having a language impairment. This is timely, in that several new clinical assessments were introduced in 2006, expanding the choice of diagnostic tests available to professionals. We will review these, as well as tests that have been used for years, in diagnosing children with language problems. For the purpose of this chapter, our review will focus on standardized tests rather than on informal assessment approaches or measures derived from language sample analysis. The perspective we will take in this review is grounded in the framework of evidence-based practice, which we briefly introduce later in the chapter.

Speech and Language Tests for Cantonese-speaking Children

Prior to 2006, only two published standardized language tests were available for use with Cantonese speaking children in Hong Kong, a Cantonese adaptation of the Reynell Developmental Language Scales (RDLS-C; Hong Kong Society for Child Health and Development, 1987) and the Hong Kong Cantonese Receptive Vocabulary Test (HKCRVT; Lee *et al.*, 1996). In addition, experimental but commercially unpublished versions of tests had been developed, such as the Preschool Language Assessment Instrument (PLAI; Blank *et al.*, 1978), which was adapted to Cantonese by Stokes and Wong (1996).

Two new standardized tests of child language were launched in 2006, the Cantonese Expressive Language Scales (CELS; Hong Kong Education and Manpower Bureau, 2006) and the Hong Kong Cantonese Oral Language Assessment Scale (HKCOLAS; T'sou *et al.*, 2006b). These tests were specifically developed for Cantonese rather than being adaptations of tests originally designed for English-speaking children. Moreover, these are the first standardized language tests designed for use with school-age children up to age 12. Each of these tests is described next. A list of standardized speech and language assessments for Cantonese-speaking children is presented in Table 6.1.

Table 6.1 List of speech and language assessments for Cantonese-speaking children

Abbreviation	*Assessment*	*Age range*	*Reference*
Language tests			
CELS	Cantonese Expressive Language Scales	6–12 years	Hong Kong Education and Manpower Bureau (2006)
HKCOLAS	Hong Kong Cantonese Oral Language Assessment Scale	5–12 years	T'sou *et al.* (2006b)
HKCRVT	Hong Kong Cantonese Receptive Vocabulary Test	2–6 years	Lee *et al.* (1996)
RDLS-C	Reynell Developmental Language Scales, Cantonese (Hong Kong) version	1–7 years	Hong Kong Society for Child Health and Development (1987)
Speech tests			
CBSPT	Cantonese Basic Speech Perception Test	3 years to adult	Lee (2006)
CSPT	Cantonese Segmental Phonology Test	2–6 years	So (1993)
HKCAT	Hong Kong Cantonese Articulation Test	2 years to adult	T'sou *et al.* (2006a)
Parent-report measures			
DLSS	Developmental Language Screening Scale	3 years	Lee *et al.* (1985)
MBCDI	MacArthur-Bates Communicative Development Inventories (Cantonese version)	8–30 months	Tardif *et al.* (in press)

RDLS-C

The RDLS was first published in the UK (Reynell, 1977) and then revised (Reynell & Huntley, 1985), before being completely redesigned and renormed (Edwards *et al.*, 1997). Versions have also been developed for use in the USA and in several European countries. The Cantonese version developed in Hong Kong (RDLS-C; Hong Kong Society for Child Health and Development, 1987) contains two subscales: a verbal comprehension subscale containing 67 items for a total of 67 points, and an expressive language subscale containing 29 items for a total of 73 points. The test can be administered in about 30 minutes. Test norms were based on 1081 children between 1 and 7 years of age. Although 56–118 children were sampled in each six-month age group, normative data are reported in three-month age bands. This has been the test of choice in many research studies of Hong Kong children's language development, presumably because it was the only broad-based, norm-referenced test of language development up to 2006. Language age scores on two subscales of the RDLS-C have been shown to be significantly correlated (all $p < 0.05$) with chronological age in children who are developing language normally (verbal comprehension and age, $r = 0.73$; expressive language and age, $r = 0.65$; $n = 71$) and those with developmental delay (verbal comprehension and age, $r = 0.81$; expressive language and age, $r = 0.79$; $n = 45$) (Au *et al.*, 2004).

HKCRVT

The HKCRVT (Lee *et al.*, 1996) was modeled on two widely used tests of receptive vocabulary of English, the Peabody Picture Vocabulary Test (USA) and the British Picture Vocabulary Scales (UK). The HKCRVT contains three training items and 100 test items, each of which tests a single item of receptive vocabulary. A four-choice, picture-pointing format is used, with each picture plate depicting the target word and phonological, semantic and unrelated distractors. The normative sample was based on 609 children between ages 1;10 (year;month) and 6;1, with 17–61 children represented in each three-month age band, with normative data being reported for each age band (Cheung *et al.*, 1997). The children were selected from a random sample of Maternal and Child Health Centers and kindergartens in Hong Kong; however, it was not reported whether children with language difficulties or other conditions were included in the normative sample. Children's scores increased steadily from a mean of 28.1 (SD = 13.6) in the earliest age group, to a mean of 91.7 (SD = 5.7) in the oldest group.

PLAI

A third test, an experimental version of a Cantonese adaptation of the PLAI, had also been reported (Stokes & Wong, 1996). Like the previous tests, the PLAI was originally developed for English-speaking children

(Blank *et al.*, 1978). This receptive language measure was designed to 'tap a child's ability to respond to teacher-talk' (Blank *et al.*, 1978: 76). The Cantonese adaptation of the test was administered to 277 children between 3 and 5 years of age using a stratified random sampling procedure. Although the authors reported acceptable levels of concurrent validity with the RDLS-C, they identified a number of problematic test items and as a result, recommended that modifications be made to the test.

CELS

The CELS (Hong Kong Education and Manpower Bureau, 2006) was developed 'to assist both teachers and speech therapists in identifying and diagnosing the speech and language problems of pupils' (Hong Kong SAR Government Information Centre, 2006a) and 'to help determine accurate therapy goals' (Hong Kong Education and Manpower Bureau, 2006). The CELS is a test of expressive language only and consists of two subscales: sentence structures and narration skills. Test norms were based on 1324 children between ages 6;0 and 12;11, with 116–235 children represented in each one-year age band. For the sentence structures subscale, normative data are presented for each six-month age band; however, the sample size of each of these subgroups is not reported. For each measure in the narration skills subscale, normative data are presented for one-year subgroups.

HKCOLAS

The HKCOLAS (T'sou *et al.*, 2006b) was designed to assess children's comprehension and production of vocabulary, grammar and narrative skills for the purpose of 'diagnosing language impairment of Hong Kong Cantonese-speaking preprimary and primary school children' (HKCOLAS website, 2006) and requires about 75–90 minutes to administer (T'sou *et al.*, 2006b, User's Manual: 3-3). The test was designed to 'help to identify children with language impairments at an early stage so that timely and appropriate assistance can be offered to them' (Hong Kong SAR Government Information Centre, 2006b). Test norms were based on 1120 children between ages 4;10 and 12;1, with 138–147 children represented in each one-year age band from Primary grades 1–6, in addition to two kindergarten-age bands having 132 and 137 children, respectively. Normative data are reported for each of these subgroups. Children were randomly recruited through co-operating schools in three Hong Kong districts, with only 28 families declining the invitation to participate in the study. The resulting sample represented children in mainstream schools, including children with language, speech, fluency and voice problems, as well as other developmental disorders.

Other assessment measures

In addition to the tests reviewed in the previous sections, two parent-report measures of children's early language development have also been published: the Developmental Language Screening Scale (DLSS; Lee *et al.*, 1985, 1990; Wong *et al.*, 1992) and a Cantonese version of the MacArthur-Bates Communicative Development Inventories (MBCDI; Tardif *et al.*, in press). In addition, two tests are available for assessing speech-sound disorders in Cantonese-speaking children: the Cantonese Segmental Phonology Test (CSPT; So, 1993; So & Leung, 2004) and a new version of the Hong Kong Cantonese Articulation Test (HKCAT; T'sou *et al.*, 2006a), originally distributed in 2002. A research version of a further test was reported by Cheung and Abberton (2000), accompanied by data on 251 Cantonese-speaking children, aged 3;6–6;0, with speech-sound disorders. Finally, a test was recently developed to assess speech perception in children as young as 3;0: the Cantonese Basic Speech Perception Test (CBSPT; Lee, 2006). Data are presented on its use as a standardized clinical assessment in children with and without impaired hearing, and on its use as a screening measure.

Survey of Speech Therapists Working in Hong Kong

Before continuing our review, it would be useful to know which of these tests speech therapists[1] (STs) working in Hong Kong actually use in their clinical practice and what they think about them. To find out, we developed a brief questionnaire of 22 items and conducted a web-based survey. The questionnaire took 5–10 minutes to complete, judging from a small sample of people who completed a pilot version. In February 2007, an invitation was sent by email to 314 STs thought to be working in pediatric settings and whose contact details were held by the Division of Speech and Hearing Sciences at the University of Hong Kong. As 15 emails bounced back, it appears that 299 invitations were delivered. One week later, an email reminder was sent out, encouraging people to respond. Respondents were given a total of two weeks to complete the questionnaire. At the end of that period, the questionnaire was taken offline.

A total of 88 individuals completed the questionnaire, a response rate of 29%.[2] Sixty-two STs reported holding an undergraduate university degree (70%), while 25 reported holding a postgraduate diploma or Master's degree (28%); one individual did not respond to this question (2%). The respondents' places of work were fairly evenly distributed across the region, with 33 STs working on Hong Kong Island, 41 in Kowloon and 42 in the New Territories. Thirty-three STs reported working in nursery, daycare or preschool settings, 35 in primary and 10 in secondary schools, 16 in private practice, 16 in special schools and

21 in other settings (e.g. hospitals, specialist clinics, child assessment centers and universities); 34 STs reported working in more than one setting. Nearly all STs reported working with children with language disorders (99%) and speech disorders (93%), while a majority also reported working with children having voice (60%), fluency (55%) and hearing problems (53%). STs reported that 99% of the children they worked with spoke Cantonese, with 31% indicating they worked with children who (also) spoke English and 11% indicating they worked with children who (also) spoke Mandarin.

For our purposes, we will focus on how STs responded to the questions about their use of standardized speech and language tests. Nearly all STs (93%; $n = 82$) indicated they used standardized tests to assess children's speech and language. Of these, 95% used them for assessment and diagnosis, 55% used them to evaluate intervention progress, 51% used them for discharge and 28% used them for screening.

Table 6.2 summarizes the number and percentage of respondents who reported using a particular test, of those who use tests. Among the broad-based language tests, the RDLS-C was used by 88% of STs, followed by the HKCOLAS (32%) and the CELS (12%). The HKCRVT, being a more restricted test insofar as it only assesses a single language domain (receptive vocabulary), was reported to be used by 23% of STs. Regarding

Table 6.2 Number and percentage of speech therapists in Hong Kong who reported using a particular test, out of those who reported using standardized tests ($n = 82$)[a]

Test	*No. of STs*
RDLS-C	72[b] (88%)
HKCOLAS	26 (32%)
CELS	10 (12%)
HKCRVT	19 (23%)
HKCAT	37 (45%)
CSPT[c]	11 (13%)
DLSS	0 (0%)
Symbolic Play Test	12 (15%)
No response	1 (1%)

Note. [a]Based on 88 out of 299 STs who responded to a web-based questionnaire in 2007. [b]Of which RDLS-III = 1. [c]Six responses entered as SPT were not included (since it was unknown whether they referred to CBSPT, CSPT or Symbolic Play Test)

the speech tests, 45% of STs reported using the HKCAT, while 13% used the CSPT.

There may be a number of reasons why individual STs prefer certain tests. These include familiarity and experience with a test, ease of administration and scoring, the test's psychometric properties (e.g. validity and reliability) or correspondence between test results and clinical judgment. Any of these might explain the apparent popularity of the RDLS-C. However, it is also likely that STs use this test because it is the only broad-based test available for children under the age of five. Another possible explanation is that the test's greater reported usage may have resulted from sample bias; for example, it is possible that proportionately more STs who work with preschool children, or older children having language abilities within the range assessed by the RDLS-C, responded to the survey. Alternatively, the lower reported usage of the HKCOLAS and CELS may simply reflect the fact that they are relatively new tests, having just been published the year before the survey was done, or it may reflect a genuine preference for the older RLDS-C. In fact, however, a number of the comments STs made about the RDLS-C cast doubt on this last possibility. This is discussed further next.

When STs were asked whether there were sufficient assessment materials available for use with Cantonese-speaking children with speech and language problems, 90% responded *no*. Table 6.3 summarizes, by category, STs' observations about where the gaps and limitations were in speech and language assessment materials at the beginning of 2007. The most frequent comment made was that there was a limited choice of assessment materials available for children of preschool age. Specific limitations of the RDLS-C were also cited. For example, norms were thought to be outdated and clinicians indicated there was a tendency for the test to overestimate children's language abilities relative to their clinical judgment. Frequent comments were also made about the length of tests for school-age children and their clinical impracticality, given the work demands of school-based clinicians. There were also frequent comments regarding the lack of assessments for pragmatics, discourse, conversation, verbal reasoning, inferencing and narrative skills. Clinicians also highlighted the lack of tests for children older than 12 years of age. Limitations were also noted in assessments for children with complex communication disorders (e.g. children with multiple handicaps) and the lack of instruments appropriate for planning and evaluating intervention. Gaps and limitations in other areas also emerged, but less frequently than those above. These are listed in the bottom half of Table 6.3.

Lastly, STs were asked to suggest several things that could be done to improve the range or quality of speech and language assessments for children in Hong Kong. Table 6.4 presents a list of their responses,

Table 6.3 Hong Kong speech therapists' categorized responses to the question, 'Where do you feel the gaps and limitations currently are in speech and language assessment materials?'[a]

Category of response	*No. of responses*
Limited range of tests, particularly for preschool children	22
Outdated RDLS-C norms; tendency of test to overestimate abilities	19
Length of tests, especially for use in school settings	15
Limited coverage of assessment areas (e.g. pragmatics, discourse, conversation, verbal reasoning, inferencing, narrative)	10
Limited tests for school-aged children, particularly those over age 12	8
Lack of available tests for certain populations (e.g. children who are deaf-blind, physically disabled, cognitively impaired)	7
Lack of tests for planning and assessing intervention	6
Limited screening measures for early identification	3
Lack of curriculum-based assessments for school-aged children	3
Lack of assessments for preverbal children	3
Lack of psychometric data, particularly with regard to test validity	3
Lack of norms for Cantonese children with voice or fluency disorders	3
Lack of assessments for children with autistic spectrum disorders	2
Lack of normative data for language sample measures	2
Lack of resources for interviewing parents/caregivers	1

Note. [a]Based on 88 out of 299 STs who responded to a web-based questionnaire in 2007

grouped into categories. The responses were consistent with the gaps and limitations of current assessments outlined in the preceding paragraph. STs called for the development of a wider range of assessments than are currently available, as well as ones that have been designed around the structure and function of Cantonese and ones that are culturally appropriate to Hong Kong. STs also called for the development of new assessments based on contemporary norms, particularly for preschool children and those over the age of 12. They

Table 6.4 Hong Kong speech therapists' categorized responses to the question, 'If you could suggest 3 things that could be done to improve the range or quality of speech and language assessments for children in Hong Kong, what would they be?'[a]

Category of response	*No. of responses*
Develop a wider range of valid, research-based, culturally appropriate assessment materials	27
Develop more time-efficient assessments (e.g. HKCOLAS short form)	26
Develop assessment materials for linguistic areas not currently covered (e.g. pragmatics, comprehension, verbal reasoning skills, narratives)	25
Develop an updated, culturally appropriate test for preschool children	23
Develop assessment materials for populations not currently covered (e.g. children over age 12, children with ASD, low-functioning children)	17
Develop screening measures for children throughout the age range	9
Develop (computerized) user-friendly language sample analyses and normative data for Cantonese-speaking children	7
Conduct a workshop for Hong Kong STs to discuss assessment needs	7
Develop norms for voice and fluency features of Cantonese	5
Develop age norms for speech and language milestones in Cantonese	5
Develop assessments for preverbal children	4
Develop standardized assessments for bilingual Cantonese children	2
Develop assessment for literacy skills (e.g. reading and writing); more research needed on SLI and normal development in Cantonese; training needed in theory of test development and test validity	1 each

Note. [a]Based on 88 out of 299 STs who responded to a web-based questionnaire in 2007

pointed out the need for assessment measures in the areas of pragmatics, comprehension, narratives and verbal reasoning, as well as assessments suitable for use with special populations (e.g. children with physical or cognitive impairment).

Limitations of the survey

Although the generalizability of these findings may be limited by the response rate (29%), the results from our survey do appear to document the range of assessments currently used by Hong Kong STs, as well as illuminating where the perceived gaps in assessment are. Moreover, our findings suggest a need to examine the adequacy of the assessment instruments currently available, both in terms of fitness for purpose and clinical efficiency. It would be useful to follow up the findings of this survey by conducting a qualitative study, based on a representative sample of STs, aimed at coming to a fuller understanding of current assessment needs in Hong Kong. In fact, a number of STs who participated in the survey felt it would be useful to organize a workshop involving stakeholders (e.g. STs, university researchers, clinical managers) to discuss current assessment needs and how to go about meeting those needs.

Evaluating Test Adequacy

Having established from the survey which tests are used in clinical practice, and having summarized the views of STs regarding the state of clinical assessment in Hong Kong, we now ask how well the tests stack up when compared against well-established, external criteria for evaluating test adequacy. We propose that there are two complementary ways of doing this. One makes use of a set of standard criteria for evaluating the normative construction and psychometric adequacy of the test and the other builds on these by providing data on diagnostic accuracy for assessing the clinical usefulness of the test as a whole and on the level of the individual client or patient and which is grounded in evidence-based practice.

Psychometric review of tests

The disciplines of psychology and education developed a very useful framework for evaluating test adequacy. This framework was formalized and articulated in the Standards for Educational and Psychological Testing, jointly published by the American Educational Research Association, the American Psychological Association and the National Council on Measurement in Education in 1974 and last revised in 1999. Rebecca McCauley and Linda Swisher were the first to apply this approach to clinical assessment in the speech and language sciences in their psychometric review of 30 norm-referenced language and articulation tests (McCauley & Swisher, 1984).[3] In that paper, they evaluated the tests with respect to 10 selective, but well-established, psychometric criteria relating to the adequacy of the normative sample, the presentation of test procedures and norms, and the reliability and validity of the test. From their review of the tests available at the time, they concluded that half of them met no more than two of the 10 criteria, while only three of them met more than four criteria. The tests reviewed in 1984 most often fell short in providing evidence that they were valid and reliable.

Ten years later, Plante and Vance (1994) published a ground-breaking paper on clinical assessment. In that paper, they employed the same methodology in a psychometric evaluation of 21 preschool language tests, but importantly, went on to empirically assess the diagnostic accuracy of four language tests in differentiating children with and without specific language impairment (SLI). They reported the sensitivity and specificity of each test based on cutoff scores empirically derived from statistical analyses that maximally differentiated the groups, rather than using more traditional, but arbitrary, cutoff scores such as one or more standard deviations below the mean. Their study was followed by a series of studies examining the diagnostic accuracy of other language tests, using the same methodology, with 4- and 5-year olds (Gray *et al.*, 1999; Merrell & Plante, 1997; Perona *et al.*, 2005; Plante & Vance, 1995).

Next, we review a subset of the Cantonese tests summarized earlier using the 10 psychometric criteria employed by McCauley and Swisher (1984), Plante and Vance (1994) and, more recently, Mikucki and Larrivee (2006). We will restrict the review to the four norm-referenced language tests listed in Table 6.1: the CELS, HKCOLAS, HKCRVT and RDLS-C. Each of the criteria are described in detail in McCauley and Swisher (1984: 38–39). Due to space limitations, however, we will not reproduce them here except to say that, as in the earlier studies, several criteria consisted of more than one component, and for a test to have scored successfully on such a criterion, it had to have addressed all the components. For example, the first criterion, involving a description of the normative sample, required a specification of: (1) the sample's geographical residence, (2) socioeconomic status and (3) the number of individuals excluded on the basis of language ability.[4] Criteria 7 and 8, involving test reliability, were met only if there was evidence of statistically significant correlation coefficients of 0.90 and above.

Table 6.5 summarizes the findings of the psychometric review. The HKCOLAS met seven of the 10 criteria, while the CELS, HKCRVT and RDLS-C each met five. As with the US tests reviewed by McCauley and Swisher (1984) and Plante and Vance (1994), none of the Cantonese tests reported any information about predictive validity. Similarly, none of the Cantonese tests met the criterion for test-retest reliability and only one test (CELS) met the criterion for interexaminer reliability. Only one test, the HKCOLAS, met the concurrent validity criterion. In the next section, we argue that this is one of the most important characteristics of a test, in that it can provide practical information about the correspondence between the test results and the clinical diagnosis.

Table 6.5 Tests meeting each psychometric criterion

Criterion	*No. tests*	*Tests*[a]
1. Description of normative sample	3	HKCRVT, HKCOLAS, RDLS-C
2. Sample size	2	CELS[b], HKCOLAS
3. Item analysis	4	CELS, HKCRVT, HKCOLAS, RDLS-C
4. Means and standard deviations	3	HKCOLAS, HKCRVT, RDLS-C
5. Concurrent validity	1	HKCOLAS
6. Predictive validity	0	
7. Test-retest reliability	0	
8. Interexaminer reliability	1	CELS
9. Description of test procedures	4	CELS, HKCRVT, HKCOLAS, RDLS-C
10. Description of tester qualifications	4	CELS, HKCRVT, HKCOLAS, RDLS-C

Note. [a]Test names and abbreviations are listed in Table 6.1. [b]Narration skills subscale meets sample size standard of 100 per subgroup (re: McCauley & Swisher, 1984: 38), but whether sentence structures subscale does cannot be determined from information given in test manual

An evidence-based approach to assessment

A complementary approach to psychometric review for evaluating the diagnostic adequacy of tests can be found in the literature on evidence-based medicine (EBM). In its early days, EBM was defined as 'the conscientious, explicit and judicious use of current best evidence in making decisions about the care of individual patients' (Sackett *et al.*, 1996: 71). Straus *et al.* (2005: 1) open the third edition of their book on EBM with a definition having a slightly different emphasis, stating that 'Evidence-based medicine (EBM) requires the integration of the best research evidence with our clinical expertise and our patient's unique values and circumstances'. And, Greenhalgh (2006: 1) begins her very readable introduction to EBM by stating unapologetically that EBM involves '... the use of mathematical estimates of the risk of benefit and harm, derived from high-quality research on population samples, to inform clinical decision making in the diagnosis, investigation or management of individual patients'. What all three of these conceptualizations have in common is an emphasis on the need to establish high-quality research evidence that can (and should) be used to guide clinical practice.

EBM, which grew out of the practice of clinical epidemiology (Haynes *et al.*, 2006), has begun to take root in the allied health professions, including the speech and language sciences (Dollaghan, 2004; Johnson, 2006; Reilly, 2004), where it is commonly referred to as evidence-based practice (EBP). Professional associations have begun to compile resources documenting evidence in support of best practice. For example, the website of the American Speech-Language-Hearing Association (ASHA) contains a large resource related to EBP for its members, and the UK's Royal College of Speech and Language Therapists recently produced a set of evidence-based clinical guidelines (Taylor-Goh, 2005). Although most of what has been written under the banner of EBP is concerned with intervention efficacy and effectiveness, there is much to be gained from using the EBM framework in evaluating and judging the soundness of diagnostic tests (Guyatt & Rennie, 2002; Haynes *et al.*, 2006). According to a recent ASHA Technical Report (2004: 4–5), 'Evaluating diagnostic procedures and measures according to EBP criteria would provide a rational basis for selecting the maximally informative and cost-effective diagnostic protocols from among the hundreds of diagnostic tools that are reported or advertised each year'.

So, what are the basic tenets of an EBP approach to evaluating tests? Haynes *et al.* (2006: 275) identified what they called a *diagnostic quartet* of characteristics that lie at the heart of evidence-based assessment. They asserted that 'A valid diagnostic study:

(1) assembles an appropriate spectrum of patients;
(2) applies both the diagnostic test and reference standard to all of them;
(3) interprets each blind to the other;
(4) repeats itself in a second, independent ("test") set of patients'.

They go on to map out the methods by which screening and diagnostic tests should be evaluated and, importantly, the pitfalls that can be expected to be encountered along the way.

We are going to go out on a limb and make a barefaced admission at this point. No study of diagnostic accuracy has been published in speech and language sciences that meets all of the criteria listed. And before there is likely to be one, there are a number of important, and far from trivial, methodological points that need to be worked out. Let's consider each of the characteristics in the diagnostic quartet as they relate to diagnostic tests of speech and language, in the order they appear earlier:

(1) While it may be appropriate in screening studies to compare positive and negative screening outcomes in individuals with and without the disorder that the screen is intended to identify, it is debatable whether this should be done in diagnostic studies, where the primary question of interest is, *Is this child (specifically) language impaired?* It may be more appropriate to assess the diagnostic accuracy of the test in individuals who are referred for clinical evaluation because of a suspected problem with communication.
(2) How should the reference standard be defined? At present, there is no universally accepted gold standard for identifying an individual as SLI or even as language impaired (Leonard, 1987; Mervis & Robinson, 2005; Tager-Flusberg, 2005). One approach that has been used is that of defining the population by setting a cutoff score for the reference test. The problem with this is that the diagnostic accuracy of the reference test often has not itself been determined. Another approach that might be considered is the empirically determined epiSLI diagnostic standard of Tomblin *et al.* (1996), although this is restricted to children aged 5–6. A further approach might be to define the reference standard as clinical judgment, informed by the results of a clinical assessment.
(3) This is the most attainable of the four criteria, and yet whether assessor blinding was done, frequently goes unreported in many studies of diagnostic accuracy in speech and language testing.
(4) Replicability is a universally accepted benchmark of good research, but unfortunately there are few reports of this in diagnostic accuracy studies of speech and language measures. As an example, we are currently running a replication of an earlier study that examined the diagnostic value of a clinical measure based on children's utterance length and lexical diversity (Klee *et al.*, 2004).

The four benchmarks are a starting point for stimulating a discussion on how to evaluate diagnostic measures of children's speech and language abilities. They are discussed in greater detail in the reference sources listed at the beginning of this section.

Two very useful checklists for evaluating diagnostic tests have recently been developed in medicine. One is aimed at test developers and the other at test users. Test developers in speech and language sciences should consider using the Standards for Reporting of Diagnostic Accuracy (STARD) checklist and flow chart, which were developed 'to improve the accuracy and completeness of reporting of studies of diagnostic accuracy' (Bossuyt *et al.*, 2003a: 41). STARD appears in the authors' instructions of over 50 journals, including those of the American

Speech-Language-Hearing Association. Although the checklist was developed with medical tests in mind, it can also be used for behavioral assessments. The STARD checklist is reproduced in Table 6.6. Information regarding each of the items on the checklist may be found in a companion paper (Bossuyt *et al.*, 2003b) and on the STARD website (http://www.stard-statement.org).

We also recommend that test users (e.g. STs) consider using the Quality Assessment of Diagnostic Accuracy Studies (QUADAS) checklist for appraising the methodological quality of diagnostic tests they are considering using. The checklist, which was developed for assessing studies of diagnostic accuracy included in systematic reviews, and instructions for using it, are described in Whiting *et al.* (2003). It was developed using a formal consensus method by a panel of experts after conducting reviews of the diagnostic literature to locate potential items. The QUADAS checklist contains 14 items and is reproduced in Table 6.7. There are a number of other critical appraisal checklists available. For example, the website of the Scottish Intercollegiate Guidelines Network contains a checklist for assessing diagnostic studies, as well as checklists for evaluating the methodological quality of intervention studies (http://www.sign.ac.uk/methodology/checklists.html). Similar checklists can also be found elsewhere (e.g. Greenhalgh, 1997, 2006). It is beyond the scope of this chapter to critically appraise each of the Cantonese tests with respect to QUADAS, but interested readers are invited to do so.

Future Directions

In a recent issue of the *British Medical Journal*, the deputy editor suggested that 'while evidence based treatment is well on the way to being sorted out, evidence based diagnosis is still in the dark ages' (Delamothe, 2006). Although he was referring to the current state of affairs in medical diagnosis, the same could be said of diagnosis in the speech and language sciences worldwide.

What can be done to work towards evidence-based assessments in speech and language sciences? To take an example, one of the recurring comments made about the RDLS-C in our survey of STs was that there was a tendency for the test to overestimate children's language abilities relative to their clinical judgment. STs felt this was reason enough to suggest either that the test be updated and renormed or that a new test be developed for assessing preschool children. This may well be what is needed; after all, STs have years of experience using this test in their clinical practice. At the moment though, there is no objective, empirical data on how accurate the test is, even relative to informed clinical judgment. There is no estimate of the test's sensitivity, specificity, positive

Table 6.6 STARD checklist for reporting studies of diagnostic accuracy

Section and topic	*Item*	*Description*
Title, abstract, and keywords	1	Identify the article as a study of diagnostic accuracy (recommend MeSH heading 'sensitivity and specificity').
Introduction	2	State the research questions or study aims, such as estimating diagnostic accuracy or comparing accuracy between tests or across participant groups.
Methods		
Participants	3	Describe the study population: the inclusion and exclusion criteria and the settings and locations where the data were collected.
	4	Describe participant recruitment: was this based on presenting symptoms, results from previous tests, or the fact that the participants had received the index tests or the reference standard?
	5	Describe participant sampling: was this a consecutive series of participants defined by the selection criteria in items 3 and 4? If not, specify how participants were further selected.
	6	Describe data collection: was data collection planned before the index test and reference standard were performed (prospective study) or after (retrospective study)?
Test methods	7	Describe the reference standard and its rationale.
	8	Describe technical specifications of material and methods involved, including how and when measurements were taken, and/or cite references for index tests and reference standard.
	9	Describe definition of and rationale for the units, cutoff points and/or categories of the results of the index tests and the reference standard.
	10	Describe the number, training and expertise of the persons executing and reading the index tests and the reference standard.
	11	Describe whether or not the readers of the index tests and reference standard were blind (masked) to the results of the other test. Describe any other clinical information available to the readers.

Table 6.6 (*Continued*)

Section and topic	*Item*	*Description*
Statistical methods	12	Describe methods for calculating or comparing measures of diagnostic accuracy and the statistical methods used to quantify uncertainty (e.g. 95% confidence intervals).
	13	Describe methods for calculating test reproducibility, if done.
Results		
Participants	14	Report when study was done, including beginning and end dates of recruitment.
	15	Report clinical and demographic characteristics of the study population (e.g. age, sex, spectrum of presenting symptoms, comorbidity, current treatments, recruitment centers).
	16	Report how many participants satisfying the criteria for inclusion did or did not undergo the index tests or the reference standard, or both; describe why participants failed to receive either test (a flow diagram is strongly recommended).
Test results	17	Report time-interval between the index tests and the reference standard, and any treatment administered between.
	18	Report distribution of severity of disease (define criteria) in those with the target condition and other diagnoses in participants without the target condition.
	19	Report a cross-tabulation of the results of the index tests (including indeterminate and missing results) by the results of the reference standard; for continuous results, the distribution of the test results by the results of the reference standard.
	20	Report any adverse events from performing the index tests or the reference standard.
Estimates	21	Report estimates of diagnostic accuracy and measures of statistical uncertainty (e.g. 95% confidence intervals).
	22	Report how indeterminate results, missing data and outliers of the index tests were handled.

Table 6.6 (*Continued*)

Section and topic	*Item*	*Description*
	23	Report estimates of variability of diagnostic accuracy between subgroups of participants, readers or centers, if done.
	24	Report estimates of test reproducibility, if done.
Discussion	25	Discuss the clinical applicability of the study findings.

Source. Used with permission, Nynke Smidt and Patrick Bossuyt. Available at www.stard-statement.org

or negative predictive values, or likelihood ratios, based on research which has been designed around the diagnostic quartet of characteristics discussed by Haynes *et al.* (2006), and which fares well against the STARD and QUADAS checklists. In the absence of such evidence, what we are left with is clinical opinion. Good as this may be, clinical opinion is at the bottom of the hierarchy of evidence relative to well-designed, evidence-based studies (Greenhalgh, 2006).

The range of clinical tests available for assessing the speech and language development of Cantonese-speaking children continues to grow. The recent addition of large-scale normative tests such as the CELS, HKCOLAS and HKCAT, as well as the MBCDI parent-report measure, has resulted in more choice than ever for STs working in Hong Kong, although the choice of assessments within a particular age group remains quite limited. While each of these shows promise as a clinical assessment, none meets all of the psychometric criteria set out by McCauley and Swisher (1984) (see Table 6.5) – a situation not unlike that in the USA (cf. Mikucki & Larrivee, 2006; Plante & Vance, 1994), the UK and elsewhere. What is needed at this stage is for test developers to begin considering how to evaluate their tests using the methodological framework of EBP. If this was done, clinicians could have more confidence in the tests they use for assessing children with language difficulties.

In closing, we would like to offer some suggestions for what might be done to advance the state of clinical practice in speech and language assessment. As pointed out by the STs in our survey, there is a need for a workshop, or series of workshops, on evidence-based assessment and diagnosis, which would involve various stakeholders such as STs, clinical managers and university researchers. The purpose of the workshop(s) would be to introduce the principles of EBP as it relates to assessment and to further explore current local needs in the area of clinical assessment. Second, assuming that workshop participants confirm the findings of the survey, there is scope for new, psychometrically sound,

Table 6.7 QUADAS checklist for assessing the quality of studies of diagnostic accuracy

Item		*Yes*	*No*	*Unclear*
1	Was the spectrum of patients representative of the patients who will receive the test in practice?	( )	( )	( )
2	Were selection criteria clearly described?	( )	( )	( )
3	Is the reference standard likely to correctly classify the target condition?	( )	( )	( )
4	Is the time period between reference standard and index test short enough to be reasonably sure that the target condition did not change between the two tests?	( )	( )	( )
5	Did the whole sample or a random selection of the sample receive verification using a reference standard of diagnosis?	( )	( )	( )
6	Did patients receive the same reference standard regardless of the index test result?	( )	( )	( )
7	Was the reference standard independent of the index test (i.e. the index test did not form part of the reference standard)?	( )	( )	( )
8	Was the execution of the index test described in sufficient detail to permit replication of the test?	( )	( )	( )
9	Was the execution of the reference standard described in sufficient detail to permit its replication?	( )	( )	( )
10	Were the index test results interpreted without knowledge of the results of the reference standard?	( )	( )	( )
11	Were the reference standard results interpreted without knowledge of the results of the index test?	( )	( )	( )
12	Were the same clinical data available when test results were interpreted as would be available when the test is used in practice?	( )	( )	( )
13	Were uninterpretable/intermediate test results reported?	( )	( )	( )
14	Were withdrawals from the study explained?	( )	( )	( )

Source. Used with permission, Penny Whiting. Available in Whiting *et al.* (2003)

evidence-based assessments for preschool children, designed from the ground up for Cantonese, aimed at updating or replacing the RDLS-C. Evidence-based assessments for children over the age of 12 will also be needed eventually, but at the moment this may be limited by the lack of research that has been done with children of this age. And finally, assessments are required in areas such as prelinguistic abilities, pragmatics and (pre)literacy skills. As we alluded to earlier, we do not pretend that employing the methods of EBP will be easy, as there is still much to be worked out in terms of how to apply the diagnostic quartet of characteristics suggested by Haynes *et al.* (2006). This is a challenge that faces the field in general, but if we succeed, the result will be a new generation of evidence-based speech and language assessments.

Acknowledgements

We would like to thank the Centre for Communication Disorders at the University of Hong Kong for supporting the survey reported in this study and all the speech therapists in Hong Kong who responded to the survey. Thanks also to Dennis Bates for his technical help in implementing the web-based survey. Ethical approval to conduct the survey was granted by the University of Hong Kong Human Research Ethics Committee for Non-Clinical Faculties. We also thank Nynke Smidt and Patrick Bossuyt for permission to reproduce the STARD checklist; Penny Whiting for permission to reproduce the QUADAS checklist; Carol To and Pamela Cheung for the test information they provided; Katie Y-Y. Fong and Tammy H-M. Lau for their help with test reviews; and two anonymous reviewers.

Notes

1. This profession is sometimes referred to by other titles elsewhere, e.g. speech and language therapist in the UK and speech-language pathologist in the USA.
2. A total of 88 valid responses remained after removing 16 duplicate entries, presumably due to some respondents hitting the return key twice. Although there was no evidence of it occurring, it was not possible to control for individuals intentionally completing the web-based questionnaire more than once.
3. DeThorne and Schaefer (2004) conducted a similar psychometric review of child non-verbal IQ measures.
4. For a discussion of the issues related to (3), see McFadden (1996), who argues against the use of truncated norms, and Peña et al. (2006), who provide a counterargument.

References

American Educational Research Association, American Psychological Association & National Council on Measurement in Education (1999) *Standards for Educational and Psychological Testing*. Washington, DC: American Psychological Association.

American Speech-Language-Hearing Association (2004) *Evidence-based Practice in Communication Disorders: An Introduction* [Technical report] [Electronic Version]. On WWW at http://www.asha.org/members/deskref-journals/deskref/default. Accessed 27.2.07.

Au, Y.L.E., Ma, K.M., Sy, W.M., Lee, W.C., Leung, L.S.J., Au Yeung, Y.C., *et al.* (2004) Use of developmental language scales in Chinese children. *Brain & Development* 26, 127–129.

Blank, M., Rose, S.A. and Berlin, L.J. (1978) *Preschool Language Assessment Instrument*. Orlando, FL: Grune & Stratton.

Bossuyt, P.M., Reitsma, J.B., Bruns, D.E., Gatsonis, C.A., Glasziou, P.P., Irwig, L.M. *et al.* (2003a) Towards a complete and accurate reporting of studies of diagnostic accuracy: The STARD initiative. *British Medical Journal* 326, 41–44.

Bossuyt, P.M., Reitsma, J.B., Bruns, D.E., Gatsonis, C.A., Glasziou, P.P., Irwig, L.M. *et al.* (2003b) The STARD statement for reporting studies of diagnostic accuracy: Explanation and elaboration. *Clinical Chemistry* 49, 7–18.

Cheung, P. and Abberton, E. (2000) Patterns of phonological disability in Cantonese-speaking children in Hong Kong. *International Journal of Language & Communication Disorders* 35, 451–473.

Cheung, P.S.P., Lee, K.Y.S. and Lee, L.W.T. (1997) The development of the 'Cantonese Receptive Vocabulary Test' for children aged 2–6 in Hong Kong. *European Journal of Disorders of Communication* 32, 127–138.

Delamothe, T. (2006) Diagnosis – the next frontier. *British Medical Journal* 333, 0–f.

DeThorne, L.S. and Schaefer, B.A. (2004) A guide to child nonverbal IQ measures. *American Journal of Speech-Language Pathology* 13, 275–290.

Dollaghan, C.A. (2004) Evidence-based practice in communication disorders: What do we know, and when do we know it? *Journal of Communication Disorders* 37, 391–400.

Edwards, S., Fletcher, P., Garman, M., Hughes, A., Letts, C. and Sinka, I. (1997) *Reynell Developmental Language Scales III*. Windsor: NFER-NELSON.

Gray, S., Plante, E., Vance, R. and Henrichsen, M. (1999) The diagnostic accuracy of four vocabulary tests administered to preschool-age children. *Language, Speech, and Hearing Services in Schools* 30, 196–206.

Greenhalgh, T. (1997) How to read a paper: Papers that report diagnostic or screening tests. *British Medical Journal* 315, 540–543.

Greenhalgh, T. (2006) *How to Read a Paper: The Basics of Evidence-based Medicine* (3rd edn). Oxford: Blackwell.

Guyatt, G.H. and Rennie, D. (eds) (2002) *Users' Guides to the Medical Literature: A Manual for Evidence-based Clinical Practice*. Chicago, IL: AMA Press.

Haynes, R.B., Sackett, D.L., Guyatt, G.H. and Tugwell, P. (2006) *Clinical Epidemiology: How to do Clinical Practice Research* (3rd edn). Philadelphia, PA: Lippincott Williams & Wilkins.

HKCOLAS website (2006) *The Hong Kong Cantonese Oral Language Assessment Scale*. On WWW at http://www.rcl.cityu.edu.hk/hkcolas/. Accessed 23.2.07.

Hong Kong Education and Manpower Bureau (2006) *Cantonese Expressive Language Scales*. Hong Kong: Education and Manpower Bureau (Speech Therapy Services Section), Government of Hong Kong SAR.

Hong Kong SAR Government Information Centre (2006a) Enhanced speech therapy services for pupils [Press Release, issued 19 May 2006]. On WWW at http://www.info.gov.hk/gia/general/200605/19/P200605190108.htm. Accessed 25.10.06.

Hong Kong SAR Government Information Centre (2006b) Department of Health introduces oral Cantonese assessment tool for school children [Press Release, issued 3 March 2006]. On WWW at http://www.info.gov.hk/gia/general/200603/03/P200603030204.htm. Accessed 29.5.06.

Hong Kong Society for Child Health and Development (1987) *Manual of the Reynell Developmental Language Scales, Cantonese (Hong Kong) Version*. Hong Kong: Author.

Johnson, C.J. (2006) Getting started in evidence-based practice for childhood speech-language disorders. *American Journal of Speech-Language Pathology* 15, 20–35.

Klee, T., Stokes, S.F., Wong, A.M.Y., Fletcher, P. and Gavin, W.J. (2004) Utterance length and lexical diversity in Cantonese-speaking children with and without specific language impairment. *Journal of Speech, Language, and Hearing Research* 47, 1396–1410.

Lee, K.Y-S. (2006) *Cantonese Basic Speech Perception Test*. Hong Kong: The Chinese University of Hong Kong.

Lee, K.Y.S., Lee, L.W.T. and Cheung, P.S.P. (1996) *Hong Kong Cantonese Receptive Vocabulary Test*. Hong Kong: Hong Kong Society for Child Health and Development.

Lee, P.W.H., Luk, E.S.L., Baconshone, J., Lau, J., Wong, V. and Ko, L. (1990) The Developmental Language Screening Scale: A validation and normative study. *Hong Kong Journal of Paediatrics* 1, 7–22.

Lee, P.W.H., Luk, E.S.L., Yu, K.K. and Baconshone, J. (1985) A developmental language screening scale for use in Hong Kong. *Hong Kong Journal of Paediatrics* 2, 152–175.

Leonard, L.B. (1987) Is specific language impairment a useful construct? In S. Rosenberg (ed.) *Advances in Applied Psycholinguistics: Disorders of First-language Development* (pp. 1–39). Cambridge: Cambridge University Press.

McCauley, R.J. and Swisher, L. (1984) Psychometric review of language and articulation tests for preschool children. *Journal of Speech and Hearing Disorders* 49, 34–42.

McFadden, T.U. (1996) Creating language impairments in typically achieving children: The pitfalls of 'normal' normative sampling. *Language, Speech, and Hearing Services in Schools* 27, 3–9.

Merrell, A.W. and Plante, E. (1997) Norm-referenced test interpretation in the diagnostic process. *Language, Speech, and Hearing Services in Schools* 28, 50–58.

Mervis, C.B. and Robinson, B.F. (2005) Designing measures for profiling and genotype/phenotype studies of individuals with genetic syndromes or developmental language disorders. *Applied Psycholinguistics* 26, 41–64.

Mikucki, B.A. and Larrivee, L. (2006) Validity and reliability of twelve child language tests. Paper presented at the Annual Convention of the American Speech-Language-Hearing Association, Miami.

Peña, E.D., Spaulding, T.J. and Plante, E. (2006) The composition of normative groups and diagnostic decision making: Shooting ourselves in the foot. *American Journal of Speech-Language Pathology* 15, 247–254.

Perona, K., Plante, E. and Vance, R. (2005) Diagnostic accuracy of the Structured Photographic Expressive Language Test: Third edition (SPELT-3). *American Journal of Speech-Language Pathology* 36, 103–115.

Plante, E. and Vance, R. (1994) Selection of preschool language tests: A data-based approach. *Language, Speech, and Hearing Services in Schools* 25, 15–24.

Plante, E. and Vance, R. (1995) Diagnostic accuracy of two tests of preschool language. *American Journal of Speech-Language Pathology* 4, 70–76.

Reilly, S. (2004) The move to evidence-based practice in speech pathology. In S. Reilly, J. Douglas and J. Oates (eds) *Evidence-based Practice in Speech Pathology* (pp. 3–17). London: Whurr.

Reynell, J. (1977) *Reynell Developmental Language Scales*. Windsor: NFER.

Reynell, J. and Huntley, M. (1985) *Reynell Developmental Language Scales: Revised*. Windsor: NFER-Nelson.

Sackett, D.L., Rosenberg, W.M.C., Gray, J.A.M., Haynes, R.B. and Richardson, W.S. (1996) Evidence based medicine: What it is and what it isn't. *British Medical Journal* 312, 71–72.

So, L.K.H. (1993) *Cantonese Segmental Phonology Test*. Hong Kong: Bradford.

So, L.K.H. and Leung, C-S.S. (2004) A phonological screening tool for Cantonese-speaking children. *Child Language Teaching and Therapy* 20, 75–86.

Stokes, S.F. and Wong, A.M.Y. (1996) Validation of a Cantonese version of the Preschool Language Assessment Instrument. *Asia Pacific Journal of Speech, Language, and Hearing* 1, 75–90.

Straus, S.E., Richardson, W.S., Glasziou, P. and Haynes, R.B. (2005) *Evidence-based Medicine: How to Practice and Teach EBM* (3rd edn). Edinburgh: Elsevier Churchill Livingstone.

Tager-Flusberg, H. (2005) Designing studies to investigate the relationships between genes, environments, and developmental language disorders. *Applied Psycholinguistics* 26, 29–39.

Tardif, T., Fletcher, P., Liang, W. and Kaciroti, N. (in press) Early vocabulary development in Mandarin (Putonghua) and Cantonese. *Journal of Child Language*.

Taylor-Goh, S. (2005) *Royal College of Speech & Language Therapists Clinical Guidelines* [Electronic Version]. On WWW at http://www.rcslt.org/resources/clinicalguidelines.

Tomblin, J.B., Records, N.L. and Zhang, X. (1996) A system for the diagnosis of specific language impairment in kindergarten children. *Journal of Speech and Hearing Research* 39, 1284–1294.

T'sou, B., Lee, T.H-T., Tung, P., Cheung, P., Ng, A., To, C.K.S. *et al.* (2006a) *Hong Kong Cantonese Articulation Test*. Hong Kong: City University of Hong Kong.

T'sou, B., Lee, T.H-T., Tung, P., Man, Y., Chan, A., To, C.K.S. *et al.* (2006b) *Hong Kong Cantonese Oral Language Assessment Scale*. Hong Kong: City University of Hong Kong.

Whiting, P., Rutjes, A.W.S., Reitsma, J.B., Bossuyt, P.M.M. and Kleijnen, J. (2003) The development of QUADAS: A tool for the quality of assessment of studies of diagnostic accuracy included in systematic reviews. *BMC Medical Research Methodology* 3, 25.

Wong, V., Lee, P.W.H., Lieh-Mak, F., Yeung, C.Y., Leung, P.W.L., Luk, S.L. *et al.* (1992) Language screening in preschool Chinese children. *European Journal of Disorders of Communication* 27, 247–264.

Chapter 7

Morphological Deficit and Dyslexia Subtypes in Chinese

SINA WU, JEROME L. PACKARD and HUA SHU

Introduction

Most research published on dyslexia in English has posited problems in phonological processing as the core deficit (Ramus, 2003). However, dyslexia may manifest differently in different languages, depending on the type of orthography used in the language. In languages with alphabetic orthographies, the unit of interface between the grapheme and the spoken language is the *phoneme*, but in Chinese orthography it is the *morpheme*. Research has shown that in Chinese, sensitivity to morphemic information is critically important in reading development (Li, 2002; McBride-Chang *et al.*, 2003), and morphological awareness has also been found to be a core cognitive construct underlying Chinese dyslexia (Shu *et al.*, 2006). Given these findings, what role might we expect morphemic knowledge to play in determining Chinese dyslexia subtypes? In this chapter, we present evidence that morphological processing represents a core construct in defining subtypes in Chinese dyslexia.

Background

Research on dyslexia subtypes in alphabetic languages

In languages with alphabetic writing systems, a phonological deficit generally has been accepted as the primary cause of developmental dyslexia (see e.g. Bradley & Bryant, 1983; Ramus, 2003; Shaywitz *et al.*, 1999; Snowling, 1991; Torgesen *et al.*, 1997). For this reason, research on dyslexia subtypes has generally followed two approaches that take phonology as a core deficit. The first approach posits subtypes involving deficits in phonology plus other areas specifically related to the reading process, while the second approach posits subtypes that involve deficits in a broader range of perceptual, attentional, motoric and other cognitive abilities in addition to phonology.

One of the best-known models, the so called 'reading-specific' approach, is based on the dual-route reading model which posits the existence of a sublexical, compiled phonology route and a lexical, 'sight-word' reading route (Castles & Coltheart, 1993; Coltheart *et al.*, 2001).

Phonological dyslexia is believed to reflect impairment in the sublexical reading route, so that children with this impairment show relatively poor performance in reading phonologically regular novel words or non-words, with the ability to read irregular words remaining relatively intact. *Surface dyslexia* is thought to reflect an impairment in the lexical route, with errors of children so afflicted tending toward regularization of irregular words, while retaining the ability to read phonologically regular words or nonwords.

A related model is that of Boder (1973), who classifies children with dyslexia into one of three subtypes based on performance differences in spelling and word recognition tasks. The dysphonetic subtype involves a problem in the auditory-phonetic system, causing problems in processing phonetic and analytic-sequential stimuli. The dyseidetic subtype reflects problems learning sight-words and in processing simultaneous-gestalt stimuli. The third subtype (dysphoneidetic) consists of subjects who have a mixed pattern.

Another reading-specific deficit model is the double-deficit model of Wolf and Bowers (2000), who propose that reading disorders are due either to a core phonological deficit, or to a deficit in rapid naming or a combination of the two. A point of debate surrounding the double-deficit theory is that as rapid naming involves the retrieval and production of sounds, the rapid naming deficit might simply reduce to a core phonological deficit.

Among the more general reading deficit models, Tallal's (1980) temporal order perception theory implicates deficiencies in low-level auditory processing as the basic cause of the core phonological deficit. According to this theory, individuals with dyslexia are impaired in discriminating and sequencing rapidly presented acoustic stimuli, resulting in disturbances in auditory processing that contribute not only to problems in speech perception, but also to weaknesses in developing the phonemic awareness skills that underlie reading impairments. Another of the reading-general models, that of Bakker (1990), classifies individuals with dyslexia into a P-subtype (involving perceptual deficits), an L-subtype (involving linguistic deficits) and an M-subtype that involves a mix of the first two. In Bakker's model, the two subtypes are characterized by different degrees of hemispheric involvement in the reading process, with the right hemisphere more implicated for P-subtypes and the left hemisphere more implicated for L-subtypes.

More recently, cluster analysis has been used to support the taxonomy of subtypes in the reading-general models (Ho *et al.*, 2004; Morris *et al.*, 1998). Morris *et al.* used cluster analysis to identify seven dyslexia subtypes, with two of the seven subtypes globally deficient, and four of the remaining five subtypes showing primary deficits in phonological processing. Regarding the more general perceptual deficit dyslexia models, it has been claimed that deficits in perceptual processing are more relevant in the 'phonological' dyslexia subtypes and not relevant to the 'surface' dyslexia subtypes (see discussion in McAnally *et al.*, 2000).

Morphological awareness and dyslexia in Chinese

In the Chinese logographic orthography system, the unit of interface between the written word and spoken language is the *morpheme*, making morphological awareness a potentially more important construct in Chinese reading than in reading alphabetic orthographies. Morphological awareness in Chinese may be thought of as consisting of three types of knowledge related to reading. The first is knowledge of homophones, the second is knowledge of homographs and the third is knowledge of the morphemic structure of complex words.

Knowledge of homophones entails the insight that in Chinese, a single spoken syllable may stand for several different morphemes. Mandarin has about 7000 morphemes but only about 1200 different syllable types, and so each syllable represents on average more than five morphemes. Therefore, the syllable *shi4* for example can mean 'is' 是 'matter, affair' 事 or 'vision' (as in 視覺 *shi4jue2* vision-perceive 'visual perception'). In English, this would be akin to knowing that the spoken words 'two' and 'too' have different meanings even though they sound the same. Knowledge of homographs means being aware that a single written character in Chinese may represent different morphemes. So, for example, the character 草 *cao3* can mean either 'grass' or 'careless', as seen by its use in the words 草地 *cao3di4* grass-land 'lawn' and 潦草 *liao3cao3* hasty-careless 'careless'. This would be like an English-speaking child knowing that the single written form <bank> can mean either 'a place to deposit money' or 'edge of a river'. Knowing the morphemic structure of complex (i.e. multimorphemic) words means being aware of the contribution made by individual morphemes to the meaning of the entire word. Most Chinese words contain more than one morpheme. For example, the compound word 電視 *dian4shi4* electric-vision 'television' consists of two morphemes 電 *dian4* 'electric' and 視 *shi4* 'vision'. Because of the central role played by the morpheme in Chinese orthography, sensitivity to morphological knowledge is especially important in the development of oral and written vocabulary in Chinese, and is critically important for children learning to read and write (Li, 2002; McBride-Chang *et al.*, 2003; Packard *et al.*, 2006).

Recently, there has been an increase in research on dyslexia in Chinese, with researchers describing different properties that serve to distinguish dyslexia subtypes. Research has revealed that phonological, naming-speed and orthographic deficits are important features in Chinese children with dyslexia, as they are in alphabetic languages (Ho & Lai,

2000; Ho *et al.*, 2004). In the most comprehensive study to date on Chinese dyslexia subtypes, Ho *et al.* tested 147 primary school children with dyslexia on a number of literacy and cognitive tasks. The results showed that a rapid naming deficit and an orthographic deficit were the two most dominant types of cognitive deficits in Chinese developmental dyslexia, with each making significant unique contributions to literacy performance. Seven subtypes of dyslexia – global deficit, orthographic deficit, phonological memory deficit, mild difficulty and three other subtypes with rapid-naming-related deficits – were identified using scores on cognitive tasks as classification measures in cluster analyses. These subtypes were validated using a behavior checklist and three literacy measures. The authors proposed that instead of a phonological deficit as in English dyslexia, orthographic-related difficulties may be the crux of the problem in Chinese dyslexia.

A recent study by Shu *et al.* (2006) specifically examined the role of morphology in Chinese dyslexia. That study found that readers with dyslexia were best distinguished from age-matched controls with tasks of morphological awareness, speeded number naming and vocabulary skill, while performance on tasks of visual skills and phonological awareness failed to distinguish the groups. Path analyses further revealed that morphological awareness was the strongest consistent predictor of a variety of literacy-related skills in both the dyslexic and control groups. Because the findings of that study suggest that morphology is an important theoretical construct in Chinese dyslexia, and because of the increasingly important role that morphological awareness plays in theories of Chinese reading, it is natural to ask the question what role morphology might play in defining Chinese dyslexia subtypes. Our goal, therefore, was to investigate the function of morphology in distinguishing subtypes in Chinese dyslexia.

Tests and procedure for screening children with dyslexia

The raw data for the present study were taken from the experiment described in Shu *et al.* (2006), which is briefly recapitulated here. Two tests were used for initial participant screening. The first is the standardized Chinese character recognition test created by Wang and Tao (1993), and the second is the Chinese version of the Raven's Progressive Matrices test (Zhang & Wang, 1985). The character recognition and Raven's tests were administered in groups to 751 fifth- and sixth-grade students in two elementary schools in Beijing, China. Students who scored 1.5 grade levels below normal on character recognition and scored between the 25th and 95th percentile on the Raven's test were identified as the normal group. The difference between the two groups in the character recognition scores is significant

Table 7.1 Participants (by mean age, character recognition scores and IQ percentile)

	Reading deficit group (n = 75)		*Normal reading group* (n = 77)	
	Mean	*SD*	*Mean*	*SD*
Age (months)	143	9.5	138	8.37
Character recognition score	2189	282.4	2821	239.5
IQ (%)	47	31	53	36

($t_{150} = 14.9$, $p < 0.001$), but the difference in IQ between the two groups as measured by the Raven's test does not reach significance ($t_{150} = 1.04$, $p > 0.05$). Subjects are presented in Table 7.1.

As in Shu *et al.* (2006), a series of nine cognitive tests were administered to assess subjects' linguistic and nonlinguistic cognitive abilities (morphological awareness, rapid naming, phonological awareness, verbal short-term memory, lexical vocabulary, visual spatial test, articulatory rate, visual attention and non-verbal short-term memory). For each cognitive ability, e.g. phonological awareness, there were two separate tests (e.g. in the case of phonological awareness, phoneme deletion and onset/rime/tone discrimination). The results from that study are summarized in Table 7.2.

The first, or original measures were used to perform the cluster analysis in the present study. The second, or alternative measures allowed us to perform tests of internal validity by providing a second measurement of the same cognitive abilities. The alternative measures of cognitive ability would be used to perform a validity check on the subtypes derived via the clustering procedure. The tasks used to elicit the measures of cognitive ability are described as follows.

Morphological awareness

Morpheme production. The experimenter orally presented a two-syllable Chinese word, within which a target syllable was identified. The child was asked to produce two new words with the target syllable, one with the same meaning as the stimulus word and one with a different meaning. For example, if the experimenter presented the word 草地 *cao3di4* (grass-land 'lawn'), the child would be asked to produce a new word using 草 in which the 草 had the same meaning as it did in 草地. One acceptable answer would be 小草 *xiao3cao3* small-grass 'grass'. The child would also be asked to produce a word using 草 in which the meaning was different from its meaning in 草地. An acceptable response would be 潦草 *liao3cao3* hasty-careless 'careless'. There were 30 items, all consisting of real words.

Table 7.2 Means and standard deviations of the two groups on the 18 cognitive measures

		Dyslexic (n = 75)		*Control* (n = 77)		
		Mean	*SD*	*Mean*	*SD*	*p*
Morphological awareness						
1.	Morpheme production[b] (30)	16.05	3.32	21.08	4.56	***
2.	Morpheme judgment[b] (30)	18.51	2.74	19.7	2.5	**
Rapid naming						
3.	Number naming[c]	16.15	3.44	13.48	3.25	***
4.	Picture naming[c]	22.45	4.14	20.04	3.73	***
Phonological awareness						
5.	Phoneme deletion[c] (16)	6.73	3.68	9.69	3.49	***
6.	Onset/rime/tone judgment[b] (36)	26.28	6.70	28.68	6.69	*
Verbal short-term memory						
7.	Syllable repetition[b] (18)	7.93	1.45	8.88	2.27	**
8.	Number repetition[a] (30)	6.51	2.45	16.73	3.15	***
Lexical-vocabulary						
9.	Vocabulary[a]	6.56	2.77	9.06	2.31	***
10.	Similarity[a]	6.99	2.31	8.65	2.71	***
Visual spatial test						
11.	WISC Block design[a]	32.27	10.29	31.99	12.19	n.s.
12.	Embedded figures 2[b]	12.39	4.64	12.64	5.02	n.s.
Articulatory rate						
13.	Syllable articulation rate 1[b]	7.89	1.65	7.28	1.22	n.s.
14.	Nonsense syllable articulation rate 2[b]	6.38	1.71	5.69	1.44	n.s.
Visual attention						
15.	Nonsense letter 1[b]	41.88	20.07	31.95	11.18	n.s.
16.	Figures 2[b]	44.67	14.83	35.51	8.59	n.s.

Table 7.2 (*Continued*)

		Dyslexic (n =75)		*Control* (n =77)		
		Mean	*SD*	*Mean*	*SD*	*p*
Non-verbal short term memory						
17.	Corsi Blocks (ordered) 1[b]	8.09	1.49	8.18	1.82	n.s.
18.	Corsi Blocks (total) 2[b]	9.99	2.02	10.09	2.04	n.s.

Note. [a]Standard score; [b]raw data; [c]time in seconds. Numbers in parenthesis represent the number of items in each task. *$p < 0.05$; **$p < 0.01$; ***$p < 0.001$; n.s. = nonsignificant
Source: Data from Shu *et al.* (2006), adapted with the permission of the American Psychological Association

Morpheme judgment. A pair of two-syllable words was orally presented to children. The members of the word pair shared an identical Chinese syllable and character. The child was asked whether the meaning of the shared member was the same in the two words or not. For example, in the first member of a word pair 生詞 *sheng1ci2* unfamiliar-word 'new word', the character 生 has the same meaning as in the second word of the pair, 生人 *sheng1ren2* unfamiliar-person 'stranger' (i.e. the character represents the morpheme meaning 'unfamiliar' in both words). An example of a second word with an identical syllable/character that did not have the same meaning would be 生活 *sheng1huo2* born-live 'life'. The child's task was to judge whether the syllable in common to both words had a similar or different meaning. There were 30 items in total.

Rapid naming

Number naming. In this task, five numbers were repeated six times on a single sheet of paper. The child was then asked to say the number names in order on the sheet from beginning to end as accurately and quickly as possible. Each child named each list twice, and the score was the average naming latency across the two trials.

Picture naming. Pictures of five objects were repeated six times in random orders, on a single sheet of paper, as described for the number-naming task. As with the number-naming task, children named each list from beginning to end twice, and the average of these two times was used for subsequent analyses.

Phonological awareness

Phoneme deletion. This 16-item task was individually administered. The experimenter first presented a one-syllable real word orally and then asked the child to say the word with a given phoneme deleted. The task included deletion of both initial and final phonemes.

Onset/rime/tone judgment. This judgment test consisted of three subtests measuring onset, rime and tone, respectively. The experimenter pronounced single-syllable real words twice, and the children were then asked to write down the one syllable that was different from the other two. Every subtest comprised 12 items, for a total of 36 items.

Verbal short-term memory

Number repetition. All children were given the Chinese version of the Digit Span subtest (Wechsler, 1974), which requires repetition of digits in forward and backward conditions. Scoring procedures were based on the local norm established by Lin and Zhang (1986).

Syllable repetition. This task requires that Chinese syllables, orally presented by the experimenter (one-syllable real words), be repeated back by each child in the order in which the experimenter presented them. The length of word strings ranged from two to ten syllables. There were two word strings of each length, yielding a total possible score of 18.

Lexical vocabulary

To measure vocabulary knowledge of the children, we individually administered Chinese versions of both the Similarities and Vocabulary subtests of the revised Wechsler Intelligence Scale for Children (WISC-R; Wechsler, 1974). Scoring procedures of these tasks were based on local norms established by Lin and Zhang (1986).

Visual spatial test

WISC-R Block design. The Block design subtest of WISC-R, which requires construction of block arrays, was individually administered to each child. Scoring procedures were based on the local norm established by Lin and Zhang (1986).

Embedded figures. In this group-administered test (Zhang, 1998), children are asked to locate a simple target figure embedded within a complex background.

Articulatory rate

Syllable articulation rate. In this task, the experimenter orally presented the child with a pair of either single-syllable or two-syllable words. Children were asked simply to repeat the pairs 10 times as quickly as possible. There were four word pairs in total, and the total score on this measure consisted of the average latencies across all four items.

Nonsense syllable articulation rate. This task was similar in method and measurement to the syllable articulation task, but using nonsense words rather than real words.

Visual attention

Nonsense letter. Following the task created by Doehring (1968), children were presented with a piece of paper containing 540 nonsense letters printed on it. Children were asked to delete a reverse *z* with a pencil each time it appeared in random sequence among all of the letters. Their score consisted of the number of reverse *z*s correctly deleted minus the total of letters that were incorrectly deleted in one minute.

Figures. We used the same technique of visual search to measure children's skills in detecting a trapezoid figure. From among 540 figures, children were asked to cross out only the trapezoid figures. Total score after one minute spent on the task was again the total number of figures correctly crossed out minus those that were incorrectly crossed out.

Non-verbal short-term memory

Corsi Blocks I. Following Milner (1971), nine blocks are placed between the experimenter and the subject. In each trial, the experimenter taps certain blocks in a given sequence, and subjects are asked to tap the same blocks, in the same sequence, as those tapped by the experimenter. Points are given only if both the blocks and their sequence are remembered correctly. There are 16 trials in all, for a total possible score of 16 points.

Corsi Blocks II. As for Corsi Blocks I, except that remembering only the correct blocks, and not their sequence, is required to earn points. There are 16 trials in all, for 16 total possible points.

Cognitive deficit in Chinese dyslexia

As a first step in the investigation of dyslexia subtypes, our strategy was to determine which cognitive domains contained deficits in subjects with dyslexia and which domains did not. It can be seen in Table 7.2 that the dyslexic group and the control group are significantly different in all of the linguistic tasks, such as phonological, morphological, naming speed and vocabulary. But no significant differences in non-linguistic tasks were found between the two groups.

As one of the goals of this study was to determine in which domains children with dyslexia do and do not show abnormal performance, it was necessary to adopt a criterion for deviance. A common procedure is to set a threshold at *n* standard deviations below the mean of the control group. However, there is of course some arbitrariness in the choice of the value of *n*, and no value has been used consistently in the literature. Following Ho *et al.* (2002), we set the definition of 'deficit' to be 1.5 standard deviations below the mean of the control group. The results can be seen in Table 7.3, which gives the percentage of dyslexic and normal subjects defined as having a deficit in the different tasks,

Table 7.3 Percentage and deficit severities of dyslexic and normal subjects defined as having a deficit

Tasks	*Factors*	*Dyslexic group*		*Normal group*
		Percent with deficit	*Degree of deficit (mean z-score)*	*Percent with deficit*
Linguistic tasks	Morpheme production	96%	– 3.97	6%
	Phoneme deletion	53%	– 1.42	8%
	Number naming	45%	– 1.58	12%
	WISC-R vocabulary	39%	– 1.28	1%
	Number STM	24%	– 0.89	4%
Non-linguistic tasks	WISC-R Block design	15%	– 0.21	2%
	Syllable articulation rate	0%	– 0.35	0%
	Nonsense letter	25%	– 0.24	21%
	Corsi Blocks I	15%	– 0.36	10%

and gives the mean *z*-score of the dyslexic group subjects in the different tasks.

The results indicate that on the linguistic tasks, the dyslexic group ranges from 24% (for verbal short-term memory) to 96% (for morpheme production) of the group having a deficit, compared to the normal group's range of 1% to 12%. The degree of deficit measure also shows that the linguistic deficits of children with dyslexia (ranging from – 0.89 to – 3.97) were much more severe than the nonlinguistic deficits (ranging from – 0.21 to – 0.36). Table 7.3 further reveals that, compared with the percentage of children with dyslexia with phonological (53%) and naming speed (45%) problems, the largest proportion (96%) of children with dyslexia had morphological problems, and the degree of morphological deficit in the children with dyslexia was more severe (– 3.97) than the degree of other deficits.

As previous studies have reported that most children with dyslexia possess more than one deficit, we analyzed the relationship between the number and degree of deficits in children with dyslexia. Given that the mean *z*-score of the dyslexic group on the verbal short-term memory test (see Table 7.3) did not reach 1.00 standard deviation below the mean of the control group (− 0.89) and the proportion of subjects with a deficit was relatively small (24%), in the *z*-score analysis to follow we considered only the four factors: morphological awareness (MA), phonological awareness (PA), rapid naming (RN) and lexical vocabulary (LV). We selected the subjects who were defined as having a deficit, i.e. those who had *z*-scores below the cutoff of − 1.50 on one or more of the four factors. As seen in Table 7.4, 10 dyslexia subtypes were extracted using this method, defined by the different combinations and deficit severities of the four factors.

From Table 7.4, it can be seen that there are three subtypes (1, 2 and 3) in which children with dyslexia have only one deficit (MA, PA or RAN). The following three subtypes (4, 5 and 6) consist of children who have two deficits (MA + PA, MA + RN and MA + LV). The next three subtypes (7, 8 and 9) are those with three deficits (MA + PA + RN, MA + RN + LV and MA + PA + LV). And the last subtype (10) consists of children with dyslexia who have deficits in all four factors. These results indicate that all of the children with dyslexia in the present study have at least one cognitive deficit, and 60 out of the 75 children with dyslexia have two or more cognitive deficits. These findings further suggest the presence of significant heterogeneity within Chinese developmental dyslexia, given the wide variability in the number and combination of deficits. The results are consistent with Ho *et al.*'s (2002, 2004) findings, but the remarkable observation of the present study is that of the 10 subtypes presented in Table 7.4, no fewer than eight contain a morphological deficit. In contrast, five contain a phonological deficit and five contain a deficit in rapid naming. This provides strong preliminary evidence that a morphological deficit may be considered a primary factor in determining Chinese dyslexia subtypes.

Defining Dyslexia Subtypes more Precisely: Cluster Analysis

From the preliminary analysis based on *z*-scores presented in the previous section, it is evident that dyslexia in Chinese is a complex phenomenon consisting of a number of heterogeneous subtypes formed from different groupings of deficit factors. In an attempt to go beyond the *z*-score analysis above and distinguish the different dyslexia subtypes more clearly, we subjected the data to two methods of cluster analysis. Similar to the analyses in Morris (1998) and Ho *et al.* (2004), we first used Ward's method, followed by the *k*-means method, implemented in the following manner.

Table 7.4 Different combinations and deficit severities of the four factors

Deficit group	*Deficit type*	*Deficited factor*	*Mean MA z-score*	*Mean PA z-score*	*Mean RN z-score*	*Mean LV z-score*	*Subject* **n**
A	1	MA	**−3.83**	− 0.31	− 0.52	− 0.45	12
	2	PA	− 1.00	− **2.00**	− 0.80	− 1.00	1
	3	RN	− 0.75	0.50	− **4.45**	− 0.71	2
							Subtotal 15
B	4	MA + RN	− **3.91**	− 0.15	− **2.54**	− 0.31	11
	5	MA + PA	− **3.21**	− **2.38**	− 0.42	− 0.71	13
	6	MA + LV	− **4.08**	− 0.67	0.10	− **2.10**	6
							Subtotal 30
C	7	MA + PA + RN	− **3.79**	− **2.57**	− **3.19**	− 0.041	7
	8	MA + RN + LV	− **4.63**	− 0.83	− **3.88**	− **2.89**	4
	9	MA + PA + LV	− **5.00**	− **2.15**	− 0.56	− **2.14**	9
							Subtotal 20
D	10	All four	− **5.15**	− **2.47**	− **2.66**	− **2.91**	10
							Total 75

Note. Bolded figures denote *z*-scores below − 1.50

Method

First, the nine original quantitative measures of cognitive ability were selected as dimensions to serve as the basis for the clustering procedures: (1) morpheme production, (2) number naming, (3) phoneme deletion, (4) number repetition, (5) vocabulary similarity, (6) WISC-R Block design, (7) syllable articulation rate, (8) nonsense letter and (9) Corsi Blocks I. The alternative measures of cognitive ability would be used later to perform a validity check on the subtypes derived via the clustering procedure. If the alternative measures significantly discriminate the categories derived from the clustering procedure, this would be considered a measure of internal validity.

For the first cluster analysis, Ward's method, which does not require the number of clusters to be specified beforehand, was used to determine potential numbers of clusters. Nine different clustering solutions resulted from Ward's analysis, with the number of clusters in each solution ranging from two to ten (i.e. the first solution had two clusters, the second had three, all the way to the ninth solution, which contained 10 clusters of subjects).

For the second cluster analysis, the *k*-means method was used. As the *k*-means method requires the number of clusters to be specified beforehand, we performed nine *k*-means analyses – one for each of the solutions found through the Ward's analysis. So the first *k*-means analysis specified a two-cluster solution, the second specified a three-cluster solution, and so on, with the ninth *k*-means analysis specifying a 10-cluster solution. For each of the nine *k*-means analyses, cluster centroids were directly generated (i.e. seeded) using mean values for subjects on the nine quantitative variables obtained via the Ward's analysis.

Next, the membership of subjects in the two sets of nine solutions (i.e. the nine solutions formed by Ward's analysis and the nine solutions formed by *k*-means analyses) was compared for consistency, i.e. for joint set membership. We determined the final number of clusters by using the cluster solution that had the highest degree of consistency between the Ward's and *k*-means analyses. The consistency between the Ward's and *k*-means analyses was found to be highest with the solution that contained nine clusters. That consistency was found to range from 72% to 90% joint set membership. Subjects that did not naturally fall into one of the nine clusters were placed into clusters by visual inspection.

As the nine clusters are based on the consistency between the two different methods of clustering, in order to assess how well the respective dimensions (morpheme production, number naming, etc.) discriminate the clusters, we performed independent ANOVAs on each of the nine dimensions, with subject score on each respective dimension as the dependent variable, and the nine clusters listed as independent variables. The resulting F values from the ANOVAs performed on each dimension are: morpheme: $F(8,143) = 25.33$, $p < 0.001$; rapid naming: $F(8,143) = 15.48$; $p < 0.001$; phoneme $F(8,143) = 16.33$, $p < 0.001$; verbal STM: $F(8,143) = 14.84$, $p < 0.001$; vocabulary: $F(8,143) = 22.16$, $p < 0.001$; spatial: $F(8,143) = 24.19$, $p < 0.001$; articulation rate: $F(8,143) = 17.33$, $p < 0.001$; attention: $F(8,143) = 13.96$, $p < 0.001$; non-verbal STM: $F(8,143) = 4.09$, $p < 0.001$. The significance of the F test in each case indicates that the dimensions do indeed provide good discrimination among clusters.

The number of subjects in each subtype (i.e. cluster) is 17 in subtype one, 24 in subtype two, 31 in subtype three, 24 in subtype four, 15 in subtype five, three in subtype six, 19 in subtype seven, six in subtype eight and 13 in subtype nine. Observing that subtypes six and eight contained only three and six subjects, respectively, we eliminated those two subtypes from consideration, leaving seven remaining subtypes containing a total of 143 subjects, or 94% of the original subject population.

Cluster analysis results

Clustering yielded seven reliable subtypes – including two nondisabled subtypes and five reading-disabled subtypes – representing 94% of the original sample. We collapsed the two nondisabled groups NDIS1 and NDIS2 into a single nondisabled group NDIS due to their similar configuration, thereby reducing the total number of groups to six (five plus the single NDIS group). The profiles of the six groups are shown in Figure 7.1, with the nine quantitative variables plotted on the x-axis, and the mean z-score of the subjects within groups on those variables plotted on the y-axis. The corresponding numerical values are provided in Table 7.5.

The profiles of the six derived subtypes are quite distinct, allowing us to label them according to the preponderance of deficit factors that seemed to best characterize the subtype. The subtype labels used were global (GLO), spatial (SPA), morphological-phonological-short-term memory (MPS), global language (GLO-L), morphological-rapid naming-short-term memory (MRS) and nondisabled (NDIS).

The performance of the subjects in the GLO subtype on eight of the cognitive measures is below normal. The subjects in the SPA subtype perform normally on all the linguistic measures and show only a slight deficit in two of the nonlinguistic measures, namely spatial and articulation rate. The MPS subtype shows deficits on both linguistic and nonlinguistic measures, especially on morphological awareness, phonological awareness and short term memory on both verbal and non-verbal measures. The GLO-L subtype shows deficits on all five linguistic measures and a slight deficit on articulation rate. The MRS subtype shows a deficiency on morphological, rapid naming and short-term

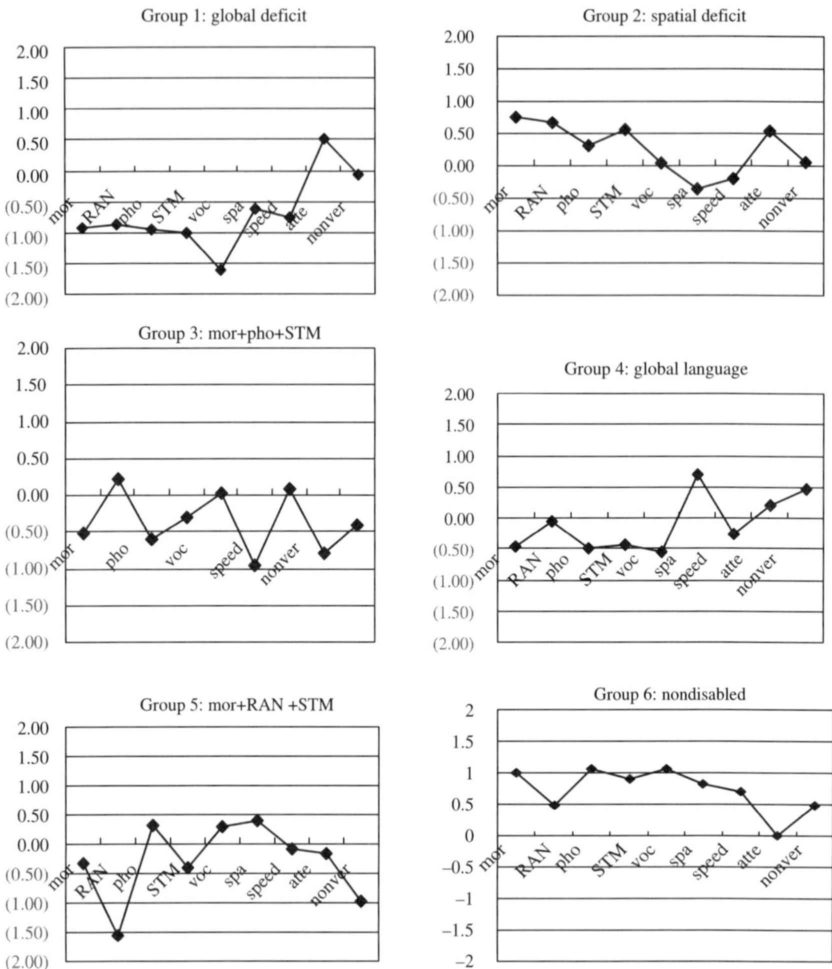

Figure 7.1 Configurations of six subtypes.
Note. mor, morphology; RAN, rapid naming; pho, phonology; STM, short-term memory; voc, vocabulary; spa, visual spatial test; speed, articulatory rate; atte, visual attention; nonver, non-verbal short-term memory.

memory measures (verbal and non-verbal measures), but manifests normally on phonological and vocabulary measures. In addition, the MRS subtype also shows a slight deficit on articulation and attention measures. For the NDIS group, performance on all of the nine cognitive measures is above normal.

The mean character recognition scores of each of the six subtypes are seen in the last line of Table 7.5. An analysis of variance (ANOVA)

Table 7.5 Summary of z-scores and standard deviations of the different subtypes on the cognitive measures

Cognitive measures	*GLO mean (SD)*	*SPA mean (SD)*	*MPS mean (SD)*	*GLO-L Mean (SD)*	*MRS mean (SD)*	*NDIS mean (SD)*
Morphological	*−0.93 (0.77)*	0.75 *(0.48)*	*−0.52 (0.69)*	*−0.47 (0.61)*	*−0.33 (0.67)*	1.00 *(0.67)*
Rapid naming	*−0.87 (1.07)*	0.67 *(0.49)*	0.23 *(0.66)*	*−0.02 (0.63)*	*−1.56 (0.96)*	0.48 *(0.66)*
Phonological	*−0.96 (0.64)*	0.31 *(0.88)*	*−0.59 (0.65)*	*−0.49 (0.76)*	0.32 *(0.87)*	1.07 *(0.51)*
Verbal STM	*−0.99 (0.56)*	0.56 *(0.72)*	*−0.31 (0.77)*	*−0.42 (0.66)*	*−0.40 (0.54)*	0.91 *(1.01)*
Vocabulary	*−1.62 (0.69)*	0.04 *(0.53)*	0.03 *(0.52)*	*−0.54 (0.71)*	0.29 *(0.56)*	1.07 (0.67)
Spatial	*−0.63 (0.83)*	*−0.36 (0.57)*	*−0.97 (0.58)*	0.70 *(0.69)*	0.40 *(0.8)*	0.83 *(0.76)*
Articulation rate	*−0.76 (1)*	*−0.20 (0.93)*	0.09 *(0.88)*	*−0.26 (0.71)*	*−0.09 (1.18)*	0.70 *(0.86)*
Attention	0.51 *(1.35)*	0.54 *(0.89)*	*−0.79 (0.68)*	0.20 *(0.78)*	*−0.16 (0.92)*	0.01 *(0.85)*
Non-verbal STM	*−0.06 (0.81)*	0.06 *(1.06)*	*−0.40 (1.07)*	0.47 *(0.73)*	*−0.97 (0.84)*	0.48 *(0.76)*
Character recognition	2005	2768	2422	2283	2358	2880

Note. Cognitive measure scores below the group mean, i.e. those with negative z-score values, are italicized and underlined performed with the character recognition scores as the dependent variable and the six subtypes as independent variables was significant ($F(5,137) = 26.95$, $p < 0.001$), indicating that the members of the six groups differ significantly in their ability to recognize characters.

Of the reading-disabled subtypes, two were globally deficient in language skills, whereas two of the three reading-disabled subtypes displayed a relative weakness in morphological awareness and variations in rapid serial naming and verbal short-term memory. The remaining disabled subtype was impaired on spatial processing. It is obvious that all of the six subtypes showed multiple deficits. This is consistent with previous results (Ho *et al.*, 2002, 2004; Morris *et al.*, 1998), but contrasts with English-speaking children with dyslexia. The most common deficit in Chinese children with dyslexia is clearly morphological.

Validation of Subtypes

Validation I

To obtain measures of internal validity for the six obtained dyslexia subtypes, we used the alternative measures of the nine cognitive abilities. As an initial step in determining internal validity, we needed to demonstrate that the clusters were derived from measures that truly tapped the underlying constructs represented by the nine cognitive abilities. Thus, our first step was to determine whether our measures of the nine original cognitive abilities were correlated with the alternative measures of the nine original cognitive abilities. We therefore calculated the Pearson's correlation coefficient between the original and alternative measures, with the result seen in Table 7.6.

As seen in Table 7.6, the two measures of the nine cognitive factors are all significantly correlated, with all pairs of measures except the morphological pair showing fairly strong internal consistency. The relatively low (albeit significant) correlation between the two morphological tasks could be due to the fact that in the morpheme production task, participants were required to produce two words, while in the morpheme judgment task, they are required to judge which choice is correct between two choices. As the chance of being correct in the morpheme judgment task is 0.5, the difference in likelihood of getting a correct answer in the two morphological tasks probably decreases the correlation between two tasks.

Validation II

Our next step was to provide an additional measure of internal validity by performing a multivariate analysis of variance (MANOVA) using the alternative measures of the nine cognitive abilities. If the six dyslexia subtypes formed by cluster analysis based on the original

Table 7.6 Internal validity correlation measures

Validity measures	*Correlation coefficient*
Morpheme production – morpheme judgment	0.35*
Rapid digit naming – rapid picture naming	0.66*
Phoneme deletion – initial/final/tone judgment	0.54*
Digit STM – character STM	0.60*
Lexical vocabulary – vocabulary similarity	0.60*
Block design – embedded figures	0.69*
Word production – nonsense word production	0.56*
Figures – letters	0.62*
Corsi Blocks I – Corsi Blocks II	0.65*

Note. *$p < 0.01$

measures of the nine cognitive abilities are valid, then the alternative cognitive measures should also, in general, successfully discriminate the six subtypes. The subtypes should differ especially when they do not share deficits in given cognitive measures. We therefore performed a MANOVA using the nine alternative cognitive ability measures as dependent variables and the six subtypes derived via cluster analysis as independent variables.

The omnibus MANOVA was significant ($F(54,758) = 5.77$, $p < 0.001$), indicating that the six subtypes do collectively differ in their values on the nine alternative cognitive ability scores. As the omnibus MANOVA provides no information on the degree of distinctiveness among the six individual subtypes on the nine scores, we also performed nine individual univariate ANOVAs, one with each of the nine alternative cognitive ability measures as a dependent variable and the six subtypes as independent variables. This analysis revealed that the differences among the six subtypes for the five linguistic alternative measures of the cognitive abilities were all significant (morphology: $F(5,137) = 4.05$, $p < 0.01$; RAN: $F(5,137) = 7.17$, $p < 0.001$; phonology: $F(5,137) = 10.88$, $p < 0.001$; lexical vocabulary: $F(5,137) = 13.07$, $p < 0.001$; VSTM: $F(5,137) = 5.22$, $p < 0.001$), suggesting that the dyslexia subtypes evidence an acceptable degree of internal validity because it was the alternate measures of the cognitive abilities that were used to confirm subtype clusters derived using the original cognitive ability scores. For the nonlinguistic cognitive abilities, the differences among the subtypes were significant only for spatial: $F(5,137) = 19.05$, $p < 0.001$, and non-verbal

STM: $F(5,137) = 3.80$, $p < 0.01$. For the nonlinguistic cognitive abilities articulatory rate and visual attention, the differences among the subtypes were not significant ($F(5,137) = 2.21$, $p > 0.05$ and $F(5,137) = 1.81$, $p > 0.05$, respectively).

To further verify the internal validity of the subtypes derived through the clustering procedure, we performed planned pairwise comparisons (adjusted for multiple comparisons using the LSD method) between all but the articulatory rate and visual attention cognitive abilities, as those cognitive abilities were not significantly different in the ANOVAs. Because the dyslexia subtypes were derived via cluster analysis by similarities in the groupings of the nine original cognitive measures, in general the planned pairwise comparisons should show differences between subtypes when they do not have a similar deficit pattern in the cognitive measures, and should show no differences between subtypes when they have a similar pattern. A dyslexia subtype is considered to contain a deficit within a cognitive ability if the mean score on the cognitive ability for the subtype is below the mean score for the cognitive ability over all six subtypes. This is most easily seen in Table 7.5, where cognitive ability scores below the mean have negative *z*-score values.

The means, standard deviations and planned pairwise comparison results of the MANOVA are seen in Table 7.7. For the morphological task, the paired comparisons found that none of the differences among the four subtypes (GLO, MPS, GLO-L and MRS) were significant (all paired comparisons $p > 0.09$), presumably because each of the four subtypes contains a deficit in morphological processing (as seen in Table 7.5, in which all have a negative *z*-score on 'morphology'). The SPA and NDIS subtypes performed significantly better than the GLO, MPS and GLO-L groups (the difference between the SPA and those three groups is significant at the $p < 0.05$ level; the difference between the NDIS and those three groups is significant at the $p < 0.01$ level), but the SPA and NDIS subtypes were not significantly different from the MRS subtypes (SPA: $p = 0.24$; NDIS: $p = 0.1$), presumably because the SPA and NDIS subtypes pattern similarly in not containing a morphological deficit, as seen in Table 7.5.

For the rapid-naming task, the GLO subtype was not significantly different from the GLO-L and MRS subtypes (all $p > 0.09$). Note that these are the three subtypes that possess a naming deficit, as seen in Table 7.5. Further, the SPA, MPS and NDIS subtypes were not significantly different (all $p > 0.12$). These are the only subtypes that do not evince a naming deficit, as seen in Table 7.5.

On the phonology task, the MPS subtype approached significance but did not differ ($p = 0.06$), and the GLO-L subtype did not differ from the MPS and GLO subtypes ($p = 0.34$). The latter three subtypes pattern similarly in containing a phonological processing deficit in the cluster

Table 7.7 Results of MANOVA (means, standard deviations and pairwise comparison results)

Tasks	*Possible score*	*Subtypes*					
		GLO	*SPA*	*MPS*	*GLO-L*	*MRS*	*NDIS*
Morphology	64						
Mean (SD)		17.53^{a} (2.35)	20.04^{c} (2.27)	18.74^{a,b} (2.36)	18.42^{a,d} (2.59)	19.07^{a,c} (3.17)	20.34^{c} (2.5)
RAN (RT)							
Mean (SD)		23.97^{a} (3.53)	19.46^{c} (3.06)	20.98^{b,c} (3.53)	22.31^{a,b} (4.73)	24.45^{a} (4.58)	19.47^{c} (3.26)
Phonology	36						
Mean (SD)		21.29^{a} (7.25)	29.83^{b,d} (6.37)	24.74^{a,c} (6.39)	26.25^{c} (5.98)	26.60^{b,c} (6.1)	32.41^{d} (3.0)
Vocabulary	30						
Mean (SD)		8.00^{a} (3.29)	13.33^{b} (3.70)	11.38^{c} (3.33)	10.79^{c} (3.17)	12.86^{b,c} (2.74)	15.19^{d} (3.05)
VSTM	18						
Mean (SD)		7.35^{a} (1.27)	9.16^{b,d} (1.99)	7.80^{a,c} (1.44)	7.87^{a,c} (1.59)	8.33^{a,b} (1.54)	9.47^{d} (2.44)
Spatial							
Mean (SD)		10.29^{a,b} (4.40)	11.21^{a} (2.70)	8.35^{b} (2.80)	14.58^{d} (4.89)	13.0^{a,d} (4.16)	16.91^{c} (3.95)
Articulation rate	45						
Mean (SD)		6.00 (0.96)	6.54 (2.3)	6.06 (1.47)	6.23 (1.38)	5.98 (1.19)	5.25 (1.27)

Table 7.7 (*Continued*)

Tasks	*Possible score*	*Subtypes*					
		GLO	*SPA*	*MPS*	*GLO-L*	*MRS*	*NDIS*
Attention							
Mean (SD)		44.94 (15.08)	38.71 (11.19)	34.77 (9.93)	40.25 (11.83)	38.80 (6.67)	39.84 (12.75)
Non-verbal STM							
Mean (SD)		$9.59^{b,d}$ (1.33)	$10.38^{a,b}$ (1.95)	$9.42^{b,e}$ (2.03)	$10.33^{b,c}$ (1.66)	$8.67^{d,e}$ (2.58)	$10.84^{a,c}$ (1.80)

Note. Identical superscripts in the same row indicate the means are not significantly different $p > 0.05$. Pairwise comparisons not performed for articulation rate and attention because larger ANOVA not significant overall for these factors analysis (as seen from their negative mean *z*-scores in Table 7.5). The SPA subtype and the NDIS group did not differ ($p = 0.10$), and although the MRS subtype performed significantly worse than the NDIS group ($p < 0.01$), it did not differ from the SPA subtype ($p = 0.09$). None of these groups had a deficit in phonological processing, as seen in Table 7.5.

On the vocabulary similarity task, the GLO subtype significantly differed from all other groups (MPS: $p = 0.001$; GLO-L: $p < 0.01$; MRS: $p < 0.01$; SPA: $p < 0.01$; NDIS: $p < 0.01$) and was one of only two groups (the other being GLO-L) that had a deficit in vocabulary. The GLO-L subtype did not differ from the MPS or the MRS subtypes (MPS: $p = 0.5$; MRS: $p = 0.06$), but scored significantly lower than the NDIS and SPA groups (NDIS: $p < 0.001$; SPA: $p < 0.01$).

On the verbal short-term memory task, there were no significant differences among the GLO, MPS, GLO-L and MRS subtypes (all $p > 0.13$), and all manifested a STM deficit in the cluster analysis. The difference between the SPA and NDIS groups was not significant ($p = 0.54$), which comports with the fact that these are the two groups that did not have a short-term memory deficit.

On the spatial task, the SPA subtype was significantly lower than the GLO-L and NDIS groups (GLO-L: $p < 0.01$, NDIS: $p < 0.001$). It was also lower than the MRS subtype, but that difference did not reach significance ($p = 0.16$). The SPA subtype score was not significantly different from the GLO subtype ($p = 0.45$), but the SPA score was significantly higher than that of the MPS subtype ($p < 0.01$), even though the only groups with a spatial deficit were GLO, SPA and MPS. In fact, it is evident from the results of the cluster analysis that the MPS subtype possesses the greatest degree of spatial deficit of all groups.

On non-verbal short-term memory, the differences among GLO, MPS and MRS were not significant ($p > 0.17$). The differences among SPA, GLO-L and NDIS were also not significant ($p > 0.32$), but those three all scored significantly higher than MRS ($p < 0.01$). This comports with the fact that the MRS subtype scored lowest on non-verbal short-term memory. In addition, the GLO, SPA, MPS and GLO-L subtypes did not significantly differ ($p > 0.19$). In the cluster analysis, although the GLO and MPS subtypes had a deficit in non-verbal short-term memory, it was significantly less than the NV-STM deficit in the MRS group.

Summarizing these validation findings, it is evident that the ANOVA results based on the nine alternative cognitive measures are by-and-large compatible with the cluster analysis results based on the nine original cognitive measures, demonstrating that the dyslexia subtypes derived using cluster analysis possess an acceptable degree of internal validity.

Discussion and Conclusion

In this study, we found that the primary determinants of dyslexia subtypes in Chinese are deficits in the linguistic factors that underlie the reading process. Among these, deficits in phonology, speeded naming and short-term memory had been amply demonstrated in past research. The present research goes a step further in finding the greatest deficit to be morphological in nature, surpassing the degree of phonological and speeded naming deficit. Furthermore, the morphological factor was found to include virtually all children classified as having dyslexia, and within that group, the degree of morphological deficit was found to be greater than the degree of deficit in other cognitive domains. Our finding of the unique status of morphological deficit in defining Chinese dyslexia subtypes exemplifies the critical role morphology plays in Chinese reading.

In our preliminary analysis (summarized in Table 7.3), we found that 15% of subjects with dyslexia possessed a unitary morphological deficit compared with those possessing a deficit solely in phonology or rapid naming (less than 1% and 2%, respectively), and that 96% of children with dyslexia had some sort of morphological deficit. Furthermore, in our cluster analysis, four of the derived subtypes (GLO, MPS, GLO-L and MRS) consisted of different combinations of deficit in morphology, phonology, rapid naming and short-term memory, and none of the subtypes contained a deficit in phonology, rapid naming and short-term memory without also containing a deficit in morphology, indicating a point of similarity between the *z*-score and cluster analyses. This result is consistent with the work of Ho *et al.* (2002, 2004), who found that sub-par performance in rapid naming was the most common type of cognitive deficit, with orthographic deficit as the next most prevalent type. Based on this finding, the authors proposed that instead of a phonological deficit as in English dyslexia, orthography-related difficulties may be the basic underlying problem in Chinese developmental dyslexia. The present research results go beyond the Ho *et al.* findings by offering evidence that dyslexia in Chinese is primarily morphological in nature, in combination with deficits in phonology and an array of other cognitive deficits.

This finding makes sense when we consider the critical role played by morphology in the development of Chinese reading. In order to become a fluent reader, a child must discover the basic internal logic of a writing system's relationship between printed form and meaning (Li *et al.*, 2001). In Chinese orthography, that form-meaning relationship is primarily mediated via the morpheme rather than the phoneme, and children who command the metalinguistic knowledge underlying this fact are likely to acquire reading skills more quickly (Packard, 2002).

A single Chinese character may represent a number of different morphemes. For example, the single character 別 may represent the very different verbs 'fasten' or 'leave', depending upon whether it occurs in the word 別針 *bie2zhen1* fasten-pin 'safety pin' or the word 告別 *gao4bie2* notify-leave 'bid farewell'. Being able to distinguish the different morphemes represented by homographs requires sophisticated knowledge on the part of the child, because it means the child has gained an awareness of the complex nature of entries in the Chinese mental lexicon. As the average character may represent several different morphemes and because morphemes are individuated and identified with the help of characters, it makes sense that the awareness of morphemes and the ability to cognitively manipulate them would constitute a critical factor for a child learning how to read Chinese.

The importance of the morpheme in Chinese reading is further heightened by the nature of morpheme combination as a primary word formation device (Packard, 2000). Morphemes in Chinese words tend to retain their default phonological form when they are combined, making their participation in word formation remarkably straightforward. So, if a child by knowing the words 公雞 (*gong1ji1* male-chicken 'rooster'), 母雞 (*mu3ji1* female-chicken 'hen') and 野雞 (*ye3ji1* wild-chicken 'pheasant') is able to infer that words containing the character 雞 and have the sound *ji1* are likely to be related to 'chicken', it makes the child's task of learning to read Chinese all that much easier. It also makes character combinations that children can say but have not formally learned – such as 雞蛋 *ji1dan4* chicken-egg 'egg' and 雞翅膀 *ji1chi4bang3* chicken-wing 'chicken wing' – easier to learn to read and write.

In conclusion, although linguistic factors play an important role in explaining dyslexia in both English and Chinese, the present study has shown that the specific linguistic factors most relevant in explaining dyslexia critically depends on the type of writing system that a language employs. In English, with its heavy reliance on grapheme-to-phoneme-conversion (GPC) rules, phonology is the strongest explanatory variable in the determination of dyslexia subtypes (Morris, 1998). In Chinese, on the other hand, with less reliance on GPC rules and greater salience of individual morphemes, morphological factors are more important in the determination of dyslexia subtypes, as the results of the present study clearly show. In this study, we have demonstrated that morphology, in addition to other linguistic and cognitive factors, is important in Chinese reading and must be considered in concert with other factors in explaining dyslexia and dyslexia subtypes in Chinese.

References

Bakker, D.J. (1990) *Neuropsychological Treatment of Dyslexia*. New York: Oxford University Press.

Boder, E. (1973) Developmental dyslexia: A diagnostic approach based on three atypical reading-spelling patterns. *Developmental Medicine and Child Neurology* 15, 663–687.

Bradley, L. and Bryant, P.E. (1983) Categorizing sounds and learning to read: A causal connection. *Nature* 30, 419–421.

Castles, A. and Coltheart, M. (1993) Varieties of developmental dyslexia. *Cognition* 47, 149–180.

Coltheart, M., Rastle, K., Perry, C., Langdon, R. and Ziegler, J. (2001) DRC: A dual route cascaded model of visual word recognition and reading aloud. *Psychological Review* 108, 204–256.

Doehring, D.G. (1968) *Patterns of Impairment in Specific Reading Disability*. Bloomington, IN: Indiana University Press.

Ho, C.S.H., Chan, D.W.O., Lee, S.H., Tsang, S.M. and Luan, V.H. (2004) Cognitive profiling and preliminary subtyping in Chinese developmental dyslexia. *Cognition* 91, 43–75.

Ho, C.S., Chan, D.W. and Tsang, S.M. (2002) The cognitive profile and multiple-deficit hypotheses in Chinese developmental dyslexia. *Developmental Psychology* 38, 543–553.

Ho, C.S.H. and Lai, D.N.C. (2000) Naming-speed deficits and phonological memory deficits in Chinese developmental dyslexia. *Learning and Individual Differences* 11, 173–186.

Li, W. (2002) Facets of metalinguistic awareness that contribute to Chinese literacy. In W. Li, J. Gaffney and J. Packard (eds) *Chinese Children's Reading Acquisition* (pp. 87–105). Boston, MA: Kluwer Academic.

Li, W., Anderson, R.C., Nagy, W.E. and Zhang, H. (2001) Facets of metalinguistic awareness that contribute to Chinese literacy. In W. Li, J.S. Gaffney and J.L. Packard (eds) *Chinese Children's Reading Acquisition: Theoretical and Pedagogical Issues* (pp. 87–106). Boston, MA: Kluwer Academic.

Lin, C.D. and Zhang, H.C. (1986) *The Chinese Revision of WISC-R*. Beijing: Beijing Teachers College Press. [In Chinese.]

McAnally, K., Castles, A. and Stuart, G. (2000) Visual and auditory processing impairments in subtypes of developmental dyslexia: A discussion. *Journal of Developmental and Physical Disabilities* 12, 145–156.

McBride-Chang, C., Shu, H., Zhou, A., Wat, C.P. and Wagner, R.K. (2003) Morphological awareness uniquely predicts young children's Chinese character recognition. *Journal of Educational Psychology* 95, 743–751.

Milner, B. (1971) Interhemispheric differences in the localization of psychological processes in man. *British Medical Bulletin* 27, 272–277.

Morris, R.D., Stuebing, K.K., Fletcher, J.M., Shaywitz, S.E., Lyon, G.R., Shankweiler, D.P. *et al.* (1998) Subtypes of reading disability: Variability around a phonological core. *Journal of Educational Psychology* 90, 347–373.

Packard, J.L. (2002) Metalinguistic awareness as a critical construct. In W. Li, J. Gaffney and J. Packard (eds) *Chinese Children's Reading Acquisition* (pp. 107–111). Boston, MA: Kluwer Academic.

Packard, J.L. (2000) *The Morphology of Chinese*. Cambridge: Cambridge University Press.

Packard, J.L., Chen, X., Li, W., Wu, X., Gaffney, J.S., Li, H. and Anderson, R. C. (2006) Explicit instruction in orthographic structure and word morphology helps Chinese children learn to write characters. *Reading and Writing* 19, 457–487.

Ramus, F. (2003) Developmental dyslexia: Specific phonological deficit or general sensorimotor dysfunction? *Current Opinion in Neurobiology* 13, 212–218.

Shaywitz, S.E., Fletcher, J.M., Holahan, J.M., Shneider A.E., Marchione, K.E., Stuebing, K.K. *et al.* (1999) Persistence of dyslexia: The Connecticut longitudinal study of adolescence. *Pediatrics* 104, 1351–1359.

Shu, H., McBride-Chang, C., Wu, S. and Liu, H. (2006) Understanding Chinese developmental dyslexia: Morphological awareness as a core cognitive construct. *Journal of Educational Psychology* 98, 122–133.

Snowling, M. (1991) Developmental reading disorders. *Journal of Child Psychology and Psychiatry* 32, 49–77.

Tallal, P. (1980) Auditory temporal perception, phonics, and reading disabilities in children. *Brain and Language* 9, 182–198.

Torgesen, J.K., Wagner, R.K. and Rashotte, C.A. (1997) Contributions of phonological awareness and rapid automatic naming ability to the growth of word-reading skills in second to fifth-grade children. *Scientific Studies of Reading* 1, 161–185.

Wang, X.L. and Tao, B.P. (1993) *Chinese Character Recognition Test Battery and Assessment Scale for Primary School Children*. Shanghai: Shanghai Education Press.

Wechsler, D. (1974) *Wechsler Intelligence Scale for Children-Revised*. San Antonio, TX: Psychological Corporation.

Wolf, M. and Bowers, P. (2000) The question of naming-speed deficits in developmental reading disabilities: An introduction to the double-deficit hypothesis. *Journal of Learning Disabilities* 33, 322–324.

Zhang, C. (1998) A study of cognitive profiles of Chinese learners' reading disability. *Acta Psychologica Sinica* 30, 50–55.

Zhang, H. and Wang, X. (1985) 瑞文標準推理測驗手冊. [*Raven's Standardized IQ Reasoning Test*.] Beijing: Department of Psychology, Beijing Normal University Press.

Chapter 8

Developmental Dyslexia in Chinese: Behavioral, Genetic and Neuropsychological Issues

KATHRIN KLINGEBIEL and BRENDAN S. WEEKES

Introduction

Developmental dyslexia is a specific and significant impairment to reading ability that cannot be explained by deficits in general intelligence, learning opportunity, general motivation or sensory acuity (Critchley, 1970; World Health Organization, 1993). Between 5% and 10% of school-aged children have specific difficulties in learning to read. Dyslexia is observed across different languages (for a summary, see Smythe *et al.*, 2004) including Chinese (Chan & Siegel, 2001; Ho *et al.*, 1999, 2000, 2002; Leong, 1999; Woo & Hoosain, 1984; Yin & Weekes, 2003; Zhang *et al.*, 1996), and the prevalence of dyslexia among children using different languages in the USA (English, Japanese and Chinese) is comparable (Stevenson *et al.*, 1982). In China, Zhang *et al.* estimated that between 4.5% and 8.0% of children had dyslexia, although Yin and Weekes reported a slightly lower prevalence of 4%.

The early belief was that dyslexia should only be observed in languages with an alphabet (Maketa, 1968; Seymour, 1986). This was under the assumption that phonological awareness is necessary to acquire an alphabet. It is known that phonological awareness is correlated with children's success in reading (Read *et al.*, 1986). If this view is correct, then the association between phonological awareness and reading and writing problems in Chinese may be minimal because the logographic writing system contains few systematic relationships between script and sound (Stevenson, 1984). However, current opinions on dyslexia in Chinese acknowledge greater systematic relationships between the features of the script as well as the phonological and the morphological properties of the language (Ho & Bryant, 1997a, 1997b; Leong, 1999, 2006; Perfetti *et al.*, 2005). This has led to several new hypotheses about dyslexia in Chinese.

The aim in this chapter is to review some of the causes, characteristics and consequences of dyslexia, including the cognitive, genetic and neuropsychological factors that are involved. However, prior to the review, the authors emphasize a rejection of the view that dyslexia has a common cause across languages or individuals. For example, reading difficulties in Chinese have been assumed to result from visual deficits only (Woo & Hoosain, 1984). Instead, the argument will be that properties of a language environment shape the patterns of reading and writing difficulties within that language. Most current research is conducted in alphabetic languages, such as English, French and German, wherein knowledge of the mappings between print and sound is essential to master literacy and arguably, knowledge about the mappings between print and meaning are not necessary for fluent reading and writing. However, even though reading acquisition in all languages requires a child to learn the mapping between orthography (symbol system) and phonology (articulation) as well as semantics (meaning), the division of labor that is required to acquire literacy will depend on the nature of the script. Problems in the representation and the use of phonological information will inevitably lead to issues in reading acquisition for alphabetic scripts, as the primary task is to learn the mappings between orthography and phonology. However, the division of labor may differ within alphabetic scripts, depending on the consistency of print-to-sound mapping, e.g. English versus Turkish (see Frith *et al.*, 1995; Goswami & Bryant, 1990). One theory of dyslexia predicts that individuals with reading and writing problems in all languages will have phonological deficits (Ziegler & Goswami, 2005; Ziegler *et al.*, 2003). However, the authors feel that even if the hypothesis of a phonological deficit can explain dyslexia in languages with alphabetic scripts, the possibility that it can explain reading and writing problems in languages with nonalphabetic script remains an open question.

Although the extant literature is minimal, it will be demonstrated that the focus of current research activity on dyslexia in Chinese does not focus on the feasibility of dyslexia as a problem for Chinese speakers. Instead, this research focuses on issues concerning the ways that dyslexia across scripts (see e.g. Landerl *et al.*, 1997; Weekes, 2006; Ziegler & Goswami, 2005) and neuroimaging studies of dyslexia across different languages (Paulesu *et al.*, 2001; Siok *et al.*, 2004) can be explained. Dyslexia in Chinese may have different causes within individuals. Other research ponders on the existence of subtypes in dyslexia in Chinese, as prevalent in other languages (Ho *et al.*, 2004). These research findings show that deficits in analyzing and representing the phonological structures of speech lead to difficulties in mastering the systematic relationships between print and sound. However, these are not the only factors involved in explaining reading and writing difficulties in Chinese. It will be argued that any further progress towards understanding the most likely factors (cognitive, genetic and neuropsychological) that may lead to developmental dyslexia in different Chinese speakers will require a conceptual framework that can accommodate extant reading and writing problems in Chinese. In addition, new predictions will be generated to explain the factors that might lead to dyslexia in Chinese. This approach has been fruitful in understanding dyslexia in English during the past 30 years (Coltheart, 1978, 2006; Manis *et al.*, 1996).

This chapter is divided into three parts. First, research will be reviewed, examining the cognitive factors that are important for the development of literacy in Chinese and hence, may predict reading and writing problems. This is necessary to understand the phenotypes of dyslexia that may be observed in different Chinese-speaking environments (Hong Kong, Mainland China, Singapore and Taiwan) as these might depend on the type of script and the different instruction methods that are used in each language environment. The focus will be on dyslexia in Putonghua speakers from Mainland China. One feature of instruction in Mainland China is a teaching method that uses an alphabetic script called *pinyin*. Pinyin is taught to preliterate speakers for enhancement of character learning and is routine for schools throughout China (but is not used in Hong Kong). Reading and writing problems appear to worsen when learning pinyin in comparison to symbolic characters. This suggests that the type of script has an impact on the phenotype of dyslexia within Putonghua speakers (Yin & Weekes, 2003). In the second part of the chapter, a cognitive framework of reading and writing in Chinese will be described. This framework will be outlined in detail because progress in assessment and treatment of dyslexia renders it necessary (Weekes & Coltheart, 1996), and also because cognitive models stimulate ideas about the causes of dyslexia. For example, the framework allows explanations for possible genetic and neuropsychological causes of subtypes in dyslexia in Chinese (Bates *et al.*, 2006; Coltheart, 2006; Coltheart *et al.*, 2001). In the final part of the chapter, this framework will be linked to current research on dyslexia in Chinese by reviewing recent findings in genetic and neuropsychological factors for other languages and generating predictions for the likely phenotype of dyslexia in Chinese. The main objective is to illustrate the necessity of a cognitive model for the interpretation of data from studies that investigate dyslexia in Chinese and not to support a universal theory of dyslexia. Finally, the conclusion will be that research findings on developmental dyslexia in Chinese can only be interpreted meaningfully in terms of a cognitive framework for reading and writing *in Chinese*.

Acquiring Literacy in Chinese

Research over the past 20 years has increased the understanding of factors that predict the normal acquisition of literacy in Chinese. However, there are debates over factors that are critical for reading success. One debate concerns the relative importance of visual, orthographic and phonological knowledge in learning to read and write in Chinese. This is not only a question about the acquisition of literacy in Chinese, but is also an issue in research on literacy in alphabetic languages (Ziegler & Goswami, 2005).

Factors affecting reading development in Chinese

Some researchers claim that phonological awareness has a major impact on the acquisition of literacy in alphabetic languages (Bradley & Bryant, 1978, 1983). Aside from that, does it also impact the acquisition of literacy in Chinese? Phonological awareness refers to words that are units of sound. However, since units of sound are mapped to print in different ways across scripts, it is not always obvious which way to compare phonological awareness across languages. There are different levels of phonological awareness, including: syllable, onset-rime as well as phoneme awareness. Syllable awareness is the understanding that spoken words are made-up of syllables. All syllables can be divided into an onset and a rime. The onset of a syllable is the initial consonant or the consonant cluster preceding a vowel. The rime consists of the vowel and the remaining consonants. Phonemes are all the segments in a syllable. For example, the word 銀行 *yin2hang2* 'bank' consists of two syllables, 銀 *yin2* and 行 *hang2*. The spoken syllable 行 *hang2* has the onset *h* and the rime *ang* with three phonemes *h*, *a* and *ng*. Additionally, the reader needs to consider the different tones used in Putonghua. Using the example of 銀行 *yin2hang2* again, the second tone (rising tone) is used in both syllables.

Syllable awareness seems to precede intrasyllabic awareness of onset and rime and this in turn appears to precede awareness of phonemes in English (Treiman & Zukowski, 1991). One question is whether syllable awareness also precedes phoneme awareness in Chinese. Research with children that are learning to read Chinese suggests that phonological awareness at the level of onset and rime is related to early Chinese reading skills (Ho & Bryant, 1997a, 1997b; McBride-Chang & Ho, 2000; Siok & Fletcher, 2001). For example, when learning to read in Chinese, some children appear to use phonetic radical cues spontaneously to read new characters. These cues appear to diminish the memory load that is required for memorizing a large number of characters (Ho & Bryant, 1997a, 1997b).

Other studies on reading development in Chinese show that the understanding of phonological structure in speech and manipulation of sounds and lexical tones are related to early reading skills (Ho & Bryant, 1997a, 1997b; Shu *et al.*, 2003; Siok & Fletcher, 2001). For example, Ho and Bryant (1997a) conducted a four-year longitudinal study in Hong Kong to examine relationships between the phonological skills of Chinese children and their success in character reading. At the age of three, before they could read, 100 children were tested on visual and phonological skills. Their findings showed that prereading phonological skills significantly predicted the reading performance of children in Chinese for the ensuing two and three years, after controlling for the effects of age, IQ and mother's education. Thus, understanding correspondences between print and sound determines the ability of children in learning characters, the equivalence of learning to read in alphabetic scripts (Ho & Bryant, 1997b; Siok & Fletcher). Note that for these studies, the authors examined phonological skills in Chinese children by having them read pinyin, which is an alphabetic script. Rapid automated naming ability is also correlated with reading acquisition in Chinese (Chow *et al.*, 2005; see also Smythe *et al.*, 2004). This may be attributed to Chinese as a logographic language, whereby characters are taught by rote instruction.

Hu and Catts (1998) reported that rapid naming was important for Chinese reading development in Taiwan. However, Chow *et al.* (2005) found that the importance of rapid automated naming in reading Chinese words faded with reading development, as more of the variance in subsequent Chinese word reading abilities was explained through previous word reading experience.

There is a debate about the relative importance of phonological and visual skills in learning to read characters. Studies conducted in Taiwan by Huang and Hanley (1994) suggested that phonological knowledge that was tested before entering school was a better predictor than early visual knowledge of character reading one year later. However, when they singled out the effects in differences for reading experiences before entering school, phonological skills no longer predicted the development of character reading abilities. Huang and Hanley (1995) reported that visual skills were related to reading abilities in Taiwanese children. They also reported that phonological skills were significantly correlated with reading abilities of children in the United Kingdom, but not in Hong Kong and Taiwan. Chinese children may learn to acquire new characters through visual memorization *only*, as most characters do not conform to grapheme-phoneme correspondence rules. Language instructors in Hong Kong, Taiwan and Mainland China make use of pictograph features that associate with meanings at a visual form level and focus on visual dimensions of characters in teaching. Of particular interest are the findings of Tan *et al.* (2001) who reported that motor and supplementary motor areas were active during silent reading in Chinese-speaking adults and argued that this implicated visual-orthographic analysis and the close connections between reading and writing in the development of literacy in Chinese.

Hu and Catts (1998) conducted a study with 50 first graders in Taiwan. Phonological awareness was measured using an oddity task in which half of the trials required children to contrast the stimulus according to word onsets (e.g. *bi, ban, hou*) and the other half required children to contrast stimulus words in accordance to rimes in the words (e.g. *ta, po, ma*). Visual processing skills were measured by a memory task that consisted of random shapes. Children were required to read characters as an index of their reading skills. In contrast to Huang and Hanley (1995), Hu and Catts found that performance on the phonological awareness task, but not the visual task, was related to reading skill. Ho and Bryant (1997a, 1997b) reported that visual measures predicted reading only in children aged three to four years old, whereas phonological measures predicted reading in children aged five to seven years old (in Hong Kong). They suggested that Chinese-speaking children (in Hong Kong) initially learned to read characters on a visual or logographic basis, but when they recognized more characters, they attended to the phonetic components in characters.

Other studies suggest that visual skills may not be as important for older children reading Chinese (e.g. McBride-Chang and Chang's study [1995], with fifth graders). Siok and Fletcher (2001) collected data in Beijing and found that visual skills predicted reading success in lower-school grades, whereas pinyin knowledge and the ability to discriminate homophonic characters predicted reading success and onset-rime awareness in Grades 2, 3, and 5, but not phonemic awareness. In higher grades, tone awareness also correlated with reading and pinyin knowledge. Siok and Fletcher suggested that learning to read in Chinese progresses from a logographic to an orthographic-phonological phase. Chow *et al.* (2005) investigated the relations between phonological processing in the native language (Chinese) and early reading abilities in Chinese and English using a longitudinal study. Their results showed that phonological awareness explained significant variance in Chinese reading, even when visual skills were controlled. They also found that phonological awareness and particularly, syllable deletion were strong predictors of Chinese and English reading abilities. Rapid naming did not predict subsequent abilities in reading words for their study.

In addition to the differences in language environments (Taiwan, Mainland China and Hong Kong) across the studies, an important reason for the conflicting results may be in the methods for measuring phonological awareness. Huang and Hanley (1995) focused on children's phonemic awareness, whereas Ho and Bryant (1997a) used tasks that were centered on syllabic and onset-rime sensitivity (see also Shu *et al.*, 2003; Siok & Fletcher, 2001). It is quite plausible that syllable awareness and onset-rime awareness are better predictors of reading success in Chinese than sensitivity to the phoneme structure because the Chinese writing system maps to speech at the syllable and not the phoneme level. As Chinese script does not contain symbols that represent phonemes, it may be difficult for Chinese children to develop phonemic awareness.

It would, therefore, not be surprising that phonological awareness has little effect on the acquisition of literacy in Chinese (Cheung *et al.*, 2001). Instead, onset and rime awareness may be better predictors of reading ability in Chinese only when an appropriate task is used (Ho & Bryant, 1997a; Hu & Catts, 1998; So & Siegel, 1997).

Different results across studies may account for variability in the methods for teaching instruction. Subsyllabic awareness may become more important if an alphabetic script is used to teach reading. McBride-Chang *et al.* (2004) compared syllable and phoneme onset awareness in kindergarten and first grade children across language environments in Toronto, Hong Kong and Xian (Mainland China) using the same tasks. As discussed previously, Chinese has a simple syllable structure compared to English. For example, consonant clusters are rare. A syllable in Chinese consists of an optional initial consonant (onset) followed by a final element, or rime, made-up of an obligatory nuclear vowel, one or more optional vowels and an optional consonant. Although the initial consonant is always a single phoneme, there are no clear boundaries within the rime at the phoneme level. McBride-Chang *et al.* found that development of phonological awareness in different orthographies is influenced by both the writing system as well as the method of teaching instruction. Syllable awareness was a relatively strong predictor of character reading in Xian and Hong Kong, but phoneme onset awareness was the stronger predictor in English reading. It did not predict performance for Chinese speakers. The differences between children in Hong Kong and Xian were also observed, with onset-rime awareness as a predictor of literacy achievement in Xian. These findings suggest that pinyin, which is used in Xian only, might promote phonological awareness at the phoneme onset (subsyllabic) level, in addition to the syllable level.

Some theorists have argued that phonological and orthographic knowledge facilitates each other during the acquisition of literacy in English (Ehri, 1991). In addition, the relationship between these levels of awareness is reciprocal rather than processing by stages. An area of interest examines the possibility of phonological and orthographic factors having an interactive relationship during the acquisition of literacy in Chinese. Similar to Ehri's (1992) suggestion for English, Chinese children may first learn to read at the logographic phase by forming arbitrary connections between visual cues and meanings in addition to the pronunciation of characters. Visual skills may, therefore, be particularly important in reading during the initial stages of literacy acquisition. Learning to read in Chinese then progresses from a visual phase to a phonological phase, as in the case for alphabetical scripts, and finally progresses to the orthographic stage where whole-word knowledge is built over time (Ho *et al.*, 2004). It is noteworthy that orthographic knowledge in English seems to contribute to skilled word recognition in older children over and above the effects of phonological factors, suggesting that this may be the ultimate goal of literacy (Cunningham *et al.*, 2001).

Ho and Bryant (1997a) found that visual measures predicted Chinese word reading in 3- to 4-year-old children. When learning to read characters, they suggested that Chinese children may begin to realize that some stroke patterns recur in different characters, such as 口 *kou3* in 釦 *kou4*, 只 *zhi3* and 吃 *chi1*, and stroke patterns are often associated with semantic categories (e.g. the radical component) and with pronunciations (such as the phonetic component). Chinese children are not typically taught the phonetic component of characters. Instead, they may learn these script-sound regularities implicitly through reading a number of characters. Ehri (1992) also suggested a visual-phonological route for the second phase, in which children begin to read words on the basis of rudimentary connections between spelling patterns and pronunciations. Similar to this, Ho *et al.* (2004) proposed a 'cipher stage' where children gradually discover the orthographic regularities of characters that allow them to read unknown characters and reduce the memory burden for memorizing each character individually. The third phase can be called the 'orthographic stage' (Ho *et al.*, 1999), where character parts or whole characters are processed automatically as a whole unit. Should the theory of developmental stages for learning to read in Chinese be correct, then there may be more than one cause or stage for arrested development, leading to the possibility of different subtypes of reading and writing problems in Chinese.

Factors that are unique to reading in Chinese

Although there may be some similarities between the stages of literacy acquisition in English and Chinese, a universal model of learning to read in Chinese is not viable unless it incorporates the idiosyncratic linguistic properties of the Chinese script. For example, tone awareness is a phonological skill that is important for learning to read in Chinese. Every syllable in the Chinese languages (Mandarin, Cantonese and other dialects) is differentiated according to tones. This allows a child with intact tone awareness to distinguish 清 (*qing1*, first tone, meaning clear) from 請 (*qing3*, third tone, meaning please). So and Siegel (1997) reported that tone awareness was a better predictor of Chinese reading skills (in Hong Kong) than rime awareness among children in the first to fourth grades. They also reported that in comparison with normal readers, poor readers in Chinese had greater difficulties with tones. Li *et al.* (2001) also reported that tone awareness predicted reading proficiency for children in the first and fourth grades (see also Siok & Fletcher, 2001). Semantic radical components are another unique feature in Chinese characters. Shu and Anderson (1997) first proposed that regularity in morphemic structure is obvious to Chinese readers because about 89% of the Chinese characters represent unique morphemes. In addition, characters are often presented in combination with their meaning in elementary school. Li *et al.* showed that in the first and fourth grades, good readers outperformed poor readers on morphological awareness tasks. Ku and Anderson (2001) found that morphological awareness developed with grade level and was strongly related to reading abilities, slightly higher for Chinese-speaking students than for English-speaking students. In Mainland China, Shu *et al.* (2003) analyzed the characters taught in elementary textbooks prepared by the Ministry of Education and found that by the end of the sixth grade, Chinese children learned about 2500 visually complex characters. Of these, 72% were semantic compounds. Therefore, characters usually provide young readers with visually distinct and reliable cues to meanings.

Shu *et al.* (2006) argued that morphological awareness was the strongest predictor for a variety of literacy-related skills (visual, phonological, speed number naming and vocabulary) for reading difficulties in the fifth and sixth grades. Shu *et al.* proposed that there were reasons to focus on morphological awareness as a critical component of learning to read in Chinese. They pointed out that the semantic radical is directly linked to meaning in 80% of the characters. Chinese is also relatively semantically transparent and vocabulary is built by combining morphemes via compounding. Shu *et al.* suggested that the young reader may have to use morphological information to understand characters because homophony is prevalent in Chinese. When a child encounters an unknown character while reading a passage, they retrieve the meaning of text via morphological knowledge in the character. Children who are good readers in Chinese show better awareness of morphological structure in characters and use semantic radical information to derive the meanings of unfamiliar characters (Shu & Anderson, 1997) even if this level of analysis is not explicitly taught (Wu *et al.*, 1999).

Predicting developmental dyslexia in Chinese

Given the understanding of literacy development in Chinese, some researchers have started to isolate the likely developmental causes of failures to acquire literacy in Chinese. It is widely accepted that phonological processing impairments may be a precursor to dyslexia in alphabetic languages. One unifying hypothesis therefore, suggests that dyslexic children have specific impairments in representing, storing and retrieving phonological information (Ramus, 2003). As previously argued, this view of dyslexia predicts that phonological deficits should be similar for individuals with dyslexia in different countries, regardless of the type of language used (see examples in Paulesu *et al.*, 2001; Ziegler *et al.*, 2003).

Wydell and Butterworth (1999) agree with the view that learning the mappings between orthography and phonology is critical for developing literacy. However, in explaining a pattern of dyslexia for a biscriptal reader with impairment in reading English, but not Japanese, they argued that the orthographic grain size (which refers to the size of orthographic and phonological units) as well as the orthographic transparency of the script (which refers to the predictability of mappings between orthography and phonology) are the key issues for understanding the process of learning to read and write and explaining dyslexia. They argued that children who are learning transparent orthographies, such as Greek, Finnish, German, Italian, Spanish and Turkish, would show a lower incidence of developmental dyslexia because print-to-sound translation in these languages is mostly transparent (one to one). Orthographies that operate at coarse grain sizes, for example, logographs and syllabaries (such as Japanese mora) will also show a relatively low incidence of developmental phonological dyslexia because subsyllabic processing will not be required for learning to read. By contrast, children learning to read in English, which contains many examples of inconsistent mappings between orthography and phonology at the subsyllabic level, will show a relatively high incidence of dyslexia.

Ziegler and Goswami (2005) argued in their Psycholinguistic Grain Size Theory for a universal cause of dyslexia that was based only on arrested phonological development. They suggested that success at phonological recoding means that a reader needs to find shared grain sizes in the symbol system (orthography) and phonology of their language to correctly map the two domains. They proposed that the incidence of developmental dyslexia will be similar across consistent and inconsistent orthographies, but its manifestation might differ according to the orthographic consistency of a script. The incidence of developmental dyslexia will also not be reduced in any simple way by coarse grain sizes, as phonological awareness of subsyllabic units may still be necessary for the acquisition of the characters or symbols used in coarse grain-size orthographies (see also Siok & Fletcher, 2001). They pointed out that inconsistent orthographies force the reading system to develop multiple grain-size mappings and argue that phonological, rather than orthographic deficits underlie developmental dyslexia in all languages that were studied. To support their views, they argued that children with dyslexia are often not worse at orthographic access with whole words (Grainger *et al.*, 2003), but always worse when computing sublexical phonology, even in languages as different as Korean, German, Dutch, Hebrew and Italian (Kim & Davis, 2004; see Smythe *et al.*, 2004 for a review).

There is evidence that children with dyslexia in Chinese are deficient in phonological processing which is compatible with the phonological deficit hypothesis. Ho *et al.* (2000) reported that dyslexic children (ages 7–10) perform significantly less well in both word and nonword repetition compared to children with normal achievements of the same age or reading level. This suggests that Chinese children with dyslexia may have difficulties in retaining sounds in short-term memory. These children also performed significantly worse than controls in onset and rime detection tasks, indicating that Chinese children with dyslexia may be less sensitive to the structure of sound. Consistent with this suggestion, clinical observations by Lam and Cheung (1996) found that one third of children having early language or phonological problems were later found to have reading and writing disabilities. In both studies, children with dyslexia were poor in phonological skills and they achieved similar reading levels to the younger readers. This suggests that phonological deficits are implicated, but may not necessarily be a cause of dyslexia in Chinese. Ho *et al.* (2000) also pointed out that dyslexic children relied more on visual strategies and employed compensatory strategies when reading, such as using the context of the text. Yin and Weekes (2003) reported that children with dyslexia in Mainland China were more likely to have problems when learning pinyin than characters. Pinyin requires knowledge of subsyllabic mappings between orthography and phonology, specifically at the level of onset and rime. This finding is compatible with Ho and Bryant (1997b), who suggested that knowledge in the sound of phonetic components is crucial to the long-term learning of orthography to phonology conversion (OPC) mappings in Chinese.

Ho and Ma (1999) investigated 15 Chinese dyslexic children in Hong Kong, who were approximately eight years old. They received five days of intensive training in phonological strategies. A comparable group received no training. They found that Chinese children normally used the phonetic components of characters for sound cues in reading, but dyslexic readers were less likely to use phonological strategies. Then they trained the dyslexic children in a five-day intensive program in phonological reading strategies and found that there was significant improvement in their reading performances. However, the children with dyslexia had particular difficulties in learning irregular characters. Ho and Ma proposed that children with dyslexia lacked knowledge on spontaneous usage of phonetic components in a character. Direct teaching of script-sound regularities in Chinese and sound cues could help dyslexic readers to acquire literacy in Chinese.

Ho *et al.* (2002) profiled dyslexic children in China. They examined visual processing, phonological processing, orthographic processing and rapid naming for Chinese dyslexic children in Hong Kong, comparing them to both age-level and reading-level controls. Ho *et al.* reported that a rapid naming deficit was the most dominant cognitive deficit in children with dyslexia, suggesting that Chinese children with dyslexia have particular difficulties in automation and the building-up of orthographic representations.

Ho *et al.* (2004) repeated the Ho *et al.* (2002) study design, but used a larger sample size. One hundred and forty-seven Primary school children with dyslexia were tested. They found that in addition to the dominant deficit in rapid naming, an orthographical deficit was a predictor of dyslexia. The authors suggested that orthographic and rapid naming deficits are an inter-related problem in developing orthographic knowledge and representation. They also proposed that phonological deficits were not the main reasons for dyslexia in Chinese. However, Ho *et al.* (2004) had also postulated that the inadequate functioning of orthographic processors and a weak linkage between orthographic and phonological processors were reflected in a low naming speed for dyslexic children.

Why would sublexical phonological processing skills have an impact on the development of literacy across languages? One possibility is a perceptual problem. Tallal (1984) suggested that a possible reason for the phonological deficit in dyslexia is that dyslexic children have problems in processing low-level auditory information. When pure tones are presented in rapid succession, individuals with dyslexia have trouble distinguishing the differences (Tallal, 1980). They also need a longer inter-stimulus interval (ISI) to separate two sounds in gap detection (McCroskey & Kidder, 1980) and are less sensitive to changes in amplitude (Menell *et al.*, 1999) and the frequency of acoustic stimuli (Witton *et al.*, 1998). This finding not only supports a link between impaired auditory resolution and poor reading, but also suggests that psychoacoustic difficulties are largely retained through adulthood and may be the source of prolonged reading difficulties (Meng *et al.*, 2005). Event-related potentials (ERP) studies show some abnormality in auditory and phonological processing for dyslexic subjects. In one study, individuals with dyslexia showed significantly smaller mismatch negativity (MMN) in perceiving oddball (in terms of acoustic frequency) sounds (Baldeweg *et al.*, 1999). However, perceptual difficulties are not limited to phonological processing. Witton *et al.* (1998) found that sensitivity to dynamic visual as well as auditory stimuli predicted nonword reading performance in both dyslexic and normal readers. It is also widely accepted now that visual processing abilities in the magnocellular visual system, including motion detection, can be impaired in children with dyslexia

(Eden *et al.*, 1996; Eden & Zeffiro, 1996; Stein & Walsh, 1997) as shown in the performances for the Ternus test (Cestnick & Coltheart, 1999). Reports of similar difficulties in Chinese speakers are also emerging (Meng *et al.*, 2005; Siok *et al.*, 2004).

Interim summary

All Chinese speakers must learn a large number of characters to become literate. Most characters represent a monosyllable that is homophonous with other characters. The prevalence of homophony in spoken Chinese suggests that phonological awareness might be imperative for distinguishing the meaning of Chinese words during vocabulary development. However, in addition to phonological processing, orthographic skills and morphological awareness are important in understanding the acquisition of reading and writing skills in Chinese. An intriguing hypothesis is that literacy helps language learners to distinguish the homophonous syllables in Chinese and thus leads to better vocabulary development (Yin & Weekes, 2003). In other words, literacy in Chinese might enhance phonological awareness of spoken words and then bootstrap subsequent character learning, unlike in English where development of literacy seems to depend primarily on phonological awareness.

Phonological processing is not only important for learning to read, but is accessed early in the identification process for Chinese characters during skilled reading. Perfetti *et al.* (2005) report on several experiments conducted with skilled adult readers, showing that phonology is accessed during character identification. At the same time, the graphic form of a character is disambiguated before the meaning of the character is accessed. Ziegler *et al.* (2000) also report experiments that demonstrated phonological frequency (syllable) effects in processing written Chinese. Characters with high phonological frequency were processed faster than characters with a low phonological frequency. Ziegler *et al.* subsequently argued for a universal phonological principle in which phonological information is routinely activated during skilled word identification. In contrast, Tan *et al.* (2000) argued that the ability to read Chinese is related to writing skills and the relationship between phonological awareness and Chinese reading is weaker than in alphabetic languages. Instead, they proposed a role for logographic writing in reading development that is mediated by interacting mechanisms. These are orthographic awareness, which facilitates development of effective links among visual symbols, phonology and semantics, as well as a mechanism that involves the establishment of motor programs that lead to the formation of long-term motor memories for characters. In the next section, current models of word recognition and oral reading in English and Chinese will be presented. The purpose is to test the utility of these models by questioning each of their roles in explaining dyslexia in Chinese.

Cognitive Models of Reading and Writing

Several different models of reading and writing in English have been proposed. Connectionist models and symbolic models can be distinguished. *Connectionist models* propose a network that reflects systematic relationships between orthographic and phonological word forms. *Symbolic models* propose regions of knowledge that are determined by independent procedures. The most famous symbolic model of reading is Coltheart *et al.*'s (2001) 'dual-route' model (also known as the 'multi' or 'triple route' model). Coltheart *et al.* assume several pathways. One is the *lexical semantic pathway*, for reading out loud known words. The second is a *direct lexical pathway* that allows readers to read words without understanding the meaning of the word. A third pathway is the *non-lexical grapheme-to-phoneme route*, which is assumed mandatory for reading regular and unknown words. One cannot read irregular words correctly using this route, but only pronounce regular grapheme-phoneme correspondence. A different model that is based on the connectionist principles of subsymbolic processing was proposed by Plaut *et al.* (1996). They assume bidirectional pathways for reading. Their model avoids whole-word representations in favor of subword components (such as onset, vowel and coda positions). Plaut *et al.* also assumed separate *semantic* and *phonological pathways*, the semantic pathway associating with word meanings and the phonological pathway connecting graphemes and phonemes in English.

Both models assume that there are at least two pathways available for mapping print to sound in English. The main difference between the models is that the dual-route model assumes an independent direct lexical and semantic pathway, whereas connectionist models do not. While Plaut *et al.* (1996) do not assume a grapheme-to-phoneme connection is needed to read nonwords, Coltheart *et al.* (2001) assume rules are required to link grapheme and phoneme representations. They are necessary to allow the correct pronunciation of nonwords in English by skilled readers. In Plaut *et al.*'s model, nonword reading is achieved via the phonological pathway that reads novel letter strings by analogy with subword representations (onset, vowel and coda). The Plaut *et al.* model does not contain lexical whole-word representations and instead, reads all letter strings via subword components only.

How do these models explain reading and writing in Chinese? The logographic nature of Chinese characters makes it likely that lexical knowledge, such as orthographic and phonological knowledge, is essential for reading characters correctly. Plaut *et al.*'s (1996) model does not contain lexical representations, but only subword components, which make it difficult for the model to explain oral reading in Chinese even though functional units, such as the rime, might be important for reading both alphabetic and nonalphabetical scripts. On the other hand, the non-lexical pathway in Coltheart *et al.*'s (2001) model will also be redundant for oral reading in Chinese because there are no graphemes in Chinese. As printed letters are not used to convey the pronunciation of words in Chinese, mappings between orthography and phonology are opaque, unlike the grapheme-phoneme-correspondence in alphabetic scripts. As argued earlier, the mappings between orthography and meanings in many characters are relatively transparent, whereas mappings between orthography and meaning in alphabetic scripts are opaque. However, it is now known that it is possible to read out loud a character via a nonsemantic pathway, such as the pathway postulated in the Coltheart *et al.*'s model.

Yin and Weekes (2003) proposed a framework for understanding developmental dyslexia in Chinese derived from a cognitive neuropsychological account of reading and writing. Yin and Weekes argued that normal oral reading in Chinese proceeds via two pathways: a *lexical semantic* pathway and a *nonsemantic* pathway. The lexical semantic pathway connects orthographic representations to phonological representations via semantic information that allows reading for meaning. The nonsemantic pathway links orthographic and phonological representations directly. The nonsemantic pathway can be referred to as a direct lexical pathway, as proposed within the Coltheart *et al.* (2001) model. This framework for reading and writing in Chinese assumes that a character will normally be processed in both pathways.

Shu *et al.* (2005) criticized this framework by stating that it is not clear that the model is applicable to Chinese developmental dyslexia and the model is limited by its failure to address the causes of dyslexia. They also claim that the model does not specify the factors that may cause developmental delays. They propose that examining the ways that phonological and semantic representations are formed in normal reading and specifying their relationships with orthographic representations may help answer this question. Therefore, a similar, but more detailed framework for understanding developmental dyslexia is proposed in Figure 8.1.

The framework in Figure 8.1 assumes three independent levels of representation, the *orthographic representation*, *semantic representation* and *phonological representation*. Since the framework has bidirectional routes, it can describe development of both reading and writing processes in a morphosyllabic language, such as Chinese. In normal reading and writing, all three representations work together. The level of orthographic

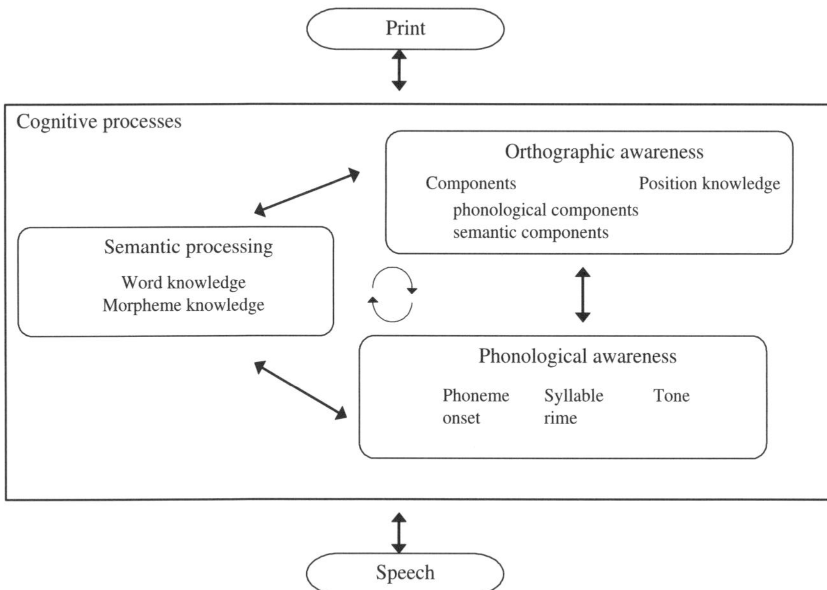

Figure 8.1 Model of reading and writing development in Chinese

representation contains the different components in Chinese characters. The term 'radical' is intentionally not used, and in its place 'component' is utilized instead. This is because all components and not only radicals are assumed for inclusion at this level of representation. Components can be divided further into phonological and semantic components with the latter having an individual linkage with semantic representations.

The semantic representation contains morpheme and word knowledge. It is noted that debate continues on representations of polymorphemic Chinese words. For example, Zhang and Peng (1992) claim that the morphological structure of compound words is explicitly represented in the lexical system. This assumption is similar to the multilevel interactive-activation model proposed by Taft (1994), although in that framework, the two levels of representations are arranged in a hierarchical relationship with phonological and orthographic lexicons. In other models, such as Taft *et al.* (1999), the status of whole-word representations has changed. Taft *et al.* suggest that whole-word phonological and orthographic representations should be replaced with a set of modality-free units called *lemmas*. Lemmas are connected to orthographic, phonological and semantic units and correspond to bound morphemes, free morphemes and polymorphemic words. It assumes that whole-word and morphemic representations are minimally present in the semantic system. Morphemic and whole-word representations are semantic in nature and arranged at the same level in the semantic system. This is consistent with Zhou and Marslen-Wilson (2000) who assume phonological and orthographic representations of polymorphemic words are 'represented as the combinations of the form representations of their constituents, without additional whole-word representations of compounds at these levels'.

The phonological representation consists of phonemes, syllable level, including onset and rime level and tone level. Even though phoneme awareness is less likely to predict Chinese reading problems, it may still be important because without phoneme awareness, one may not be able to distinguish syllables, such as *cheng4* (e.g. 稱) and *deng4* (e.g. 鄧). A linear structure between phonemes is assumed, syllable representation (including onset and rime) and tonal information, each one independent on one dimension for phonological representation. Law and Or (2001) have proposed a multitiered structure in the phonological representation and suggest that the structure of phonological representations is non-linear. They also refer to autosegmental phonology (Goldsmith, 1976; Leben, 1973; Yip, 1980) including the *segmental features* (such as consonant and vowels) as being independent of *suprasegmental features* (such as tone).

In the normal oral reading of Chinese characters, the orthographic representation reflects character components. It automatically connects components with semantic features in the semantic representation and phonological representations where syllable articulation and tone are activated. When a character is presented, the lexical semantic pathway activates the target character and other characters that are related in meaning. It is assumed that the same components are activated during normal writing to dictation and given the bidirectional connections assumed in the framework shown in Figure 8.1, this model can also be applied to the development of orthographic, phonological and semantic knowledge used in writing as well as reading. Note that these components are assumed in cognitive models of skilled writing, such as those that have been proposed by Law and Or (2001). Bidirectional connections also allow a developmental sequence in stages to emerge from knowledge of strokes to character-sound representations and higher-level orthographic and morphological knowledge.

Interim summary

The framework in Figure 8.1 describes and designs predictions with respect to phenotypes of dyslexia in Chinese. It interprets data from studies of possible causes for dyslexia within individual Chinese speakers. It is a unified framework that incorporates unique features of the Chinese language and allows the inclusion of behavioral, genetic and neuropsychological phenomena obtained from studies of Chinese-speaking individuals.

Failure to specify the mechanisms that are used to learn to read in Chinese is weakness in the framework. It is believed that computational theories of reading in Chinese offer the potential of providing a more potent account of dyslexia because they incorporate a learning mechanism. For example, the computational Lexical Constituency model of oral reading in Chinese described by Perfetti *et al.* (2005) contains interlinked constituents at the orthographic, semantic and phonology levels. In addition, Perfetti *et al.* assume a radical input level, containing 146 units and four possible spatial relationships between radicals within a Chinese character (left-right such as 悅 *yue4*, top-bottom such as 安 *an1*, closed-outside-inside such as 國 *guo2* and open-outside-inside such as 周 *zhou1*). Just as the framework in Figure 8.1, the Lexical Constituency model has direct links between orthographic and semantic units, allowing the retrieval of character meaning without activating the phonological level. On the phonological level, the model assumes a syllable representation, whereby each syllable is coded into onset, vowel and tone. The model only represents syllables of Mandarin with five tones. Perfetti *et al.* point out that the phonological level is a distributed representation lacking within-level linkages, in contrast to the orthographic and semantic levels. At the character level, meaning is a localized representation with each of the 204 units corresponding to a unique meaning of a single character. Each orthographic character unit has three connections: one to onset, one to vowel and one to tone. At this stage, a computational model does not exist for skilled reading in Chinese that offers a theoretical account of reading development. The Lexical Constituency model only simulates skilled reading. However, the parameters of the model allow for an explanation of reading and writing impairments for Chinese, including developmental and acquired dyslexia (for a further discussion of these theoretical issues, see Chapter 11 of this volume).

Future Directions

In the final part of this chapter, the direction for questions that will likely better guide the understanding of dyslexia in Chinese with a focus on biological factors, including genetic and neurological factors, will be suggested. In doing so, the importance of adopting a cognitive framework to generate hypotheses and guide progress in the understanding of dyslexia will be highlighted.

Genetics in reading disorder

Reading and writing behaviors are a recent notion in cultural history. However, it is important to look for genetic factors that might have an influence on the development of reading and writing. As Coltheart (2006) points out, the genes that affect the learning of word meanings by a child and the ability to read familiar words and nonwords, presumably have a basic biological function that is literacy dependent. It has been shown that no single gene is attributed to learning to read or for dyslexia in English, but a number of different risk loci have been identified (Fisher & DeFries, 2002), including potential sites on chromosomes 2, 6, 15 and 18. These loci are believed to be responsible for normal variation in reading skills across the population as well as in individuals with dyslexia (Grigorenko *et al.*, 2006).

For many years, it has been known that reading difficulties tend to run in families (see example in Orton, 1937). Early evidence from twin studies suggested that dyslexia is influenced by genetic factors. Zerbin-Rudin (1967) reported 100% concordance for dyslexia in monozygotic (MZ) twins, but only 52% concordance in dizygotic (DZ) twins. Stanovich *et al.* (1997) identified one potentially biologically based factor, the 'core phonological deficit', while the other factor, print exposure, was due to a shared or unique environmental influence. Gayán and Olson (2001) also reported genetic influences on deficits in phoneme awareness tasks and phonological decoding ability which can be taken as evidence for shared genetic influences on reading and reading-related skills. Longitudinal findings from Hayiou-Thomas *et al.* (2006) further show that individuals with speech and language impairment have family members with reading problems, suggesting that there is a possible etiological relationship between language and literacy. Moreover, non-verbal ability measured at 4.5 years old is related to reading at 7 years old and this relationship is influenced by shared genetic contributions. However, none of the extant studies were designed to allow any inference from correlation to causation (Hayiou-Thomas *et al.*, 2006).

Castles and colleagues (Castles *et al.*, 1999, 2006) argued that there is the possibility for distinct sets of genes that exert control over the acquisition of different components in the reading system. They postulate that in dual-route terms, some genes might influence only the ability to acquire non-lexical reading skills, whereas others might influence the ability to acquire lexical reading skills. Castles *et al.* (1999) analyzed a group of 322 twins (MZ and DZ). Both groups consisted of patients with phonological and surface dyslexia. For children with phonological dyslexia, the estimated heritability component was highly significant ($r = 0.67$), while the shared environmental influence was smaller ($r = 0.27$). For the children with surface dyslexia, the shared environment influence was relatively large ($r = 0.63$), while the genetic influence was smaller ($r = 0.30$). Similar heritability estimates have been reported in other studies (Gayán & Olson, 2001).

Castles *et al.* (2006) later found additive genetic effects for 73% of the variance in lexical reading (measured by irregular word reading), 71% of the variance in non-lexical reading (measured by nonword reading) and 61% in regular word reading, which is assumed to reflect both lexical and non-lexical processing. These findings are consistent with those of Gayán and Olson (2003), who reported heritability estimates of 0.87 for 'orthographic' and 0.80 for 'phonological' reading and 1–5% of insignificant shared environment effects for orthographic and phonological readings in their sample. Tiu *et al.* (2004) and others found that genetic effects increase after the age of nine. Shared environment exerts a significant influence on early reading.

Castles *et al.* (2006) echo Gayán and Olson (2003) in proposing two independent genetic influences for lexical and non-lexical reading. They highlight the importance of selecting and defining a phenotype of dyslexia, which provides an illustration for the ways in which psychological models can inform genetic studies. They argue that it is important to measure precise phenotypes that are derived from well-specified cognitive models of reading, in order to explain the genetic and environmental influences. Castles *et al.* examined genetic and environmental contributions to irregular word reading and nonword reading in a large sample of adult twins, where reading disability was not a factor. Their data indicated that in addition to shared genetic effects on reading irregular words, nonword independent genetic factors also had an influence on lexical and non-lexical reading ability. In terms of the framework in Figure 8.1, delays in the nonsemantic pathway and the semantic pathway could cause developmental deep and surface dyslexia (Shu *et al.*, 2005; see also Chapter 7 of this volume). Furthermore, the complementary genetic components of dyslexia provide information on the independence of these two pathways.

Few genetic studies are conducted on languages other than English. Most studies on the genetics of reading disorders are conducted in Europe, the USA and Australia. One exception is a study by Grigorenko and colleagues (2006) who looked at children (sibling pairs) from Bagamoyo in Tanzania that were learning to read Swahili. They found heritability estimates for reading and reading-related behaviors comparable with those found in samples from developed countries. There are no similar studies for Chinese-speaking countries. There are also very few studies on writing disorders, however Bates *et al.* (2006) propose a unified genetic model for literacy.

Nation (2006) points out that rather than a single gene leading to dyslexia, existing studies demonstrate that expression of dyslexia is more likely to be influenced by a number of different susceptibility loci operating in a probabilistic manner, in interaction with multiple environmental risks and protective factors. The relationship between genotype and phenotype is, therefore, likely to be complex and interactive. The science of developmental cognitive genetics holds promise for increasing understanding of the complexities in reading development and reading disorders (Nation, 2006). Future research needs to investigate the ways that different components of reading models are influenced by genetic factors. There should also be attention paid to the connection between cognitive reading models and genetic data, which should help uncover the causal pathways to success and failure in children that are learning to read and write.

Brain activation in reading disorder

The universal theory of dyslexia allows for a biological origin in dyslexia across languages, perhaps one that is focused on perceptual impairment. This perceptual weakness may have a biological predisposition that is exposed in genetic linkage and becomes manifest due to neurological abnormality (see Paulesu *et al.*, 2001). Functional brain imaging studies of adult subjects with dyslexia from different cultures and languages (English, French, Italian) find the same abnormal patterns of brain activity during implicit reading (Marino *et al.*, 2004). This suggests common neurobiological causes for dyslexia regardless of a person's spoken language (Marino *et al.*). Neuroscientific research has explored several hypotheses about dyslexia, each related to a perceptual or motor disorder. Some believe that dyslexia is caused by visual processing problems due to magnocellular abnormality impairment (Facoetti *et al.*, 2003), binocular vision abnormalities (Evans *et al.*, 1996) or low-level impairments in transient visual system (Goulandris & Snowling, 1991; Lovegrove *et al.*, 1986). There is evidence that the visual magnocellular system in some children with dyslexia is less sensitive (Amitay *et al.*, 2003; Chase & Stein, 2003). A developmental decrease in right ventral stream activity indicates a decreasing reliance on non-lexical form recognition systems for word identification. It also provides support for Orton's theory (1937) that learning to read requires children to disengage visual representations in the posterior right hemisphere that interfere with word identification (Johansson, 2006). Other perceptual factors include the cerebellar hypothesis, the visual ('magnosystem') theory and the temporal processing theory (see Habib, 2000 for a review). Impaired reading of alphabetic scripts is associated with dysfunction in the left temporal brain regions that perform phonemic analysis and conversion of written symbols from phonological units of speech, such as grapheme-phoneme conversion. Perceptual processing of phonological information in dyslexia appears to have a neurological correlation. However, this biological correlation does not necessarily need to be perceptual, but linked instead to cognitive processing of phonological information.

Activity in the left posterior superior temporal sulcus is associated with the maturation of phonological processing abilities in young readers (Balsamo *et al.*, 2002; Simos *et al.*, 2001). In readers between the ages of six and 22 years, reading is associated with increased activity in the left hemisphere middle temporal and inferior frontal gyri and decreased activity in right inferotemporal areas (Turkeltaub *et al.*, 2003). These results extend evidence that posterior language areas mature earlier than anterior ones (Balsamo *et al.*, 2002; Simos *et al.*, 2001). Paulesu *et al.* (1996) using positron emission tomography (PET), reported five compensated adult developmental dyslexic subjects, who were impaired in phonological processing, including rhyming, short-term memory and Spoonerism tasks, to have associations with reduced brain activity in the left hemisphere. McCrory *et al.* (2005) reported that dyslexic subjects, who were impaired for reading, spelling and naming speed and matched for age and IQ with controls, showed reduced left occipitotemporal activity during word reading and picture naming, even with intact behavioral performance during scanning. McCrory *et al.* suggested this area might act as an interface in the retrieval of phonology from visual input.

A meta-analysis of neuroimaging studies on reading across writing systems indicates that writing systems utilize a common network of regions in word processing, but localization within regions differs across writing systems (Bolger *et al.*, 2005). Paulesu *et al.* (2001) compared English, French and Italian subjects with dyslexia and controls. They found that explicit and implicit reading showed the same reduced activity in the left hemisphere region for dyslexic subjects from all language groups, with the maximum peak in the middle temporal gyrus and additional peaks in both inferior and superior temporal as well as middle occipital gyri. Paulesu *et al.* concluded there may be a universal neurobiological basis for dyslexia. Variations in reading performance among dyslexic subjects from different countries are due to different orthographies, not neurological function.

Neuroimaging studies on dyslexia in Chinese can be based on hypotheses derived from studies of dyslexia in alphabetic (European) languages and knowledge about brain activity during normal reading in Chinese. There are three regions in the brain that are of interest in Chinese reading, involving orthographic, semantic and phonological processing. In an fMRI study on character recognition, Tan *et al.* (2000) found that reading was characterized by extensive activation of neural systems with strong left lateralization in the frontal and temporal cortices and right lateralization in the visual systems, parietal lobe and cerebellum. The location of peak activity in the frontal regions coincided for all character types and the left frontal activations were modulated by ease of semantic retrieval (Tan *et al.*, 2000). Tan *et al.* (2001) reported strong activity in motor and supplementary motor areas during silent reading with Chinese adults. This may be the consequence of visual-orthographic analysis and the close connection in reading and writing for Chinese reading development. The right hemisphere cortical regions are relatively more implemented during the reading of Chinese compared to English, suggesting that the left middle frontal area co-ordinates and integrates the intensive visuospatial analysis that is demanded by the configuration of logographs and semantic (or phonological) analysis required by the task (Tan *et al.*, 2001). Chen *et al.* (2002) concluded that both alphabetic and nonalphabetic scripts (Chinese characters versus alphabetic pinyin symbols) activate a common brain network for reading, after using fMRI to test dual brain processing routes in reading Chinese character and pinyin. Siok *et al.* (2004) showed that in Chinese readers, dyslexia is associated with reduced activity in the left middle frontal gyrus, which is important for working memory in visuospatial and verbal information and co-ordinates cognitive resources as a central executive system (Courtney *et al.*, 1998). Two regions in the right hemisphere differed from normal readers who showed stronger activity in the right mid-inferior frontal gyrus, whereas impaired readers showed stronger activity in the right inferior occipital cortex. Right mid-inferior frontal regions contribute to fluent Chinese reading (Tan *et al.*, 2001) and the increased activity of right inferior occipital gyrus is known to be involved in the processing of Chinese characters (Tan *et al.*, 2000). This suggests that impaired Chinese readers struggle with visuospatial analysis of printed characters, which is consistent with the idea that cognitive strategies for reading development fine tune the cortex (Tan *et al.*, 2003). However, visuospatial analysis may not be the only factor that is important for dyslexia in Chinese. Meng *et al.* (2005) reported that Chinese dyslexic children have deficits in auditory temporal processing using ERP, as well as linguistic processing. Auditory and temporal processing is, therefore, important to reading development in logographic writing systems as it is in alphabetic writing systems. These findings tend to support a universal neurobiological basis for dyslexia as suggested by Paulesu *et al.* (2001) and merits further research attention.

For future research, it is suggested that a cognitive reading model is necessary as a baseline. For orthographic representations, an interesting question would be, is there a word form area in Chinese, and if so, where is it located? Recent studies in other languages suggest a location for the word form area in the parieto-occipital junction (Cohen *et al.*, 2000, 2002). The semantic representation could be located in the temporal lobes, the phonological representation in Boca's area or in other frontal brain regions. A connection from semantics to phonological representations might be found between the temporal and frontal regions. These could be the clues towards more knowledge on reading and writing disabilities in

Chinese. However, a reading model for Chinese is necessary to gain more knowledge on biological constraints in dyslexia.

Conclusion

The development of literacy in Chinese involves many of the linguistic and cognitive processes that are necessary in other languages. These include phonological and orthographic awareness as well as unique knowledge of the morphological features depicted in characters. These may emerge at different stages of development and have a reciprocal influence during development. Although phonological awareness may not extend to phoneme knowledge beyond the onset of a syllable in Chinese, the awareness of subsyllabic properties, such as the rime, appear as the key to development of literacy. Moreover, awareness of the suprasegmental features of Chinese syllables, including tone, may be vital. Dyslexia in Chinese reflects specific problems with the acquisition of processes that depend upon these levels of awareness leading to the possibility of subtypes in developmental dyslexia in Chinese. The framework in Figure 8.1 can accommodate subtypes by assuming that components do not develop normally in children with dyslexia. For future studies in Chinese, there is the need to examine the extent that biological factors explain problems in the development of these processes.

A genetic predisposition to development of phonological awareness that is identified in European languages suggests a genetic correlate for rime or tone awareness may also be found in Chinese-speaking children. Similarly, visual and auditory processing problems in children with dyslexia could be observed in studies of individuals with dyslexia in Chinese. However, eliciting the most interest for understanding dyslexia in Chinese is not the existence of a universal basis for dyslexia across languages, but the circumstances that inherited or perceptual impairments will lead to dyslexia in Chinese. For example, future genetic studies could investigate the possibility of phonological awareness at the level of onset and rime as a biological marker in children with dyslexia. Biological factors may determine whether a child is at risk for dyslexia. However, the phenotype of dyslexia will depend on the spoken language. Therefore, research requires a framework for reading in Chinese to make predictions about the locus of impairment in dyslexia and interpret data meaningfully.

References

Amitay, S., Ben-Yehudah, G., Banai, K. and Ahissar, M. (2002) Disabled readers suffer from visual and auditory impairments but not from a specific magnocellular deficit. *Brain* 125, 2272–2285.

Baldeweg, T., Richardson, A., Watkins, S., Foale, C. and Gruzelier, J. (1999) Impaired auditory frequency discrimination in dyslexia detected with mismatch evoked potentials. *Annals of Neurology* 45, 495–503.

Balsamo, L.M., Xu, B., Grandin, C.B., Petrella, J.R., Braniecki, S.H., Elliott, T.K. *et al.* (2002) A functional magnetic resonance imaging study of left hemisphere language dominance in children. *Archives of Neurology* 59, 1168–1174.

Bates, T.C., Castles, A., Luciano, M., Wright, M.J., Coltheart, M. and Martin, N.G. (2006) Genetic and environmental bases of reading & spelling: A unified genetic dual route model. *Reading and Writing* 20, 147–171.

Bolger, D.J., Perfetti, C.A. and Schneider, W. (2005) Cross-cultural effect on the brain revisited: Universal structures plus writing system variation. *Human Brain Mapping* 25, 93–104.

Bradley, L. and Bryant, P. (1978) Difficulties in auditory organization as a possible cause of reading backwardness. *Nature* 271, 746–747.

Bradley, L. and Bryant, P.E. (1983) Categorizing sounds and learning to read: A causal connection. *Nature* 300, 419–421.

Castles, A., Bates, T., Coltheart, M., Luciano, M. and Martin, N.G. (2006) Cognitive modelling and the behaviour genetics of reading. *Journal of Research in Reading* 29, 92–103.

Castles, A., Datta, H., Gayan, J. and Olson, R.K. (1999) Genetic influences on subtypes of developmental dyslexia. *Journal of Experimental Child Psychology* 72, 73–94.

Cestnick, L. and Coltheart, M. (1999) The relationship between language processing and visual processing in developmental dyslexia. *Cognition* 71, 231–255.

Chan, C.K.K. and Siegel, L.S. (2001) Phonological processing in reading Chinese among normally achieving and poor readers. *Journal of Experimental Child Psychology* 80, 23–43.

Chase, C. and Stein, J. (2003) Visual magnocellular deficits in dyslexia. *Brain* 126, e2.

Chen, Y., Fu, S., Iversen, S.D., Smith, S.M. and Matthews, P.M. (2002) Testing for dual brain processing routes in reading: A direct contrast of Chinese character and pinyin reading using fMRI. *Journal of Cognitive Neuroscience* 14, 1088–1098.

Cheung, H., Chen, H.C., Lai, C.Y., Wong, O.C. and Hills, M. (2001) The development of phonological awareness: Effects of spoken language experience and orthography. *Cognition* 81, 227–241.

Chow, B.W.Y., McBride-Chang, C. and Burgess, S. (2005) Phonological processing skills and early reading abilities in Hong Kong Chinese kindergarteners learning to read English as a second language. *Journal of Educational Psychology* 97, 81–87.

Cohen, L., Dehaene, S., Naccache, L., Lehericy, S., Dehaene-Lambertz, G., Henaff, M.A. *et al.* (2000) The visual word form area: spatial and temporal characterization of an initial stage of reading in normal subjects and posterior split-brain patients. *Brain* 123, 291–307.

Cohen, L., Lehericy, S., Chochon, F., Lemer, C., Rivaud, S. and Dehaene, S. (2002) Language-specific tuning of visual cortex? Functional properties of the visual word form area. *Brain* 125, 1054–1069.

Coltheart, M. (1978) Lexical access in simple reading tasks. In G. Underwood (ed.) *Strategies for Information Processing* (pp. 151–216). New York: Academic Press.

Coltheart, M. (1996) Phonological dyslexia: Past and future issues. *Cognitive Neuropsychology* 13, 749–762.

Coltheart, M. (2006) The genetics of learning to read. *Journal Research in Reading* 29, 124–132.

Coltheart, M., Rastle, K., Perry, C., Langdon, R. and Ziegler, J. (2001) DRC: A dual route cascaded model of visual word recognition and reading aloud. *Psychological Review* 108, 204–256.

Courtney, S.M., Petit, L., Maisog, J.M., Ungerleider, L.G. and Haxby, J.V. (1998) An area specialized for spatial working memory in human frontal cortex. *Science* 279, 1347–1351.

Critchley, M. (1970) *The Dyslexic Child*. London: Heinemann Medical Books.

Cunningham, A., Perry, K. and Stanovich, K.E. (2001) Converging evidence for the concept of orthographic processing. *Reading & Writing: An Interdisciplinary Journal* 14, 549–568.

Eden, G.F., VanMeter, J.W., Rumsey, J.W., Maisog, J. and Zeffiro, T.A. (1996) Abnormal processing of visual motion in dyslexia revealed by functional brain imaging. *Nature* 348, 66–69.

Eden, G.F. and Zeffiro, T.A. (1996) The visual deficit theory of developmental dyslexia. *NeuroImage* 4, S108–S117.

Ehri, L.C. (1991) Learning to read and spell words. In L. Rieben and C.A. Perfetti (eds) *Learning to Read: Basic Research and its Implications* (pp. 57–73). Mahwah, NJ: Erlbaum.

Ehri, L.C. (1992) Reconceptualising the development of sight word reading and its relationship to recoding. In P.B. Gough, L.C. Ehri and R. Treiman (eds) *Reading Acquisition* (pp. 107–143). Hillsdale, NJ: Erlbaum.

Evans, B.J.W., Drasdo, N. and Richards, I.L. (1996) Dyslexia, the link with visual deficits. *Ophthalmic and Physiological Optics* 16, 3–10.

Facoetti, A., Lorusso, M.L., Paganoni, P., Cattaneo, C., Galli, R., Umiltà C., *et al.* (2003) Auditory and visual automatic attention deficits in developmental dyslexia. *Cognitive Brain Research* 16, 185–191.

Frith, U., Landerl, K. and Frith, C. (1995) Dyslexia and verbal fluency: More evidence for a phonological deficit. *Dyslexia: An International Journal of Research and Practice* 1, 2–11.

Fisher, S.E. and DeFries, J.C. (2002) Developmental dyslexia: Genetic dissection of a complex cognitive trait. *Nature Revue Neuroscience* 3, 767–780.

Gayán, J. and Olson, R.K. (2001) Genetic and environmental influences on orthographic and phonological skills in children with reading disabilities. *Developmental Neuropsychology* 20, 487–511.

Gayán, J. and Olson, R.K. (2003) Genetic and environmental influences on individual differences in printed word recognition. *Journal of Experimental Child Psychology* 84, 97–123.

Goldsmith, J.A. (1976) *Autosegmental Phonology*. Bloomington, IN: Indiana University Linguistic Club.

Goswami, U. and Bryant, P.E. (1990) *Phonological Skills and Learning to Read*. Hillsdale, NJ: Erlbaum.

Goulandris, A. and Snowling, M. (1991) Visual memory deficits: A plausible cause of developmental dyslexia? Evidence from a single case study. *Cognitive Neuropsychology* 8, 127–154.

Grainger, J., Bouttevin, S., Truc, C., Bastien, M. and Ziegler, J.C. (2003) Word superiority pseudoword superiority and learning to read: A comparison of dyslexic and normal readers. *Brain & Language* 87, 432–440.

Grigorenko, E.L., Ngorosho, D., Jukes, M. and Bundy, D. (2006) Reading in able and disabled readers from around the world: Same or different? An illustration from a study of reading-related processes in a Swahili sample of siblings. *Journal of Research in Reading* 29, 104–123.

Habib, M. (2000) The neurological basis of developmental dyslexia: An overview and working hypothesis. *Brain* 123, 2373–2399.

Hayiou-Thomas, M.E., Harlaar, N., Dale, P.S. and Plomin, R. (2006) Genetic and environmental mediation of the prediction from preschool language and nonverbal ability to 7-year reading. *Journal of Research in Reading* 29, 50–74.

Ho, C.S.H. and Bryant, P. (1997a) Phonological skills are important in learning to read Chinese. *Developmental Psychology* 33, 946–951.

Ho, C.S.H. and Bryant, P. (1997b) Learning to read Chinese beyond the logographic phase. *Reading Research Quarterly* 32, 276–289.

Ho, C., Chan, D., Lee, S.H., Tsang, S. M. and Luan, V.H. (2004) Cognitive profiling and preliminary subtyping in Chinese developmental dyslexia. *Cognition* 91, 43–75.

Ho, C.S.H., Chan, D.W.O., Tsang, S.M. and Lee, S.H. (2002) The cognitive profile and multiple-deficit hypothesis in Chinese developmental dyslexia. *Developmental Psychology* 38, 543–553.

Ho, C.S.H. and Ma, R.N.L. (1999) Training in phonological strategies improves Chinese dyslexic children's character reading skills. *Journal of Research in Reading* 22, 131–142.

Ho, C.S.H., Law, T.P.S. and Ng, P.M. (2000) The phonological deficit hypothesis in Chinese developmental dyslexia. *Reading and Writing: An Interdisciplinary Journal* 13, 57–79.

Ho, C.S.H., Wong, W.L. and Chan, W.S. (1999) The use of orthographic analogies in learning to read Chinese. *Journal of Child Psychology and Psychiatry* 40, 393–403.

Hu, C.F. and Catts, H.W. (1998) The role of phonological processing in early reading ability: What we can learn from Chinese. *Scientific Studies of Reading* 2, 55–79.

Huang, H.S. and Hanley, J.R. (1994) Phonological awareness, visual skills and Chinese reading acquisition in first graders: A longitudinal study in Taiwan. In H.W. Chang, J.T. Huang, C.W. Hue and O.J.L. Tzeng (eds) *Advances in the Study of Chinese Language Processing. Volume 1: Selected Writings from the Sixth International Symposium on Cognitive Aspects of the Chinese Language* (pp. 235–342). Department of Psychology, National Taiwan University.

Huang, H.S. and Hanley, J.R. (1995) Phonological awareness and visual skills in learning to read Chinese and English. *Cognition* 59, 119–147.

Johansson, B.B. (2006) Cultural and linguistic influence on brain organization for language and possible consequences for dyslexia: A review. *Annals of Dyslexia* 56, 13–50.

Kim, J. and Davis, C. (2004) Characteristics of poor readers of Korean Hangul: Auditory, visual and phonological processing. *Reading and Writing* 17, 153–185.

Ku, Y-M. and Anderson, R.C. (2001) Chinese children's incidental learning of word meanings. *Contemporary Educational Psychology* 26, 249–266.

Lam, C.C.C. and Cheung, P.S.P. (1996) Early developmental problems as indicators for specific learning disabilities among Chinese children. Paper presented at the 47th Annual Conference of the Orton Dyslexia Society, Boston, November.

Landerl, K., Wimmer, H. and Frith, U. (1997) The impact of orthographic consistency on dyslexia: A German-English comparison. *Cognition* 63, 315–334.

Law, S.P. and Or, B. (2001) A case study of acquired dyslexia and dysgraphia in Cantonese: Evidence for nonsemantic pathways for reading and writing Chinese. *Cognitive Neuropsychology* 18, 729–748.
Leben, W. (1973) Suprasegmental phonology. Unpublished doctoral dissertation, MIT, Massachusetts.
Leong, C.K. (1999) What can we learn from dyslexia in Chinese? In I. Lundberg, F.I. Tønnessen and I. Austad (eds) *Dyslexia: Advances in Theory and Practice* (pp. 117–139). Dordrecht: Kluwer.
Leong, C.K. (2006) Making explicit children's implicit epilanguage in learning to read Chinese. In P. Li, L.H. Tan, E. Bates and O. Tzeng (eds) *Handbook of East Asian Psycholinguistics, Volume 1: Chinese Psycholinguistics* (pp. 70–80). Cambridge: Cambridge University Press.
Li, W., Anderson, R.C., Nagy, W.E. and Zhang, H. (2001) Facets of metalinguistic awareness that contribute to Chinese literacy. In W. Li, J.S. Gaffney and J.L. Packard (eds) *Chinese Children's Reading Acquisition: Theoretical and Paedagogical Issues* (pp. 87–106). Boston, MA: Kluwer Academic.
Lovegrove, W., Martin, F. and Slaghuis, W. (1986) A theoretical and experimental case for a visual deficit in specific reading disability. *Cognitive Neuropsychology* 3, 225–267.
Maketa, K. (1968) The rarity of reading disability in Japanese children. *American Journal of Orthopsychiatry* 38, 599–614.
Manis, F.R., Seidenberg, M.S., Doi, L.M., McBride-Chang, C. and Pedersen, A. (1996) On the basis of two subtypes of developmental dyslexia. *Cognition* 58, 157–195.
Marino, C., Giorda, R., Vanzin, L., Nobile, M., Lorusso, M.L., Baschirotto, C. *et al.* (2004) A Locus on 15q15-15qter influences dyslexia: Further support from a transmission/disequilibrium study in an Italian speaking population. *Journal of Medical Genetics* 41, 42–47.
McBride-Chang, C., Bialystok, E., Chong, K.K.Y. and Li, Y.P. (2004) Levels of phonological awareness in three cultures. *Journal of Experimental Child Psychology* 89, 93–111.
McBride-Chang, C. and Chang, L. (1995) Memory, print exposure, and metacognition: Components of reading in Chinese children. *International Journal of Psychology* 30, 607–616.
McBride-Chang, C. and Ho, C.S.H. (2000) Developmental issues in Chinese children's character acquisition. *Journal of Educational Psychology* 92, 50–55.
McCrory, E.J., Mechelli, A., Frith, U. and Price, C.J. (2005) More than words: A common neural basis for reading and naming deficits in developmental dyslexia? *Brain* 128, 261–267.
McCroskey, R.L. and Kidder, H.C. (1980) Auditory fusion among learning disabled, reading disabled, and normal children. *Journal of Learning Disabilities* 13, 18–25.
Menell, P., McAnally, K. and Stein, J. (1999) Psychophysical sensitivity and physiological response to amplitude modulation in adult dyslexic listeners. *Journal of Speech & Hearing Research* 42, 797–803.
Meng, X., Sai, X., Wang, C., Wang, J., Sha, S. and Zhou, X. (2005) Auditory and speech processing and reading development in Chinese school children: Behavioural and ERP evidence. *Dyslexia* 11, 292–310.
Nation, K. (2006) Reading and genetics: An introduction. *Journal of Research in Reading* 29, 1–10.
Orton, S.T. (1937) *Reading, Writing and Speech Problems in Children*. New York: Norton.

Paulesu, E., Demonet, J., Fazio, F., McCrory, E., Chanoine, V., Brunswick, N. *et al.* (2001) Dyslexia: Cultural diversity and biological unity. *Science* 291, 2165–2167.

Paulesu, E., Frith, U., Snowling, M., Gallagher, A., Morton, J., Richard, S.J. *et al.* (1996) Is developmental dyslexia a disconnection syndrome? Evidence from PET scanning. *Brain* 119, 143–157.

Perfetti, C.A., Liu, Y. and Tan, L.H. (2005) The Lexical Constituency Model: Some implications of research on Chinese for general theories of reading. *Psychological Review* 112, 43–59.

Plaut, D.C., McClelland, J.D., Seidenberg, M.S. and Patterson, K. (1996) Understanding normal and impaired word reading: Computational principles in quasi-regular domains. *Psychological Review* 103, 56–115.

Ramus, F. (2003) Developmental dyslexia: Specific phonological deficit or general sensorimotor dysfunction? *Current Opinion in Neurobiology* 13, 212–218.

Read, C.A., Zhang, Y., Nie, H. and Ding, B. (1986) The ability to manipulate speech sounds depends on knowing the alphabetic reading. *Cognition* 24, 31–44.

Seymour, P.H.K. (1986) *Cognitive Analysis of Dyslexia*. London: Routledge & Kegan Paul.

Shu, H. and Anderson, R.C. (1997) Role of radical awareness in the character and word acquisition of Chinese children. *Reading Research Quarterly* 32, 78–89.

Shu, H., Chen, X., Anderson, R.C., Wu, N. and Xuan, Y. (2003) Properties of school Chinese: Implications for learning to read. *Child Development* 74, 27–47.

Shu, H., Meng, X., Chen, X., Luan, H. and Cao, F. (2005) The subtypes of developmental dyslexia in Chinese: Evidence from three cases. *Dyslexia* 11, 311–329.

Shu, H., Wu, S., McBride-Chang, C. and Liu, H. (2006) Understanding Chinese developmental dyslexia: Morphological awareness as a core cognitive construct. *Journal of Educational Psychology* 98, 122–133.

Simos, P.G., Breier, J.I., Fletcher, J.M., Foorman, B.R., Mouzaki, A. and Papanicolaou, A.C. (2001) Age-related changes in regional brain activation during phonological decoding and printed word recognition. *Developmental Neuropsychology* 19, 191–210.

Siok, W.T. and Fletcher, P. (2001) The role of phonological awareness and visual-orthographic skills in Chinese reading acquisition. *Developmental Psychology* 37, 886–899.

Siok, W.T., Perfetti, C.A., Jin, Z. and Tan, L.H. (2004) Biological abnormality of impaired reading is constrained by culture. *Nature* 431, 71–76.

Smythe, I., Everatt, J. and Salter, R. (eds) (2004) *The International Book of Dyslexia*. Chichester: John Wiley.

So, D. and Siegel, L.S. (1997) Learning to read Chinese: Semantic, syntactic, phonological and working memory skills in normally achieving and poor Chinese readers. *Reading and Writing* 9, 1–21.

Stanovich, K.E., Siegel, L.S. and Gottardo, A. (1997) Converging evidence for phonological and surface subtypes of reading disability. *Journal of Educational Psychology* 89, 114–127.

Stein, J. and Walsh, V. (1997) To see but not to read: The magnocellular theory of dyslexia. *Trends in Neuroscience* 20, 147–151.

Stevenson, H.W. (1984) Orthography and reading disabilities. *Journal of Learning Disabilities* 17, 296–301.

Stevenson, H.W., Stigler, J.W., Lucker, G.W., Lee, S.Y., Hsu, C.C. and Kitamura, S. (1982) Reading disabilities: The case of Chinese, Japanese and English. *Child Development* 53, 1164–1181.

Taft, M. (1994) Interactive-activation as a framework for understanding morphological processing. *Language and Cognitive Processes* 9, 271–294.

Taft, M., Liu, Y. and Zhu, X. (1999) Morphemic processing in reading Chinese. In J. Wang, A.W. Inhoff and H.C. Chen (eds) *Graphonomics: Contemporary Research in Handwriting* (pp. 321–327). Amsterdam: Elsevier Science.

Tallal, P. (1980) Auditory temporal perception, phonics, and reading disabilities in children. *Brain and Language* 9, 182–198.

Tallal, P. (1984) Temporal or phonetic processing deficit in dyslexia? That is the question. *Applied Psycholinguistics* 5, 167–169.

Tan, L.H., Liu, H.L., Perfetti, C.A., Spinks, J.A., Fox, P. and Gao, J.H. (2001) Neural systems underlying Chinese logograph reading. *NeuroImage* 13, 836–846.

Tan, L.H., Spinks, J.A., Feng, C.M., Siok, W.T., Perfetti, C.A., Xiong, J. *et al.* (2003) Neural systems of second language reading are shaped by native language. *Human Brain Mapping* 18, 158–166.

Tan, L.H., Spinks, J.A., Gao, J.H., Liu, A., Perfetti, C.A., Xiong, J. *et al.* (2000) Brain activation in the processing of Chinese characters and words: A functional MRI study. *Human Brain Mapping* 10, 16–27.

Tiu, R.D., Wadsworth, S.J., Olson, R.K. and DeFries, J.C. (2004) Causal models of reading disability: A twin study. *Twin Research* 7, 275–283.

Treiman, R. and Zukowski, A. (1991) Levels of phonological awareness. In S.A. Brady and D.P. Shankweiler (eds) *Phonological Processes in Literacy: A Tribute to Isabelle Y. Liberman* (pp. 67–83). Hillsdale, NJ: Erlbaum.

Turkeltaub, P.E., Gareau, L., Flowers, D.L., Zeffiro, T.A. and Eden, G.F. (2003) Development of neural mechanisms for reading. *Nature Neuroscience* 6, 767–773.

Weekes, B. and Coltheart, M. (1996) Surface dyslexia and surface dysgraphia: Treatment studies and their theoretical implications. *Cognitive Neuropsychology* 13, 277–315.

Weekes, B.S. (2006) Deep dysgraphia: Evidence for a summation account of written word production. *Brain and Language* 99, 21–22.

Witton, C., Talcott, J.B., Hansen, P.C., Richardson, A.J., Griffiths, T.D., Rees, A. *et al.* (1998) Sensitivity to dynamic auditory and visual stimuli predicts nonword reading ability in both dyslexic and normal readers. *Current Biology* 8, 791–797.

Woo, E.Y.C. and Hoosain, R. (1984) Visual and auditory functions of Chinese dyslexics. *Psychologia* 27, 164–170.

World Health Organization (1993) *ICD-10: Classification of Mental and Behavioral Disorders* (10th rev.). Geneva: Author.

Wu, X., Li, W. and Anderson, R.C. (1999) Reading instruction in China. *Journal of Curriculum Studies* 31, 571–586.

Wydell, T.N. and Butterworth, B. (1999) An English-Japanese bilingual with monolingual dyslexia. *Cognition* 70, 273–305.

Yin, W.G. and Weekes, B.S. (2003) Dyslexia in Chinese. *Annals of Dyslexia* 53, 255–275.

Yip, M. (1980) The tonal phonology of Chinese. Unpublished doctoral dissertation, MIT, Massachusetts.

Zerbin-Rudin, E. (1967) Kongenitale Wortblindheit oder spezifische Dyslexie [Congenital wordblindness or specific dyslexia]. *Bulletin of the Orton Society* 17, 47–56.

Zhang, B.Y. and Peng, D.L. (1992) Decomposed storage in the Chinese lexicon. In H.C. Chen and O.J.L. Tzeng (eds) *Language Processing in Chinese* (pp. 131–149). Amsterdam: North-Holland.

Zhang, C., Zhang, J., Yin, R., Zhou, J. and Chang, S. (1996) Experimental research on reading disability of Chinese students. *Psychological Science* 19, 222–256.

Zhou, X. and Marslen-Wilson, W. (2000) Lexical representations of compound words: Cross-linguistic evidence. *Psychologica* 43, 47–66.

Ziegler, J.C. and Goswami, U. (2005) Reading acquisition, developmental dyslexia, and skilled reading across languages: A Psycholinguistic Grain Size Theory. *Psychological Bulletin* 131, 3–29.

Ziegler, J.C., Perry, C., Ma-Wyatt, A., Ladner, D. and Schulte-Körne, G. (2003) Developmental dyslexia in different languages: Language-specific or universal? *Journal of Experimental Child Psychology* 86, 169–193.

Ziegler, J.C., Tan, L.H., Perry, C. and Montant, M. (2000) Phonology matters: The phonological frequency effect in written Chinese. *Psychological Science* 11, 234–238.

Chapter 9
Lexical Tones Perceived by Chinese Aphasic Subjects

JIE LIANG

Introduction

Words in tonal languages not only differ in the sequence of vowels and consonants (segments), but also by word melody ('tone'). What happens when a Chinese speaker suffers a brain lesion (e.g. as a result of a stroke) in the left hemisphere, the dominant hemisphere for language processing? Packard (1986) demonstrated that left-hemisphere (LH) damaged non-fluent aphasic speakers of Chinese experience a tonal production deficit. Our own study of a Chinese speaker with left hemisphere damage also provided evidence for tonal production deficit (Liang & van Heuven, 2004).

Models of speech perception and speech production typically postulate a processing level that involves some form of phonological encoding. There is disagreement, however, on the question of whether there are separate phonological encoding systems for perception versus production (Dell *et al.*, 1997; Levelt *et al.*, 1999), or whether a single system participates in phonological encoding for both the input and output of speech (Allport, 1984; Coleman, 1998; MacKay, 1987).

If a single system participates in phonological encoding for both the input and output of speech, then we should expect individuals with tonal production deficits to produce speech perception deficits. A closely related issue is the nature of the deficit. To account for the nature of the deficit in aphasic speech, two main approaches have been developed. Some investigators suggest that language impairments can be considered indices of the 'loss' of linguistic structure, where selective or dissociable language deficits are taken as evidence of the modularity of the linguistic representation or the mechanisms underlying processing (Caplan, 1983; Caramazza, 1986; Friedmann & Grodzinsky, 1997; Grodzinsky, 2000; Hagiwara, 1995). The alternative account assumes that speech production problems result from processing limitations. Some studies show that the language difficulties of aphasic individuals are often caused by deficits in accessing and processing representations, rather than damage to the representation itself. These studies suggest a different theoretical approach, one that locates the decrement of language ability in aphasic subjects to limitations in processing capacity (Bates & Wulfeck, 1989; Blackwell & Bates, 1995; Blumstein, 1997; Blumstein & Milberg, 2000; Friederici & Frazier, 1992; Kolk, 1995).

Lexical tones in connected speech can be quite different from their citation forms. Fundamental to linguistic methodology is to distinguish between the abstract structure of an utterance, its form, and its behavioral expression, its substance. The traditional division of labor between phonology and phonetics derives from that distinction (Fischer-Jørgensen, 1975). Our question for the present study is whether there is a single phonological encoding system for perception and production and whether lexical-tone impairments in Chinese are due to a structural deficit or to acquired processing limitations that prevent individuals from effectively accessing their linguistic knowledge. We assume that listeners take more time to identify a lexical tone in connected speech than in citation form. Given a processing limitation, we should observe similar identification patterns from subjects when they are allowed more time. When the application of time pressure has no effect on the subject's performance, the problem is typically assumed to be a structural deficit. Our aim was to test this difference between abstract and substance format by examining the effect of time pressure (accuracy versus speed) on subjects' responses when identifying lexical tones presented in isolation or embedded in a carrier sentence.

Studying the breakdown of lexical tones in aphasia can provide valuable insight into the nature of tonal representation. There have been views as to whether contour tones should be considered unitary contour units or sequences of level units such as a low followed by a high and a high followed by a low. The former view assumes that contour tones found in languages such as Thai and Mandarin should be considered as single units (Abramson, 1978; Clark, 1978; Pike, 1948; Wang, 1967), while the latter view argues that contour tones are sequences of high and low targets (Duanmu, 1994; Gandour, 1974; Leben, 1973; Woo, 1969; Yip, 1991). Studying individuals who have a selective impairment among the four lexical tones or units will allow us to test theoretical assumptions regarding the specification of Chinese lexical tone representation.

Methods

We set up a three-factor experiment with listener type, stimulus type and task condition as the principal independent variables in the construction of the stimulus materials.

Participants

Fourteen aphasic participants who were native Beijing speakers from Tianjin, Peoples Republic of China, aged 31–80, were diagnosed by

Professor Zhang Banshu from Tianjin General Hospital as having non-fluent Broca's aphasia. The spoken language performance of these participants was characterized by word-finding difficulties, incomplete syntactic constructions and errors in sound production. Production studies on the tones and vowels of one of the participants, the severest case, showed that lexical tones were seriously impaired while the vowels were preserved (Liang & van Heuven, 2004). The participants' non-verbal communication was still effective, and apart from their aphasia, they were able to carry out activities of daily life without difficulty. All of them suffered from unilateral damage in the left frontal and/or parietal lobe (detailed information presented in Table 9.1) and showed normal hearing sensitivities at 0.5, 1 and 2 kHz following a pure-tone air-conduction screening. None of the participants had been diagnosed with neurological or psychiatric illness prior to brain injury. Subjects participated in this experiment during January 2002 to January 2003.

Their healthy controls were tested in September 2002. They were all native speakers of the Beijing dialect, aged between 21 and 70 (average 40 years), 17 male and 13 female. All of them were right-handed with normal hearing and at least 12 years of standard education. They participated in the experiments.

Stimuli

Sound recordings of experimental materials used in the experiments were obtained using a male native speaker of the Beijing dialect (Standard Chinese), experienced in sound recording. All the recordings were made in a sound-insulated booth at the Phonetics Laboratory, Leiden University, on digital audiotape (DAT) using a Sennheiser MKH-416 unidirectional microphone, then transferred to computer memory and downsampled to 16 kHz (16-bit amplitude resolution) by the Praat speech-processing package (Boersma & Weenink, 1996).

In the lexical condition, four high-frequency words were used, with one each having a tone from the Beijing four-tone system, 媽 麻 馬 罵 */ma1 ma2 ma3 ma4/* 'mother, hemp, horse, scold', respectively. In connected speech, tone sandhi results in categorical tone shift. For example, the low tone in Beijing dialect changes into a rising tone when followed by another low tone. When that happens, the derived rising tone is perceptually indistinguishable from the lexical rising tone (Wang & Li, 1967). In order to study the effect of context, each of the four lexical-tone stimuli was read aloud five times in isolation and five times in medial position in a fixed carrier sentence: '我說____ 這個字' [*wo3 shuo1 __ zhe4 ge0 zi4*] 'I say … this word', which took 1.5 seconds. In total, there were 40 stimuli for lexical-tone identification, i.e. four tones in two

Table 9.1 MRI or CT scan findings of the lesion site in the left hemisphere for individual subjects

Subjects	***Name***	***PYF***	***ZZL***	***XWC***	***CRY***	***HSQ***	***QCF***	***YSY***	***CH***	***ZHR***	***YJJ***	***FZJ***	***ZLJ***	***TDH***	***LKM***
	Age	39	50	68	43	47	63	69	80	31	54	50	69	56	52
	Sex	F	M	F	M	M	F	F	F	M	M	M	M	M	M
	Time after onset (months)	23	25	5	6	6	4	2	12	2	6	12	4	35	39
Frontal lobe	Precentral gyrus lower part	●			●	●				●				●	●
	Superior frontal gyrus posterior								●						
	Inferior gyrus pars triangularis	●	●			●					●		●	●	
	Broca's area pars opercularis						●	●					●		●
Parietal lobe	Postcentral gyrus lower part	●	●	●	●							●	●		
	Supramarginal anterior							●	●						
	Gyrus posterior						●								
	Posterior						●								
	Superior lobule										●				
Cingulate	Gyrus posterior			●					●						

experimental conditions (in a carrier sentence and isolation) and five repetitions of each stimulus.

Task conditions and procedure

The stimuli were randomized and presented by computer binaurally over headphones (Sony MDR-V3) at a comfortable listening level. Listeners were tested one at a time in a quiet room, and in the case of some participants, in the subject's own home. A custom-designed keyboard was used with four buttons marked with the corresponding Chinese characters (in font 72) for the tone identification. Each experimental task was preceded by a short practice session, with four practice trials for the tone identification task. The experiment lasted about 20 minutes. Reaction times (measured from the offset of the stimulus, precision 1 ms) were stored in the computer. Stimulus presentation and response collection were controlled by the E-prime software package.

The subjects' task was to decide which of the four words they heard by pressing one of the four buttons on the response keyboard each time they were presented with a stimulus. The buttons were evenly spaced across the top row on the response box; a black key for continue/start was located in the center of the bottom row. Before each part of the experiment, specific instructions were given both orally and in writing. In the first stage of the experiment, they were asked to avoid errors (no time pressure). In the second stage, the subjects were instructed not only to avoid errors but also to perform the task as quickly as they could manage (time pressure). The 40 lexical-tone stimuli, 20 in a carrier sentence and 20 in isolation were presented to the listeners twice in two blocks (once without time pressure and a second time with time pressure). When there was no time pressure, there was a fixed 3000-ms (isolated targets) or 5000-ms (targets in carrier) interstimulus interval (ISI) after the offset of the stimulus, irrespective of the reaction time. When no response was given within the ISI, the trial timed out and the next stimulus was presented. In the sections with time pressure imposed on the listener, the next stimulus started 1000 ms (in isolation) or 2000 ms (in a carrier sentence) after the response. The shorter ISI in the time-pressure condition prompted the subjects to speed up their reaction time. In the debriefing after the experiment, subjects confirmed that they had felt under time pressure; the effects of pressure are also apparent in the results: not only were reaction times much faster, but the number of timed-out responses was higher (even though the ISI had not been reduced).

Results

In this section, we report results for lexical-tone identification for each listener type. We first analyzed the data for the perception of the lexical-tone contrast. In the matter of lexical tones, we can determine whether the listener correctly identified the tone pattern intended by the speaker of the utterance. Also, we can determine how much time it takes for the listener to decide on the tonal category correctly. As the stimuli were presented for identification once with and once without emphasis on speed of response (time pressure), we predicted that listeners would trade accuracy for speed under time pressure, i.e. were prepared to gamble in the case of ambiguous stimuli in order to gain speed.

Percent correct lexical-tone identification scores were computed and submitted to a mixed analysis of variance (ANOVA) with listener type (controls, aphasic subjects) as a between-subject factor, and stimulus tone, context (carrier sentence, citation form) and time pressure (on, off) as within-subject factors. The ANOVA shows that, overall, percent correct was significantly different for time pressure ($F(2, 3468) = 24.0$, $p < 0.001$).

A similar mixed ANOVA was carried out on reaction time to lexical-tone responses. Overall, reaction time was significantly different for context ($F(2, 3468) = 17.6$, $p < 0.001$) and time pressure ($F(2, 3468) = 147.6$, $p < 0.001$). A significant interaction was found between context and time pressure ($F(2, 3468) = 29.5$, $p < 0.001$).

The correct tone identification (percent) and the associated reaction time (ms) as a function of tone type broken down by listener type is presented in Figure 9.1.

Figure 9.1 shows that the aphasic group was much worse in tone identification and much slower in their reaction time relative to the control group. In order to have a clear picture of the distribution of these data, we plotted percent correct by listener groups against the

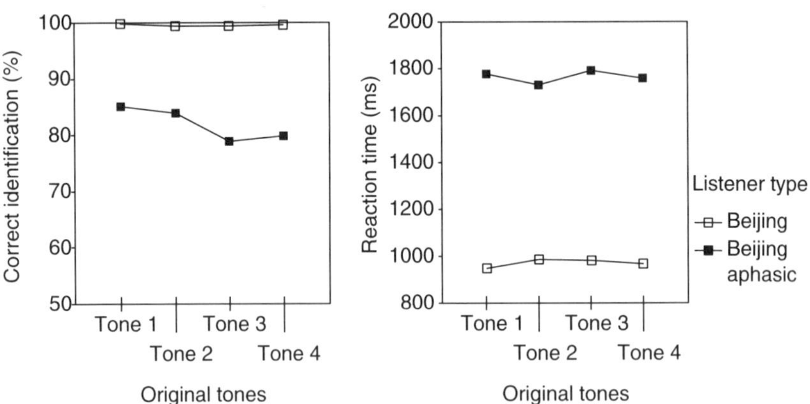

Figure 9.1 Correct tone identification (percent) and associated reaction time (ms) as a function of tone type broken down by listener type (controls versus aphasic)

associated reaction time broken down by presence versus absence of time pressure for tones in carrier sentences and in isolation. These data are presented in Figure 9.2.

The following effects can be seen in Figure 9.2:

(1) Listener type. The aphasic listeners took almost twice as long as the control listeners to identify lexical tones. The ellipse drawn around the four centroids for the aphasic group (solid line) does not overlap with the ellipse drawn around the centroids for the control group (dashed).

(2) Time pressure. Time pressure leads to considerably shorter reaction time, but has little effect on percent correct for control listeners. In contrast, time pressure reduces percent correct as well as reaction time for the aphasic group.

(3) Context. Both types of listeners took longer to identify tones in the carrier sentence than in isolation. Importantly, however, embedding the target in a carrier did not affect percent correct for either group.

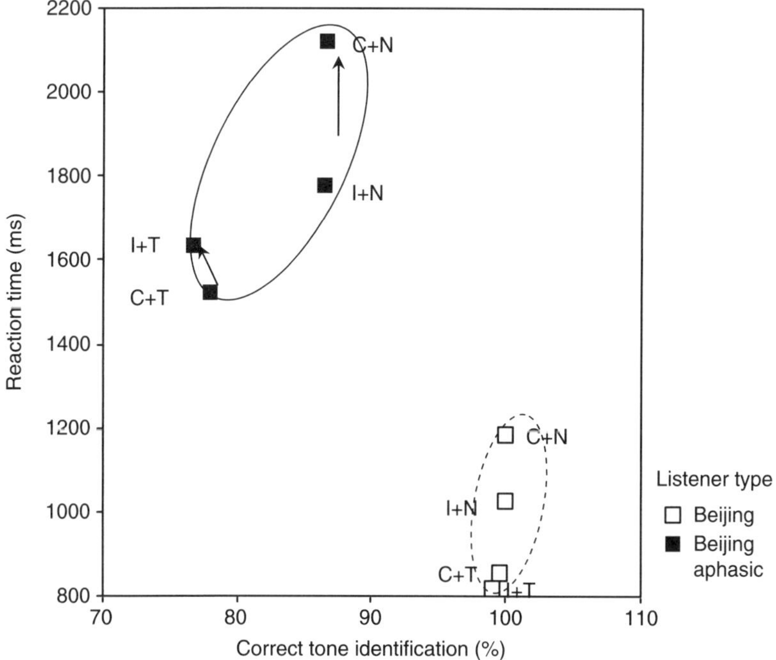

Figure 9.2 Percent correct identification of lexical tone plotted against reaction time (ms) for listener type (control versus aphasic) in two time-pressure conditions (no time pressure 'N' versus time pressure 'T') and two contexts (in carrier sentence 'C' versus isolation 'I'). Spreading ellipses were drawn around the centroids by hand

(4) Identification pattern. When there was no time pressure, the aphasic group displayed a similar identification pattern to that of the healthy listeners, who took longer to identify tones in the carrier sentence than in isolation. This pattern was reversed under time pressure.

From these findings, we conclude that compared with healthy listeners, aphasic listeners' tone identification ability was weakened (less than 90% correct regardless of time pressure), and they exhibited more difficulty out of context: they either took much longer or could not tell the difference. This was regardless of time pressure.

As a last analysis of lexical-tone identification, we collapsed the results across the four separate tones in Figure 9.3, which show the following:

(1) Aphasic listeners performed poorly, with correct identification ranging from 70% to 90%. Time pressure affected the percent of lexical-tone identification, especially in the case of Tone 3, and did not affect Tone 1 identification as much as other tones.
(2) Controls identified tones almost perfectly with no less than 99.3% correct regardless of time pressure.

Clear, tone identification is easy for controls. Therefore, we will not analyze the perceptual confusion structure for these listeners further. However, a tone-confusion analysis for the aphasic listeners is informative. The pattern of lexical-tone confusion for Beijing aphasic listeners broken down by context (carrier versus isolation) and time pressure (presence versus absence of time pressure) is presented in Table 9.2.

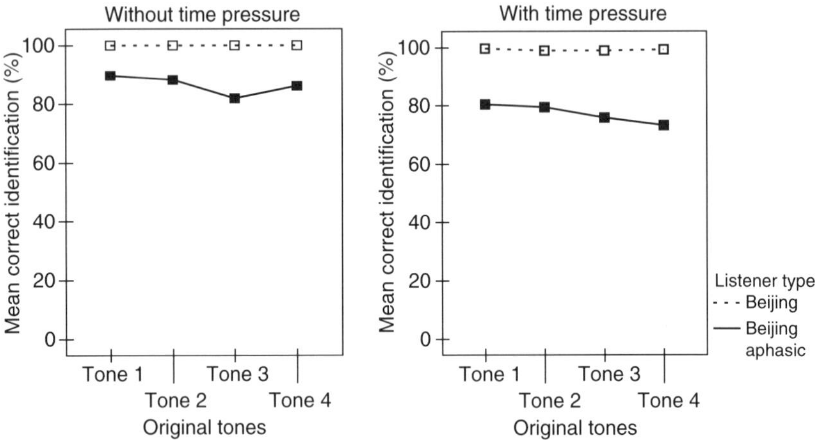

Figure 9.3 Correct tone identification (percent) as a function of tone type broken down by listener type (control versus aphasic) without time pressure (left panel) and with time pressure (right panel)

Table 9.2 Confusion matrices of tone identification by Beijing aphasic listeners broken down by presence versus absence of time pressure for tones in carrier sentences and in isolation

			Responses							
			In carrier sentence				*In isolation*			
Listener type	*Time pressure*	*Tones*	*Tone 1*	*Tone 2*	*Tone 3*	*Tone 4*	*Tone 1*	*Tone 2*	*Tone 3*	*Tone 4*
Beijing aphasic subject	No	Tone 1	**88.1**	7.5	3.0	1.5	**91.3**	1.4	7.2	
		Tone 2	4.5	**87.9**	4.5	3.0	1.4	**88.6**	**10.0**	
		Tone 3	8.8	1.5	**83.8**	5.9	8.6	7.1	**80.0**	4.3
		Tone 4	4.5	4.5	4.5	**86.6**	8.6	5.7		**85.7**
	Yes	Tone 1	**82.4**	8.8	7.4	1.5	**78.5**	4.6	9.2	7.7
		Tone 2	7.8	**73.4**	7.8	**10.9**	7.4	**85.3**	5.9	1.5
		Tone 3	9.0	**10.4**	**74.6**	6.0	**12.1**	4.5	**77.3**	6.1
		Tone 4	**12.5**	6.3		**81.3**	7.5	**10.4**	**16.4**	**65.7**

Note. Bold numbers on shaded background are correct responses; other bold numbers identify confusions (≥ 10%)

The aphasic listeners have an even spread of tone confusions across the four different types of tone. Only in seven cases are tones confused by more than 10% of trials or participants. Without time pressure, tone confusion was observed only once for tones in isolation (Tone2 > Tone 1) and never for tones in a carrier sentence. With time pressure, confusion was more widespread, affecting perception of Tones 2, 3 and 4, but never Tone 1. Thus, we found evidence of a selective impairment among the four lexical tones.

In order to characterize the performance of the two listener groups, we determined receiver operating characteristic (ROC) curves for each individual in each of the two groups (aphasic subjects versus controls) with and without time pressure, and broken down for presence versus absence of context. As ROC analysis applies to dichotomies only, the responses were analyzed in terms of four binary oppositions: Tone 1 versus not Tone 1, Tone 2 versus not Tone 2, Tone 3 versus not Tone 3, and Tone 4 versus not Tone 4. We computed d'-values as a measure of detectability of each lexical tone among its competitors (with standard correction for perfect scores and zero false alarms). Figure 9.4 plots the d'-scores averaged over the four tones.

The d′-values were submitted to a mixed ANOVA. Significant effects were found for time pressure ($F(1, 42) = 62.4$, $p < 0.001$) and for listener type ($F(1, 42) = 47.8$, $p < 0.001$). In addition, the second-order interaction between time pressure and listener type was significant ($F(1, 42) = 40.9$, $p < 0.001$), as was the third-order interaction between time pressure, listener type and context ($F(1, 42) = 5.8$, $p = 0.02$). Again, the results show that the controls were more sensitive to lexical tones than the aphasic listeners, regardless of time pressure and context.

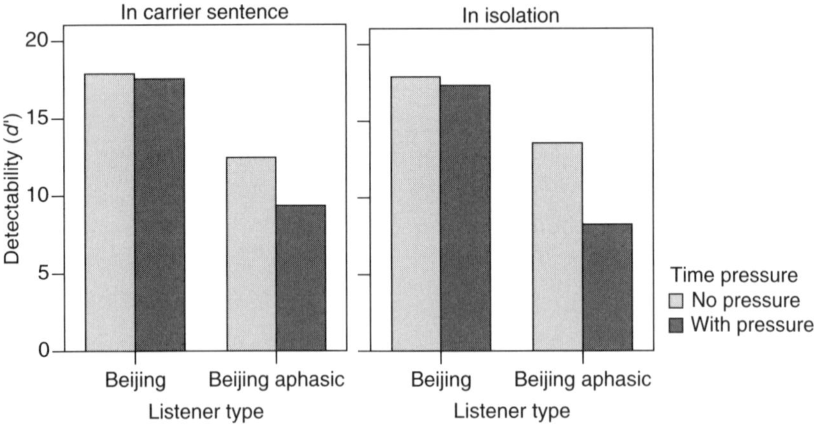

Figure 9.4 Detectability measure (d') for listener type broken down by presence versus absence of time pressure

Discussion

The findings show that non-fluent Chinese aphasic speakers are impaired in tone perception. They take almost twice as long as controls to identify lexical tones and their performance was reduced by 10–20% compared to controls. That is to say, the percentage of aphasic speakers' correct tone recognition was substantially worse and they required much more time to make a decision than the control group.

These findings are consistent with previous research in Chinese and in other languages. For instance, in case studies of a Chinese aphasic subject with a left hemisphere intracerebral stroke, lexical-tone perception was impaired (Naeser & Chan, 1980; see also Eng *et al.*, 1996). In analyses of the impairments in our aphasic participants, the main outcome is preserved status for Tone 1. Next, we discuss the results in detail in terms of the effects of time pressure, context and tonal impairments.

As stated in the Introduction, the nature of tonal impairment is still a matter of debate, and this debate is focused on whether performance is constrained by structural or processing limitations. We assumed that if there was a limitation problem, the aphasic subjects would behave in the same way as the healthy group given sufficient time. However, relaxing time constraints had little impact on performance for the aphasic group. Tone identifications for healthy listeners' under time pressure and without time pressure differed in reaction time (about 200–300 ms), but did not differ in percentage correct performance (over 99%). This indicates that time pressure had no impact on accuracy of lexical-tone identification.

Compared with healthy controls, we found the aphasic listeners' identification was reduced by about 10% when there was no time pressure. This indicates that the aphasic listeners could not process tones as well as healthy controls even with sufficient time. In addition, without time pressure, performances in terms of both reaction time and percentage correct were compromised. Therefore, the findings show that aphasic listeners' impairments involved both structural deficits and processing limitations.

We found healthy listeners' tone identification in different contexts (in isolation or in a carrier sentence) differed only in reaction time, but not percentage correct (both almost perfect) when there was no time pressure. We interpret this as evidence that context slows identification. The finding that listeners are able to factor out the effect of tonal context is consistent with previous studies on Chinese lexical-tone identification in context (Xu, 1994). Again, our findings support the assumption that listeners apply phonological rules to relate the surface tone to its canonical form. Applying this rule is a more or less error-free process, but it takes time.

For aphasic listeners, we found tone identification differs only in reaction time, but not percentage correct performance when there is no time pressure. This shows that aphasic individuals were able to factor out the effect of context or they could effectively access their linguistic knowledge. Obviously, the canonical forms of the tones, the underlying representations, were more or less changed, as their identification was not as perfect as the controls even if they were allowed sufficient time.

However, for both groups, when there was time pressure, the correct percent for tones in isolation was reduced and we have no better explanation than miss-hitting as listeners traded accuracy for speed under time pressure, i.e. gambled in the case of ambiguous stimuli in order to gain speed.

Alternatively, the context factor would trigger little to no tone assimilation or tone sandhi to occur because only Tone 1 was used as context in our experiment. This also explains why the context slowed identification, but did not lead to more errors for both groups. Therefore, we can only claim that aphasic listeners were not sensitive to tone variation caused by Tone 1.

The findings show that Tone 1 was best identified (Figure 9.1). The findings from confusion patterns showed that associated error confusion ($\geq 10\%$) occurred between Tone 2 and Tone 3. These findings support the view that contour tones should be considered sequences of level units such as a low followed by a high and a high followed by a low, which can explain the patterns shared by Tone 2 and Tone 3, i.e. sequences of low followed by high (Duanmu, 1994; Gandour, 1974; Leben, 1973; Woo, 1969; Yip, 1991).

The findings from the perception experiment provide evidence for the preserved status of Tone 1. The findings are consistent with the results from our production study (Liang & van Heuven, 2004) showing that Tone 1 was preserved while other tones were damaged. Findings from both production and perception experiments favor models that assume a single system is used in phonological encoding of lexical tones for both input and output.

Conclusion

In conclusion, we provide evidence for a speech model that assumes a correspondence between the systems necessary in phonological encoding for both the input and output of speech (Allport, 1984; Coleman, 1998; MacKay, 1987). This is evidence of close correspondence between speech perception and production in Chinese aphasia. We replicated previous findings that aphasic speakers can have a selective loss of lexical-tone identification in tone languages such as Thai and Chinese (Gandour & Dardarananda, 1983; Gandour *et al.*, 2000; Hsieh *et al.*, 2001; Hughes *et al.*,

1983; Klein *et al.*, 2001; Yiu & Fok, 1995). Because in all these studies, including our own, the aphasic subjects had a lesion in the left hemisphere only, it must be the case that the lexical tones are primarily lateralized to the left hemisphere. What is novel about our results is that brain damage in the left hemisphere does not appear to make any difference to the detection of canonical shapes of tones (isolated citation forms) and assimilated forms in context.

Finally, we claim that Tone 1 has a special status in Chinese. Aphasic listeners have a fairly even spread of tone confusion among the four types of tone in the absence of time pressure. Under time pressure, there was some confusion, typically affecting the perception of Tones 2, 3 and 4, but never Tone 1. This could be a language-specific effect, but might also be observed in aphasic speakers in other tonal languages. This claim is consistent with an earlier finding of an aphasic speaker with preserved Tone 1 production that was much better than any other tone in production (Liang & van Heuven, 2004).

The effect of context suggests that all four lexical tones preceding or following the target tones should be considered in experimental designs in which a target tone goes through assimilation and/or sandhi and thus deviates from its canonical form. As for canonical tonal identification, another possible manipulation would be to see if meaning could be derived through context when the tones are close to their canonical forms (as in focal positions in the carrier sentence) versus tones that are deviated (as in non-focal positions).

References

Abramson, A.S. (1978) The phonetic plausibility of the segmentation of tones in Thai phonology. In W.U. Dressler and W. Meid (eds) *Proceedings of the 12th International Congress of Linguistics* (pp. 760–763). Innsbruck: Institut für Sprachwissenchaft der Universität Innsbruck.

Allport, D.A. (1984) Speech production and comprehension: One lexicon or two? In W. Prinz and A.F. Sanders (eds) *Cognition and Motor Processes* (pp. 209–228). Berlin: Springer-Verlag.

Bates, E. and Wulfeck, B. (1989) Comparative aphasiology: A crosslinguistic approach to language breakdown. Invited review article with peer commentary. *Aphasiology* 3, 111–142.

Blackwell, A. and Bates, E. (1995) Inducing agrammatic profile in normals: Evidence for the selective vulnerability of morphology under cognitive resource limitation. *Journal of Cognitive Neuroscience* 7, 228–257.

Blumstein, S.E. (1997) A perspective on the neurobiology of language. *Brain and Language* 60, 335–346.

Blumstein, S.E. and Milberg, W.P. (2000) Language deficits in Broca's and Wernicke's aphasia: A singular impairment. In Y. Grodzinsky and L.P. Shapiro (eds) *Language and the Brain: Representation and Processing. Foundations of Neuropsychology Series* (pp. 167–183). San Diego, CA: Academic Press.

Boersma, P. and Weenink, D. (1996) *Praat, a System for Doing Phonetics by Computer. Report 132*. University of Amsterdam: Institute of Phonetic Sciences.

Caplan, D. (1983) Syntactic competence in agrammatism: A lexical hypothesis. In M. Studdert-Kennedy (ed.) *Psychobiology of Language* (pp. 177–187). Cambridge, MA: MIT Press.

Caramazza, A. (1986) On drawing inferences about the structure of normal cognitive systems from the analysis of patterns of impaired performance: The case for single-patient studies. *Brain and Cognition* 5, 41–66.

Clark, M. (1978) A dynamic treatment of tone, with special attention to the tonal system of Igbo. Unpublished doctoral dissertation, University of Massachusetts.

Coleman, J. (1998) Cognitive reality and the phonological lexicon: A review. *Journal of Neurolinguistics* 11, 295–320.

Dell, G.S., Schwartz, M.F., Martin, N., Saffran, E.M. and Gagnon, D.A. (1997) Lexical access in aphasic and nonaphasic speakers. *Psychological Review* 104, 801–838.

Duanmu, S. (1994) Against contour tone units. *Linguistic Inquiry* 25, 555–608.

Eng, N., Obler, L.K., Harris, K.S. and Abramson, A.S. (1996) Tone perception deficits in Chinese-speaking Broca's aphasics. *Aphasiology* 10, 649–656.

Fischer-Jørgensen, E. (1975) *Trends in Phonological Theory: A Historical Introduction.* Copenhagen: Akademisk Forlag.

Friederici, A.D. and Frazier, L. (1992) Thematic analysis in agrammatic comprehension: Syntactic structures and task demands. *Brain and Language* 42, 1–29.

Friedmann, N. and Grodzinsky, Y. (1997) Tense and agreement in agrammatic production: Pruning the syntactic tree. *Brain and Language* 56, 397–425.

Gandour, J. (1974) On the representation of tone in Siamese. *UCLA Working Papers in Phonetics* 27, 118–146.

Gandour, J. and Dardarananda, R. (1983) Identification of tonal contrasts in Thai aphasic patients. *Brain and Language* 18, 98–114.

Gandour, J., Wong, D., Hsieh, L., Weinzapfel, B., Van Lancker, D. and Hutchins, G.D. (2000) A crosslinguistic PET study of tone perception. *Journal of Cognitive Neuroscience* 12, 207–222.

Grodzinsky, Y. (2000) The neurology of syntax: Language use without Broca's area. *Behavioral and Brain Science* 23, 1–71.

Hagiwara, H. (1995) The breakdown of functional categories and the economy of derivation. *Brain and Language* 50, 92–116.

Hsieh, L., Gandour, J., Wong, D. and Hutchins, G. (2001) Functional heterogeneity of inferior frontal gyrus is shaped by linguistic experience. *Brain and Language* 76, 227–252.

Hughes, C.P., Chan, J.L. and Su, M.S. (1983) Aprosodia in Chinese patients with right cerebral hemisphere lesions. *Archives of Neurology* 40, 732–736.

Klein, D., Zatorre, R., Milner, B. and Zhao, V. (2001) A cross-linguistic PET study of tone perception in Mandarin Chinese and English speakers. *NeuroImage* 13, 646–653.

Kolk, H.H.J. (1995) A time-based approach to agrammatic production. *Brain and Language* 50, 282–303.

Leben, W.R. (1973) Suprasegmental phonology. Unpublished doctoral dissertation, University of Massachusetts.

Levelt, W.J.M., Roelofs, A. and Meyer, A.S. (1999) A theory of lexical access in speech production. *Behavioral & Brain Sciences* 22, 1–75.

Liang, J. and van Heuven, V.J. (2004) Evidence for separate tonal and segmental tiers in the lexical specification of words: A case study of a brain-damaged Chinese speaker. *Brain and Language* 91, 282–293.

MacKay, D.G. (1987) *The Organization of Perception and Action: A Theory for Language and Other Cognitive Skills*. New York: Springer-Verlag.
Naeser, M.A. and Chan, W-C.S. (1980) Case study of a Chinese aphasic with the Boston Diagnostic Aphasia Exam. *Neuropsychologia* 18, 389–410.
Packard, J.L. (1986) Tone production deficits in nonfluent aphasic Chinese speech. *Brain and Language* 29, 212–223.
Pike, K.L. (1948) *Tone Languages*. Ann Arbor, MI: University of Michigan Press.
Wang, W.S-Y. (1967) Phonological features of tone. *International Journal of American Linguistics* 33, 93–105.
Wang, W.S.Y. and Li, K.P. (1967) Tone 3 in Pekinese. *Journal of Speech Hearing Research* 10, 629–636.
Woo, N. (1969) Prosody and phonology. Unpublished doctoral dissertation, University of Massachusetts.
Xu, Y. (1994) Production and perception of coarticulated tones. *Journal of the Acoustical Society of America* 95, 2240–2253.
Yip, M. (1991) *The Tonal Phonology of Chinese*. New York: Garland Press.
Yiu, E. and Fok, A. (1995) Lexical tone disruption in Cantonese aphasic speakers. *Clinical Linguistics and Phonetics* 9, 79–92.

Chapter 10

Selective Grammatical Class Deficits: Implications for the Representation of Grammatical Information in Chinese

ZAIZHU HAN and YANCHAO BI[1]

Introduction

Grammar, the rules that allow infinite sentences to be built based on a finite set of words, is an essential component of languages. Although the question on the ways that the human brain represents and processes grammatical information has attracted the attention of philosophers and linguists for centuries, most psycholinguistic studies have focused on a specific class of single words, i.e. concrete nouns. How are grammatical properties of words in various classes captured by the cognitive/neural system? How does the brain 'compute' the agreements (e.g. case, tense, grammatical gender) between words so that grammatical sentences are produced to convey a message? How do language-specific linguistic factors affect the cognitive processes? Recent development of new techniques, such as neuroimaging (e.g. Li *et al.*, 2004; Shapiro *et al.*, 2006; Tyler *et al.*, 2004) has promoted some new ways of examining such theoretical questions. Nevertheless, the most consistent and revealing evidence is derived from the study of brain-damaged individuals.

Historically, the 1970s was revolutionary for its study of patterns in the breakdowns induced by brain damage, starting with alleged 'agrammatic' speakers. Observations concluded that individuals with typical Broca's aphasia, who produced speech with poor grammatical structure and made errors on grammatical morphemes, often also had difficulty in comprehending sentences where grammatical structure interpretation was necessary. This evoked excitement among researchers and led to the proposal that there could be a functionally (possibly neurologically) independent 'grammar module' shared by language production and comprehension, and that it could be selectively impaired (see Caramazza *et al.*, 1981). Although this was captivating, the hypothesis was soon proven wrong. Individuals with various profiles, such as those with only agrammatic speech but intact comprehension, or with deficits in only one type of morphological morphemes, were reported (e.g. Bastiaanse, 1995; Miceli *et al.*, 1983; Nespoulous *et al.*, 1988). Instead of trying to find a general mechanism that underlies brain-damaged individuals who are classified as a syndrome group with 'grammatical impairment', subsequent research has focused more on the understanding of the subcomponent organization in the grammatical system by looking at single cases with specific profiles. Among them, the representation of nouns and verbs has been one of the most fundamental issues of interest.

In this chapter, the intention is not to provide a complete review of the progress in understanding grammatical processes. Instead, the focus is on a distinctive type of individual who shows varied patterns of noun/verb dissociations. In addition, the ways that the study of such patterns provides information on the representation of these two major grammatical categories in the brain will be discussed. In particular, there is an attempt to understand the contrast between the Chinese language and Indo–European languages, which might provide special insights into the issue. The chapter is organized into three sections. First, there will be a brief discussion of some specific properties in Chinese grammar and the possible ways that such properties may affect cognitive processing. This will be followed by a review of previous reports of brain-injured individuals, including Chinese speakers, exhibiting noun/verb dissociations. Finally, directions for future research will be discussed.

Chinese Grammatical System

Certain aspects of grammar are more likely to be universal across languages, such as the existence of a 'noun' and a 'verb' class. Nouns act as the objects or subjects in a sentence, while verbs act as their predicates. However, the detailed grammatical rules differ widely among languages. Packard (1993) conducted a comprehensive review of the specific characteristics of the Chinese grammatical system. Discussion for this chapter will be limited to those that are potentially significant for cognitive theory building. A marked characteristic of the Chinese language is the paucity of inflectional morphology. In languages with rich morphology such as Hungarian, for example, a noun sometimes can take up to 100 different inflectional forms. However, a Chinese word has only one form, regardless of the person, case, gender, tense or number attributes of the word. The consequences for the near absence of inflection in the cognitive system then become interesting. On the one hand, it is possible that the difference in the morphological processing mechanisms that are associated with nouns and verbs in Indo–European languages (see 'Morphosyntactic processing of nouns and verbs' for a detailed discussion) may not be visible in Chinese (refer to Shapiro & Caramazza, 2003). On the other hand, the paucity of explicit inflectional morphemes might not necessarily imply the absence of an abstract morphosyntactic processing mechanism.

In Chinese, information such as aspect and case is sometimes carried by various types of grammatical markers that are free-standing morphemes, such as classifiers, coverbs, affixations, negative markers and aspect markers (see Law & Cheng, 2002). Some of them are specific for open-class words in a certain grammatical category. For instance, between a determiner and a noun, a classifier is obligatory. Prepositions were treated by Packard as coverbs, given that they contained some attributes of verbs. Grammatical markers that are associated with verbs include aspect markers, which are used to express aspectual relations (過 */guo4/*, indicating the completion of the verbal action; 了 */le0/*, indicating the completion of the verbal action or change of the sentence situation; 着 */zhe0/* or 在 */zai4/*, indicating continuative aspect of verbal action).

The most productive morphological procedure in the formation of Chinese words is compounding. It is worth noting that the morphemes that comprise the compound could originate from various grammatical classes. These might be either the same as the compound or different from it. For example, the word 火車 (*/huo3che1/* 'train') is composed of two nominal morphemes 火 (*/huo3/* 'fire') and 車 (*/che1/* 'car'), referred to as a 'N = nn' compound. The noun 講台 (*/jiang3tai2/* 'dais'), on the other hand, consists of a verbal element 講 'speak' and a nominal element 台 'platform' (N = vn). A verbal compound example is 跳水 (*/tiao4shui3/* 'to dive'), which contains a verbal element 跳 'jump' and a nominal element 水 'water' (V = vn). Therefore, the richness of internal word structures provides opportunities to study the grammatical aspects of word composition.

Finally, relative to other languages, the word order in Chinese is more flexible. Although the common word order is subject-verb-object (SVO), this order is often changed to a focus or emphasis on the object. Furthermore, some elements, such as noun phrases and pronouns, are more frequently omitted in Chinese than in other languages. These characteristics render the evaluation of grammatical deficits in a less straightforward way for language production in Chinese speakers. The approaches that are taken include: obtaining speech, generating norms of normal speakers and delegating of tasks with highly constrained grammatical components.

Whether such linguistic differences affect the cognitive system is theoretically significant. If this is the case, what is the importance? Packard (1993) based the analysis of one single case on an agrammatic Chinese case (Chen) and compared the agrammatic speech patterns in Chinese to the common profiles observed in Western language speakers. Similar to brain-damaged individuals of Western languages, Chen's speech showed short phrases, slow speech rate, syntactic simplification, function-word omission and underemployment. However, in contrast to the frequent substitutions of functional morphemes that are observed in Western individuals with aphasia, no substitution errors were observed for this Chinese agrammatic individual. The author argues that this difference is theoretically important because there are two potential origins for the substitution errors in alphabetic languages. These include deficits at the inflectional morphology system and deficits at selecting bound morphemes. As Chinese has bound morphemes, but little inflectional morphology, the absence of substitution errors in the Chinese case indicates that the substitution errors in Western languages might originate from the inflectional system. It is common knowledge that agrammatic individuals are not homogeneous and the patterns reported by Packard could either be due to the language difference or attributed to a particular case. However, his work inspires possible ways to address the issue.

Some researchers propose that the linguistic features of Chinese might also influence the acquisition pattern of nouns and verbs. While it has been widely reported that nouns are acquired earlier than verbs in many Indo–European languages (e.g. Bornstein *et al.*, 2004), Tardif and colleagues (Tardif, 1996; Tardif *et al.*, 1997, 1999) observed a reverse trend in Chinese children. These authors attributed such differences to a set of variables, including concept imageability, linguistic status as well as the parental speech input frequency. For instance, they observed that the early-acquired verbs by Chinese children had higher imageability than those by English-speaking children, leading them to postulate that imageability affects verb learning because actions with high imageability are more easily segmented and labeled. They also proposed that Mandarin verbs tend to occur at the end of utterances without complex morphological changes, making them easier for segmentation and learning. A further observation that might underlie the verb acquisition difference is that Chinese-speaking mothers spoke more verbs to their children than English-speaking mothers.

Li *et al.* (2004) proposed that the paucity of inflectional morphology in Chinese may affect the ways that nouns and verbs are represented in the brain. Indeed, in a fMRI study where Chinese participants were asked to perform a lexical decision task on Chinese nouns and verbs, they failed to detect any difference in the neural activation between these two classes of words. This was different from the results with English speakers (e.g. Federmeier *et al.*, 2000; Shapiro *et al.*, 2006; but see Tyler *et al.*, 2004). One may argue that the lexical decision task used in their study was not sensitive to grammatical information and therefore, the null result should not be taken as evidence that Chinese nouns and verbs do not have distinguishable neural substrates. In the next section, several kinds of representations and processes in which nouns and verbs may differ and the possible ways that nouns and verbs as grammatical entities are represented in Chinese speakers will be discussed.

Selective Noun–Verb Deficits

G. B. Vico (1688–1744) began the pursuit of noun/verb representation differences through seminal work that first described a brain-damaged male with selective impairment of verbs relative to nouns (see Denes & Barba, 1998). Subsequent researchers reported similar dissociations in both directions, including more severe impairment with verbs than nouns (for instance, Berndt *et al.*, 1997a, 1997b; Breedin *et al.*, 1998; Caramazza & Hillis, 1991; Hillis & Caramazza, 1995; Hillis *et al.*, 2002; Kim & Thompson, 2000; Kohn *et al.*, 1989; Laiacona & Caramazza, 2004; McCarthy & Warrington, 1985; Miceli *et al.*, 1984, 1988; Rapp & Caramazza, 1998; Silveri & di Betta, 1997; Williams & Canter, 1997; Zingeser & Berndt, 1990) and more impairment with nouns than verbs (e.g. Laiacona & Caramazza, 2004; Miceli *et al.* 1984, 1988; Rapp & Caramazza, 1997; Robinson *et al.*, 1999; Shapiro *et al.*, 2000; Silveri & di Betta, 1997; Zingeser & Berndt, 1990).

The double dissociation between nouns and verbs has also been found in Chinese brain-damaged individuals. Bates *et al.* (1991) conducted the first group study of Chinese speakers with noun/verb production by administering an oral picture-naming task to two groups of subjects, individuals with Broca's aphasia and those with Wernicke's aphasia. They reported that the first group had more severe impairment in naming verbs/actions than nouns/objects, but the latter presented the reverse. More recently, Bi *et al.* (2005, 2007) conducted substantive investigation on a single case, ZBL, who had greater difficulty in producing nouns orally in contrast to verbs.

Does the existence of such noun/verb dissociations indicate that the lexical representations of nouns and verbs are supported by different neural substrates and therefore, can be impaired selectively? This is not necessarily true. There are at least three levels of cognitive processing in which nouns and verbs may differ, including the conceptual, lexical and grammatical processing (e.g. morphosyntactic) systems (refer to a similar position in Bates *et al.*, 1990; Laiacona & Caramazza, 2004; Shapiro & Caramazza, 2001, 2003). The grammatical dissociations observed in brain-damaged individuals were argued as attributable to any one or a combination of these levels. In the following, the abilities and ways for the noun/verb grammatical distinction to play a role in each of these cognitive systems will be discussed.

Semantic/conceptual organization of nouns and verbs

The semantic/conceptual system is the cognitive component that is most unlikely to be affected by language-specific parameters (refer to Whorf, 1956). Therefore, if the noun/verb dissociation originates from the representation and/or processing difference in the conceptual system, it is likely to be universal among all languages, including Chinese. The school of semantic/conceptual accounts reduces the cause of noun-verb dissociation to a conceptual basis. They claim that the grammatical class effects in such dissociations are due to certain conceptual differences between nouns and verbs. These include concreteness/abstractness (Marshall *et al.*, 1996a, 1996b), imageability (Bird *et al.*, 2000, 2001), semantic complexity (or specificity; Breedin *et al.*, 1998) or semantic feature compositions (e.g. Vigliocco *et al.*, 2004; Vinson *et al.*, 2003). These accounts argue that verbs tend to be more abstract or have less specific semantic representations than nouns. For example, the selective noun or verb deficits may arise from deficits in the semantic system itself, which is affected by concreteness and/or conceptual complexity. Grammatical-specific deficits of some individuals can indeed be explained by these accounts (e.g. Berndt *et al.*, 1997a; Marshall *et al.*, 1996a, 1996b), but some speakers' noun/verb dissociation persists even after the concreteness and imageability are matched between noun and verb stimuli.

The most prevailing conceptual theories are the object/action theory for the noun/verb dissociations. While nouns/verbs are terms addressing the grammatical dimensions, objects/actions are relevant in the conceptual system. As noun/verb production is usually studied by using object- and action-naming tasks, there is confound between the noun/verb dimension and the object/action dimension. Therefore, the observed noun/verb dissociation might not be grammatical, but simply the disproportionate impairment of object or action concepts, if it is assumed that the concepts of objects and actions in the semantic system are independently represented and can be selectively impaired (e.g. Damasio & Tranel, 1993; McCarthy & Warrington, 1985).[2]

There are recent theoretical accounts that specify in greater detail on the ways that the conceptual system is organized, such that nouns and verbs (objects and actions) can emerge as categories, such as the 'extended sensory/functional theory' (ESFT; Bird *et al.*, 2000, 2001) and the 'featural and unitary semantic space' (FUSS) theory (e.g. Vigliocco *et al.*, 2004; Vinson *et al.*, 2003). These theories assume that conceptual knowledge is organized by distributed, modality-specific features (such as sensory, functions, motoric, etc.), different categories of concepts (for instance, living things, artifacts, tools, body parts, actions) have different compositions of various types of features, and the higher the proportion that a concept has of a certain feature type, the more 'important' it becomes for the concept. Category-specific semantic deficit arises because of damage to one feature type, resulting in more severe impairment to the category in which that feature type is most important. For instance, in one specific model, Bird and colleagues (2000) assumed that the concepts of animate things (nouns), inanimate things (nouns), and actions (verbs) are represented by a gradual decreasing proportion of sensory features to functional features. As a result, damage to sensory features will affect animate nouns the most, inanimate nouns less and action verbs the least. Although there are reported cases that are consistent with this prediction (Bird *et al.*, 2000), showing disproportionate noun (object) deficit and also animacy effect (better with animate things than inanimate things) within the object domain, there are also cases that contradict the prediction of this theory (see discussion in Laiacona & Caramazza, 2004).

Bi *et al.* (2005, 2007) reported a Chinese-speaking case, ZBL, who showed a pattern that was opposite to ESFT predictions. ZBL suffered two strokes, and a MRI scan revealed a lesion in the territory of the left posterior cerebral artery. It involved the occipital lobe and extended into the mesial surface of the left temporal lobe and laterally into the temporal occipital junction. During the testing sessions after the acute stage, he showed mild difficulty in visual and auditory comprehension tasks and more severe deficits in oral production tasks. His naming errors were not due to any peripheral motor impairment, but instead, were predominantly semantic errors. Significantly, he was better at naming verb/action pictures orally than naming noun/object pictures ($\chi^2(1) = 7.43$, $p < 0.01$) orally. Given that the object pictures and action pictures were matched on various factors including word surface frequency, word token frequency, number of syllables, name agreement, age of acquisition and familiarity ratings (see details in Bi *et al.*, 2007), it is hard to argue that ZBL's noun/verb (object/action) oral naming differences were due to variations in the difficulty level. An attribute judgment task, where ZBL was required to decide whether an attribute of a given thing was true or false (for instance, 'a rooster has a short curly tail'), was used to examine ZBL's conceptual knowledge. The results indicated that in comparison with the control group, ZBL was impaired in attribute judgment for inanimate objects ($\chi^2(1) = 24.37$, $p < 0.0001$), but not for animate objects ($\chi^2(1) = 1.40$, $p = 0.24$). Furthermore, his performance on nonvisual features was better than his performance on visual features ($\chi^2(1) = 3.77$, $p = 0.05$). The difference was carried mainly by the inanimate objects (animate items: $\chi^2(1) = 1.26$, $p = 0.26$; inanimate items: $\chi^2(1) = 3.23$, $p = 0.07$). The reverse-animacy effect (better performance on animate things than inanimate things) was also observed in an oral picture-naming task to object pictures in a range of categories, again, after the control of various nuisance factors (lexical frequency and familiarity). The presence of the reverse-animacy effect and the disproportionate noun deficit compared with verbs for the same case, directly challenge the assumptions of ESFT.

The failure of one particular theory to account for the noun/verb (action/object) dissociation does not imply that noun and verb concepts do not differ in a systematic way. It is possible that the conceptual system is organized by modality-specific features and featural composition differences underlying noun/verb categories. The problem is the assumptions on deficit mechanisms. It is also possible that the assumptions on feature distributions should be modified (see Vigliocco *et al.*, 2004; Vinson *et al.*, 2003, for an alternative featural theory, FUSS). However, given the rich profiles of the brain-damaged cases with noun/verb dissociations that cannot be explained by existing conceptual theories, most likely, the grammatical class effects have other sources, such as the lexical and morphosyntactic processing.

Lexical organization of nouns and verbs

There is a line of evidence suggesting that the organization of the lexical system with regard to grammatical class distinction comes from cases with modality-specific grammatical deficits. Several cases have been reported to show the grammatical category-specific deficits in only one modality. For example, HW had selective difficulty in speaking verbs (oral picture naming and oral reading) and had intact ability in speaking nouns, writing both nouns and verbs (written picture naming and writing to dictation) (Caramazza & Hillis, 1991). Even when homonym pairs (e.g. 'the watch'/'to watch') were used, he was impaired when speaking the verbs ('to watch'), but not the nouns ('the watch'). Given that HW was flawless in writing tasks, his semantic knowledge of concepts was intact and his verb deficits in oral production cannot be attributed to a semantic basis. Such modality-specific selective grammatical class deficits led researchers to propose that the organization of the lexical system includes a grammatical dimension such that verbs can be selectively impaired within the phonological (output) lexicon (see also Caramazza & Hillis, 1991; Hillis *et al.*, 2002).

One might argue that the Chinese lexicon is less likely to be organized by grammatical categories because of an abundance of homographs/ homophones, the frequent nominal use of verbs and the prevalence of compounds with morphemes of various grammatical types. The observation of noun/verb dissociation at the lexical level in Chinese would be strong evidence that lexical distinctions are made along grammatical class dimensions. Indeed, there have not been any Chinese individuals documented with modality-specific selective noun or verb deficits until recently.

Han *et al.* (2005) presented a Chinese speaker, MPJ, with primary progressive aphasia, who suffered from atrophy of the left frontal and temporal lobes. He did not show significant noun/verb differences in visual comprehension (visual word-picture matching: nouns: 25/25; verbs: 22/25; $p = 0.23$) and oral word reading (nouns: 16/34; verbs: 11/34; $p = 0.22$). However, in written picture naming using the same well-matched stimulus sets that were mentioned earlier (see also Bi *et al.*, 2005, 2007, for detailed information), he wrote nouns (18/34) better than verbs (6/34) ($\chi^2(1) = 9.27$, $p < 0.01$). Such a pattern was replicated using an independent set of stimuli where nouns and verbs were matched on word frequency (nouns: 43/100; verbs: 14/100; $\chi^2(1) = 20.63$, $p < 0.001$). He was equally impaired with nouns and verbs in auditory comprehension and oral naming. However, because his performance in these two modalities was at floor, it was not certain whether the noun/verb difference was selective to the written production modality.

In a recent preliminary study, a Chinese dysgraphic case, SJS, was observed to show a noun/verb dissociation only in written naming. He was a 57-year-old, right-handed male with a college education. He demonstrated a relatively preserved ability in a variety of lexical comprehension and oral production tasks, including auditory word/picture matching (nouns: 25/25 correct; verbs: 24/25), visual word/picture matching (nouns: 25/25; verbs: 25/25) and oral picture naming (nouns: 31/34; verbs: 32/34). In contrast, he made frequent omission errors in written production tasks and showed more severe deficits for verbs than nouns, including written picture naming (nouns: 27/34; verbs: 17/34; $p < 0.05$) and writing to dictation (nouns: 30/34; verbs: 20/34; $p < 0.05$), using the same set of well matched noun/verb items that were tested on ZBL and MPJ. Such noun advantage in writing to dictation is not likely an attribute of sublexical mechanism because there is no grapheme-phoneme conversion in the writing of Chinese.

If one was to accept such modality-specific noun/verb difference as evidence for the existence of a grammatical dimension in the lexical system, how are compounds treated within such a lexical organization? As demonstrated in earlier in 'Chinese Grammatical System', Chinese compounds are quite often composed of morphemes from different grammatical classes, e.g. 開關 ('light-switch', open-close). Are words such as 'light-switch', represented in the noun 'section' or in the verb 'section'? Bates *et al.* (1991) argued that a straightforward distinction between a 'verb lexicon' and a 'noun lexicon' where compounds are treated as nouns and verbs by their composite class cannot be the full story. In their study, they found that Chinese-speaking individuals with Broca's aphasia named verb/action pictures worse than noun/object pictures. Individuals with Wernicke's aphasia named noun/object pictures worse than verb/action pictures. Most interestingly, they observed that Broca's individuals were significantly less likely to substitute the verbal element with another verb in V = vn compounds, while Wernicke's individuals were less able to substitute the nominal element with another noun in the same compound words. Based on these findings, Bates and colleagues postulated that there is a 'sublexical' level in which the grammatical category information also plays a role. Either the dissociation between verbs and nouns was due to the distinction of their sublexical level (nominal elements versus verbal elements) or that dissociation could occur both at the word level and at the sublexical level. It was further observed that the effects of the sublexical components were mostly present in Wernicke's individuals, but not in Broca's aphasic speakers. Under the assumption that the speakers with Wernicke's aphasia had more conceptual impairment than speakers with Broca's aphasia, the authors speculated that the distinction of nominal and verbal components in compounds had its roots in the semantic system.

However, subsequent studies failed to replicate the pattern described by Bates *et al.* (1991). For example, ZBL, who is described earlier with disproportionate noun deficits, was tested on three types of pictures (see Figure 10.1). The picture names corresponded to Chinese two-character compounds, including V = vn (跳水 /*tiao4shui3*/ 'to dive'), N = vn (講台 /*jiang3tai2*/ 'dais') and N = nn (火車 /*huo3che1*/ 'train'). Each type of word had 14 items. The items in the three types were matched on relevant variables including name agreement, concept agreement, familiarity, word frequency and syllable frequency. The task was oral picture naming. ZBL was better at naming V = vn pictures than N = vn pictures ($\chi^2(1) = 5.859$, $p < 0.05$), although the two classes of words had exactly the same sublexical structure. In contrast, he showed no difference between naming N = vn pictures and N = nn pictures ($\chi^2(1) < 1$) (see Figure 10.1). It seemed that only the grammatical class of the whole word, not the components, mattered. The same pattern was also observed in SJS, using this same set of stimuli, whose writing performance was affected by the grammatical class of the compound as a whole, but not its components (V = vn: 57% correct; N = vn: 79%; N = nn: 71%). As argued by Zhou *et al.* (1993), it is possible that some compounds in Bates *et al.*'s study were actually phrases and the 'sublexical' grammatical effects were lexical effects. It can also be argued that the lack of sublexical grammatical effect in ZBL and SJS were null results with the danger of Type II error. Further studies of the representation of compounds along grammatical class dimensions are necessary to resolve the issue.

Morphosyntactic processing of nouns and verbs

The grammatical category has also been proposed as a dimension along which syntactic processing and/or morphological processing of nouns

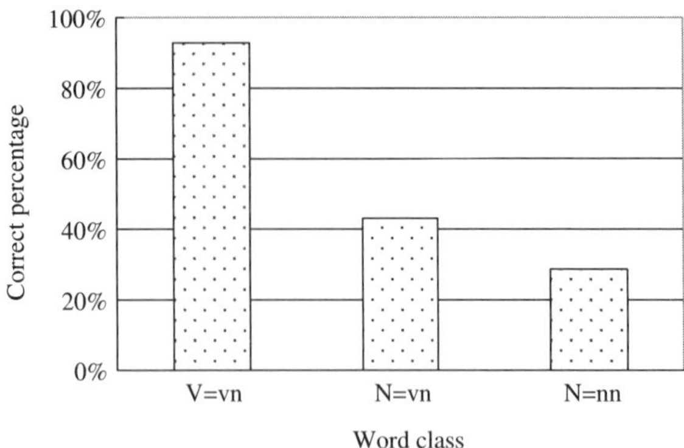

Figure 10.1 ZBL's performance as a function of grammatical word class in oral picture naming

and verbs operate differently. First, it is possible that nouns and verbs play different roles in sentence construction and a syntactic processing deficit might affect one class of words more than the other. For instance, it has been proposed that in comparison to nouns, verbs involve greater syntactic complexity in a sentence (see Berndt *et al.*, 1997a; Zingeser & Berndt, 1990, for discussion). In this case, when brain damage causes deficits of the representation and/or processing of syntactic knowledge, verbs will be more severely impaired than nouns. This syntactic account provides a reasonable interpretation of the origins for some verb-specific deficits (e.g. Kim & Thompson, 2000; Miceli *et al.*, 1984), but it has inherent difficulty in accounting for noun-specific deficits.

Morphosyntactic accounts argue that some noun/verb dissociation of speakers in picture-naming (or other single word naming) tasks can be due to the selective deficit of the morphological operation to one grammatical class. Evidence is derived from the association between picture-naming deficit of one grammatical class and the deficit in carrying morphological operations for that class. For example, JR (Shapiro *et al.*, 2000) had more difficulty in naming object pictures with nouns than in naming action pictures with verbs. When required to complete orally presented sentences with noun and verb homonyms that involved the addition/deletion of a nominal or verbal suffix (such as, 'This is a guide; these are ___'; 'This person guides, these people ___'), he was worse at producing nominal plural/singular forms than at producing verbal third-person singular/plural forms. The same pattern persisted even when pseudowords were used. For instance, JR was able to complete the sentence 'This person wugs, these people ___', but not the sentence 'These are wugs, this is a ___'. A reverse pattern was observed for the case of MR (Laiacona & Caramazza, 2004), who presented a selective deficit in processing verbal as opposed to nominal morphology. Based on these findings, it was proposed that morphosyntactic operations for nouns and verbs can be selectively impaired and it is one of the causes for the noun/verb dissociation observed in the noun/verb (object/action) naming tasks. It seems that content words are always 'inflected', even when a single word is produced in 'bare forms'.

Is it possible to explain the noun/verb dissociation of Chinese brain-damaged speakers by the grammatical processing to one particular class? On the one hand, the rare occurrence of morphological inflection on word forms in Chinese could mean that there is no comparable mechanism to be selectively impaired and to cause noun/verb dissociation in single word naming. The noun/verb dissociations in Chinese can only be explained by the conceptual and lexical account. If Chinese individuals with noun/verb dissociation have intact conceptual knowledge in both classes of words (e.g. SJS), then it becomes strong evidence for the theory that nouns and verbs are represented in the lexical system, such that they can be differentially affected.

Alternatively, it can be argued that the morphosyntactic processes for different grammatical classes have some abstract and universal properties that can be realized differently in various languages. While it is reflected by morphological inflection in Indo–European languages, the morphosyntactic process may underlie noun and verb production by other means in Chinese, for instance, by the association with the grammatical markers that were introduced in earlier in 'Chinese Grammatical System'. Information including aspects and numbers, can be expressed by certain grammatical markers, such as particles, classifiers, negative markers, etc. Some markers are related to nouns, such as determiners and classifiers, and some to verbs, such as negative markers and aspect markers. Law and Cheng (2002) developed a comprehensive 'Cloze test' to examine the production of these different types of grammatical morphemes in Cantonese aphasia. A wide range of grammatical morphemes was investigated in the test, including aspect markers, negative markers, classifiers, proforms, coverbs, particles and structural particles. They studied six fluent and four non-fluent Cantonese-speaking individuals with aphasia, along with five control participants. The participants were required to supply the missing elements of the sentences in highly constrained contexts. For example, to complete a sentence stimulus '弟弟係男仔; 妹妹係男仔' *dai4dai2hai6naam4zai2; mui4mui2__hai6naam4-zai2* 'the brother is a boy; the sister_is a boy', a negative marker 唔 *m4* is required '弟弟係男仔; 妹妹_唔係男仔' *dai4dai2hai6naam4zai2; mui4-mui2 m4 hai6naam4zai2* 'the brother is a boy; the sister isn't a boy'. They compared the relative accessibility of different grammatical morphemes between different aphasia types. The results revealed a tendency for better performance in the individuals with fluent aphasia for various morpheme types, relative to the speakers with non-fluent aphasia. However, the difference between the two groups was quantitative rather than qualitative. This is not surprising because it is now known that these 'syndrome' groups are not homogeneous and standardizing cases with different underlying deficit mechanism can be misleading.

It is proposed that further investigation along this line would be to study whether grammatical markers of one particular type can be selectively impaired by brain damage and the relationship between such categorical effects and the grammatical class effect in single word production. For instance, if a brain-damaged individual is observed to have more difficulty in producing verbs (action names) than producing nouns (object names) in picture naming or other naming tasks, the question that may be asked is whether she or he also shows a selective deficit in producing grammatical markers for verbs, e.g. aspect markers and coverbs compared to nominal grammatical markers, such as classifiers. It is known that individuals showing noun/verb dissociation do not necessarily show dissociation between nominal markers and verbal markers at the same time, given that some noun/verb dissociation may have a conceptual cause. However, it is an open issue whether a speaker with a selective deficit in grammatical markers of one class will also show more severe difficulty in single content word production in the corresponding category. If such association is prevalent, it would be evidence that is consistent with the view that morphosyntactic processes are universal and sensitive to grammatical classes. However, if cases are observed that have selective impairment to grammatical markers of one grammatical class, but intact single word production, they would suggest that lexical retrieval of content words and the corresponding grammatical markers are rather independent. It would also mean that the grammatical effects for single word naming in Chinese are not readily explained by some of the grammatical class effect in the morphosyntactic processes.

Future Directions

It has been argued that selective deficits to one grammatical class of words (nouns or verbs) displayed by individuals with brain damage offer an opportunity to study the representation and processing of grammatical knowledge in the brain. With the understanding that there are heterogeneous causes for such dissociations, the following lines are proposed for future research.

To isolate the different sources of noun/verb dissociation, the focus should be more on single cases, using tasks and test stimuli with more dimensions of manipulation. For example, using the materials of abstract nouns and verbs helps discriminate the conceptual explanation from others. Also, cross-linguistic comparisons would be particularly informative in unveiling the core, universal aspects of grammatical processing. In this context, it is crucial to integrate multiple research methods, including the cognitive neuropsychological approach with brain-damaged individuals and functional imaging and behavioral techniques with normal subjects.

Instead of finding a unified reason for the observed noun/verb dissociation in clinical settings, the goal for this line of pursuit is to answer the following questions: how is the knowledge of a word being a noun or a verb represented and processed in the brain? How is conceptual knowledge organized? How are lexical knowledge and grammatical operations integrated together? In other words, how does the brain know that a noun is a noun and use it as a noun?

Notes

1. Corresponding author.
2. Whenever we cannot distinguish these two dimensions, we acknowledge such confound by using these two sets of terms interchangeably. The major limitation of this explanation is that it is unspecified for the presentation manner of abstract nouns and abstract verbs (see Laiacona & Caramazza, 2004).

References

Bastiaanse, R. (1995) Broca's aphasia: A syntactic and/or a morphological disorder? A case study. *Brain and Language* 48, 1–32.

Bates, E., Chen, S., Tzeng, O., Li, P. and Opie, M. (1991) The noun-verb problem in Chinese. *Brain and Language* 41, 203–233.

Berndt, R., Haendiges, A., Mitchum, C. and Sandson, J. (1997a) Verb retrieval in aphasia. 2. Relationship to sentence processing. *Brain and Language* 56, 107–137.

Berndt, R., Mitchum, C., Haendiges, A. and Sandson, J. (1997b) Verb retrieval in aphasia. 1. Characterizing single word impairments. *Brain and Language* 56, 68–106.

Bi, Y., Han, Z., Shu, H. and Caramazza, A. (2005) Are verbs like inanimate objects? *Brain and Language* 95, 28–29.

Bi, Y., Han, Z., Shu, H. and Caramazza, A. (2007) Nouns, verbs, objects, actions, and the animate/inanimate effect. *Cognitive Neuropsychology* 24, 485–504.

Bird, H., Howard, D. and Franklin, S. (2000) Why is a verb like an inanimate object? Grammatical category and semantic category deficits. *Brain and Language* 72, 246–309.

Bird, H., Howard, D. and Franklin, S. (2001) Noun-verb difference? A question of semantics: A response to Shapiro and Caramazza. *Brain and Language* 76, 213–222.

Bornstein, M.H., Cote, L.R., Maital, S., Painter, K., Park, S.Y., Pascual, L. *et al.* (2004) Cross-linguistic analysis of vocabulary in young children: Spanish, Dutch, French, Hebrew, Italian, Korean, and American English. *Child Development* 75, 1115–1139.

Breedin, S., Saffran, E. and Schwartz, M. (1998) Semantic factors in verb retrieval: An effect of complexity. *Brain and Language* 63, 1–31.

Caramazza, A., Berndt, R.S., Basili, A.G. and Koller, J.J. (1981) Syntactic processing deficits in aphasia. *Cortex* 17, 333–348.

Caramazza, A. and Hillis, A.E. (1991) Lexical organization of nouns and verbs in the brain. *Nature* 349, 788–790.

Damasio, A.R. and Tranel, D. (1993) Nouns and verbs are retrieved with differently distributed neural systems. *Proceeding of the National Academy of Sciences* 90, 4957–4960.

Denes, G. and Barba, G.D. (1998) G.B. Vico, Precursor of cognitive neuropschology? The first reported case of noun-verb dissociation following brain damage. *Brain and Language* 62, 29–33.

Federmeier, K.D., Segal, J.B., Lombrozo, T. and Kutas, M. (2000) Brain response to nouns, verbs and class-ambiguous words in context. *Brain* 12, 2552–2566.

Han, Z., Shu, H., Zhang, Y. and Zhou, Y. (2005) A primary progressive aphasic patient with verb specific deficits. *Chinese Journal of Clinical Rehabilitation* 9, 58–59.

Hillis, A.E. and Caramazza, A. (1995) Representation of grammatical categories of words in the brain. *Journal of Cognitive Neuroscience* 7, 396–407.

Hillis, A.E., Wityk, R.J., Barker, P.B. and Caramazza, A. (2002) Neural regions essential for writing verbs. *Nature Neuroscience* 6, 19–20.

Kim, M. and Thompson, C. (2000) Patterns of comprehension and production of nouns and verbs in agrammatism: Implications for lexical organization. *Brain and Language* 74, 1–25.

Kohn, S., Lorch, M. and Pearson, D. (1989) Verb finding in aphasia. *Cortex* 25, 57–69.

Laiacona, M. and Caramazza, A. (2004) The noun/verb dissociation in language production: Varieties of cases. *Cognitive Neuropsychology* 21, 103–124.

Law, S.P. and Cheng, M.Y. (2002) Production of grammatical morphemes in Cantonese aphasia. *Aphasiology* 16, 693–714.

Li, P., Jin, Z. and Tan, L.H. (2004) Neural representations of nouns and verbs in Chinese: An fMRI study. *NeuroImage* 21, 1533–1541.

Marshall, J., Chiat, S., Robson, J. and Pring, T. (1996a) Calling a salad a federation: An investigation of semantic jargon. Part 2-verbs. *Journal of Neurolinguistics* 9, 251–260.

Marshall, J., Pring, T., Chiat, S. and Robson, J. (1996b) Calling a salad a federation: An investigation of semantic jargon. Part 1-nouns. *Journal of Neurolinguistics* 9, 237–250.

McCarthy, R. and Warrington, E. (1985) Category specificity in an agrammatic patient: The relative impairment of verb retrieval and comprehension. *Neuropsychologia* 23, 709–727.

Miceli, G., Mazzucchi, A., Menn, L. and Goodglass, H. (1983) Contrasting cases of Italian agrammatic aphasia without comprehension disorder. *Brain and Language* 19, 65–97.

Miceli, G., Silveri, M.C., Nocentini, U. and Caramazza, A. (1988) Patterns of dissociation in comprehension and production of nouns and verbs. *Aphasiology* 2, 351–358.

Miceli, G., Silveri, M.C., Villa, G. and Caramazza, A. (1984) On the basis for agrammatics difficulty in producing main verbs. *Cortex* 20, 207–220.

Nespoulous, J.L., Dordain, M., Perron, C., Ska, B., Bub, D., Caplan, D. *et al.* (1988) Agrammatism in sentence production without comprehension deficits:

Reduced availability of syntactic structures and/or grammatical morphemes? *Brain and Language* 33, 273–295.
Packard, J.L. (1993) *A Linguistic Investigation of Aphasic Chinese Speech.* Dordrecht: Kluwer Academic.
Rapp, B. and Caramazza, A. (1997) The modality-specific organization of grammatical categories: Evidence from impaired spoken and written sentence production. *Brain and Language* 56, 248–286.
Rapp, B. and Caramazza, A. (1998) A case of selective difficulty in writing verbs. *Neurocase* 4, 127–140.
Robinson, G., Rossor, M. and Cipolotti, L. (1999) Selective sparing of verb naming in a case of severe Alzheimer's disease. *Cortex* 35, 443–450.
Shapiro, K. and Caramazza, A. (2001) Sometimes a noun is just a noun: Comments on Bird, Howard, and Franklin (2000). *Brain and Language* 76, 202–212.
Shapiro, K. and Caramazza, A. (2003) The representation of grammatical categories in the brain. *Trends in Cognitive Sciences* 7, 201–206.
Shapiro, K., Moo, L. and Caramazza, A. (2006) Cortical signatures of noun and verb production. *Proceedings of the National Academy of Sciences* 130, 1644–1649.
Shapiro, K., Shelton, J. and Caramazza, A. (2000) Grammatical class in lexical production and morphological processing: Evidence from a case of fluent aphasia. *Cognitive Neuropsychology* 17, 665–682.
Silveri, M. and di Betta, A. (1997) Noun-verb dissociation in brain-damaged patients: Further evidence. *Neurocase* 3, 477–488.
Tardif, T. (1996) Nouns are not always learned before verbs: Evidence from Mandarin speakers' early vocabulary. *Developmental Psychology* 32, 492–504.
Tardif, T., Shatz, M. and Naigles, L. (1997) Caregiver speech and children's use of nouns versus verbs: A comparison of English, Italian, and Chinese. *Journal of Child Language* 24, 535–565.
Tardif, T., Susan, G. and Fan, X. (1999) Putting the 'noun bias' in context: A comparison of English and Mandarin. *Child Development* 70, 620–635.
Tyler, L.K., Bright, P., Fletcher, P. and Stamatakis, E.A. (2004) Neural processing of nouns and verbs: The role of inflectional morphology. *Neuropsychologia* 42, 512–523.
Vigliocco, G., Vinson, D.P., Lewis, W. and Garrett, M.F. (2004) Representation the meanings of object and action words: The featural and unitary semantic space hypothesis. *Cognitive Psychology* 48, 422–488.
Vinson, D.P., Vigliocco, G., Cappa, S. and Siri, S. (2003) The breakdown of semantic knowledge along semantic field boundaries: Insights from an empirically-driven statistical model of meaning representation. *Brain and Language* 86, 347–365.
Whorf, B. (1956) Linguistic relativity, science and linguistics. In J.B. Carroll (ed.) *Language, Thought, and Reality: Selected Writings of Benjamin Lee Whorf.* Cambridge, MA: MIT Press.
Williams, S.E. and Canter, C.J. (1997) Action-naming performance in four syndromes of aphasia. *Brain and Language* 32, 124–136.
Zhou, X.L., Ostrin, R.K. and Tyler, L.K. (1993) The noun-verb problem and Chinese aphasia: Comments on Bates *et al.* 1991. *Brain and Language* 45, 86–93.
Zingeser, L. and Berndt, R. (1990) Retrieval of nouns and verbs in agrammatism and aphasia. *Brain and Language* 39, 14–32.

Chapter 11

Acquired Reading Disorders in Chinese: Implications for Models of Reading

BRENDAN S. WEEKES, I FAN SU and WENGANG YIN

Much of the progress in our understanding of communication disorders in Indo–European languages has come from cognitive neuropsychological studies of brain damaged individuals who have selective disorders of reading (dyslexia), spelling and writing (dysgraphia). This is the cognitive neuropsychological approach to investigating reading and writing disorders first pioneered by Marshall and Newcombe (1966, 1973) and colleagues such as Coltheart (1982, 1984), Hillis and Caramazza (1995), Patterson (1990) and Patterson and Lambon Ralph (1999). Our motivation for this chapter is to review reports of individuals who have acquired dyslexia in Chinese following brain damage. Note that, unless noted, we will consider oral reading of single characters only. These reports have led to the development of a functional architecture of the normal reading system in Chinese that we describe in detail. In the final part of the chapter, we will consider whether computational models of reading can explain the extant patterns of acquired dyslexia in Chinese.

Acquired Dyslexia

There are different types of acquired dyslexia reported in the neuropsychological literature and these fall into two categories: (1) central disorders that are called surface, phonological and deep caused by problems with memory and language processing and (2) peripheral disorders that are caused by problems with vision, attention and motor control.

The classic type of peripheral dyslexia is called *pure alexia*. In 30 AD, Valerius Maximus described a man who was struck on the head by an axe and became word blind, losing his memory for letters with no other defects including preserved writing. In the late 19th century, 'word blindness' was defined by the French neurologist Dejerine as pure alexia because it is the only form of acquired dyslexia in which writing and spelling can be unaffected, i.e. alexia without agraphia. In pure alexia, single letter recognition is usually intact and the comprehension and production of spoken language is normal. Pure alexia has also been referred to as 'letter-by-letter reading' because individuals use an oral spelling strategy to recognise written words, e.g. cap → 'C', 'A', 'P'. A striking feature of pure alexia is that individuals are unable to read aloud words they have themselves just written. Individuals appear to decode words as a sequence of isolate letters without any access to the holistic process that is used by the normal reader. Letter-by-letter reading appears to arise from a disconnection that prevents the parallel mapping of abstract letter identities onto word level representations so that access to word forms becomes slow and sequential. Reading of words and nonwords is slow and reading time is a linear function of the number of letters in a letter string.

Reports of pure alexia in Chinese are rare probably because – as letters do not exist in Chinese – it is not possible to observe letter-by-letter reading. However, Yin and Butterworth (1998) reported a phenomenon called radical-by-radical reading in an individual who suffered damage to the left occipital lobe and the splenium. Their participant would read aloud the components of a character instead of the whole character itself suggesting a loss of knowledge about the orthographic form of the whole word – a type of word blindness. However, pure alexia in Chinese cannot be identical to pure alexia in alphabetic scripts.

Acquired *surface dyslexia* in alphabetic languages refers to a selective impairment when reading aloud of irregularly spelled words, particularly if items are low in word frequency, e.g. *indict*. Approximately 25% of words in English are irregular words, some of which are referred to as exception words because they contain violations of English spelling-to-sound rules. When an exception word is misread, oral reading is characterised by regularisation errors when reading the components of a word, e.g. *pint* is pronounced as though it rhymed with *mint*. In pure cases this impairment is accompanied by preserved reading of regularly spelled words and made up/invented nonwords, e.g. *zint*. Acquired surface dysgraphia refers to misspellings of irregularly spelled words, e.g. *yacht* → *yot*, together with homophone confusions in writing, e.g. writing the word *stake* when asked to write the sentence 'He had steak for dinner' (Weekes & Coltheart, 1996).

Surface dyslexia and dysgraphia are often coincident in the same individual, but each disorder can be observed in isolation (Behrmann & Bub, 1992). Surface dyslexia is most often observed in individuals who have semantic dementia (Woollams *et al.*, 2007). This brain disease results in a progressive deterioration of semantic knowledge that is due to brain atrophy in the temporal lobes. Surface dyslexia is also observed in cases of developmental dyslexia, which is a learning difficulty in individuals without known neurological abnormality (Castles & Coltheart, 1993). These individuals learn to sound out words phonetically using letter-sound rules, but have problems learning a sight vocabulary. Thus, exception words tend to be regularised in developmental surface dyslexia. Acquired and developmental surface dyslexia can be treated using a mnemonic technique to restore whole words into the lexicon (Weekes & Coltheart, 1996).

A different pattern of impairment is acquired *phonological dyslexia*, which refers to impaired reading of nonwords together with a preserved ability to read aloud irregular and regular words. There are no reported cases of phonological dyslexia where nonword reading is impaired and word reading is 100% correct, making the disorder a relative rather than absolute difficulty with nonword reading. Some individuals with phonological dyslexia are impaired at decoding letter-strings into constituent graphemes. A grapheme is a letter or string of letters that represents an individual speech sound or phoneme – e.g. the string SHOOF has the three graphemes SH, OO and F. Other individuals have difficulty assigning correct phonemes to graphemes and others have difficulty in blending together a sequence of phonemes into an integrated pronunciation. Phonological dysgraphia refers to poor spelling of non-words accompanied by preserved spelling of irregular and regular words. Phonological dyslexia also occurs in developmental dyslexia (Castles & Coltheart, 1993). These children have trouble with the phonic side of reading – that is, in learning to sound out words by letter-sound rules. They have less trouble with developing a sight vocabulary. Phonological dyslexia can be treated using training methods that are focussed on learning phonic letter-to-sound rules (de Partz, 1986; de Partz *et al.*, 1992). Deep dyslexia is a severe form of phonological dyslexia where individuals produce semantic errors, e.g. *arm* read as *finger*; visual errors, e.g. *bus* read as *brush*; and morphological errors, e.g. *run* read as *running*. All individuals with deep dyslexia have left-hemisphere damage sufficient to produce aphasia (Broca's). Deep dyslexics read concrete (highly imageable) words, e.g. *tulip*, better than abstract words, e.g. *idea*. Reading of nonwords and function words (and, or) is impossible. Deep dysgraphic individuals produce analogous errors in spelling, e.g. *symphony* → *orchestra* (Raman & Weekes, 2005b).

The difference between phonological dyslexia and deep dyslexia is subtle. In both disorders, nonword reading is impaired relative to word reading. Also some phonological dyslexic individuals show the same pattern of impairment as deep dyslexic individuals, i.e. poor reading of abstract words compared to concrete words and function words compared to content words. However, phonological and deep dyslexia are distinct reading disorders because individuals with phonological dyslexia do not make semantic errors when reading aloud. There is evidence that deep dyslexia, but not phonological dyslexia, results from reading via the intact right hemisphere following extensive left hemisphere damage (Weekes *et al.*, 1997b). According to the right hemisphere hypothesis, semantic errors are not produced in phonological dyslexia because activation in the left hemisphere is sufficient to inhibit these errors. Phonological and deep dyslexia are debilitating conditions. Nevertheless, they respond well to intensive treatment focussed on learning phonic letter-to-sound rules.

The patterns of central acquired dyslexia and dysgraphia reported in English are also observed in other languages including Arabic (Beland & Mimouni, 2001), Dutch (Diesfeldt, 1992), Finnish (Laine *et al.*, 1990), French (Beland & Mimouni, 2001; Cardebat *et al.*, 1991; Goldblum, 1985; Majerus *et al.*, 2001; Valdois *et al.*, 1995), Japanese (Fushimi *et al.*, 2003; Patterson *et al.*, 1995, 1998), Italian (Angelelli *et al.*, 2004; Luzzi *et al.*, 2003; Miceli & Caramazza, 1993; Miozzo & de Bastiani, 2002) and Spanish (Ardilla, 1991; Cuetos, 1993; Cuetos & Labos, 2001; Cuetos *et al.*, 1995, 2003; Iribarren *et al.*, 2001; Ruiz *et al.*, 1994). Although the characteristics of reading and writing disorders vary across scripts, these reports reveal dissociable symptoms of dyslexia and dysgraphia (see Weekes [2005] for further examples).

Acquired Dyslexia in Chinese

Several patterns of acquired dyslexia in Chinese have been reported (Law, 2004; Law & Or, 2000, 2001; Weekes & Chen, 1999; Yin & Butterworth, 1992). Yin and Butterworth report aphasic Mandarin speakers with cerebrovascular disease who displayed patterns of impaired and preserved oral reading that resembled features of deep and surface dyslexia in other languages. For example, one group showed a tendency to produce semantic errors on reading tasks and produced more errors to low-imageability characters compared to high-imageability characters matched for word frequency. Some individuals who they termed deep dyslexic produced semantic errors when reading aloud. For example, ZSP, a 36-year-old male, produced semantic errors such as reading 風 *feng* meaning 'wind' as 刮 *gua* meaning 'blow'; visual errors 木 *mu* meaning 'wood' as 才 *cai* meaning 'just'; mixed-target with errors sharing a signific 狗 *gou* meaning 'dog' as 豬 *zhu* meaning 'pig'. There was also a pattern of better reading of nouns than verbs and function words (a grammatical class effect).

Other dyslexic individuals produced 'regularisation' or more precisely legitimate alternative reading of component (LARC) errors when they read irregular characters aloud. A LARC error in Chinese is an incorrect pronunciation of an irregular character that is appropriate in other characters containing the same component. So, for example, if 秤 *cheng* is read as 平 *ping*, this is a LARC error. Chinese surface dyslexic individuals also tend to read homographic heterophones out of word context as reported in Law (2004). Homographic heterophones are phonologically ambiguous characters similar to the words wind, read and lead. This pattern of reading errors suggests that characters are read without semantic support (cf. Patterson & Hodges, 1992). Yin and Butterworth (1992) reported a positive association between semantic impairment and production of LARC errors, suggesting that lexical-semantic knowledge has an impact on the ability to read irregular characters in Chinese. This makes intuitive sense given the relationship between orthography and phonology is arbitrary for most characters so, unlike reading aloud in alphabetic scripts, knowing the name of components will not automatically afford the pronunciation of the character.

Weekes and Chen (1999) also reported a Chinese speaker with surface dyslexia. Following the results of Yin and Butterworth (1992), they formulated a hypothesis about their subject's reading based on reports of an association between surface dyslexia and lexical-semantic impairment in Chinese and other languages. Weekes and Chen reasoned that the correct reading of irregular, low frequency, abstract characters requires support from semantic memory, and LARC errors are the result of loss of semantic support from the lexical-semantic pathway used to read in Chinese. This hypothesis was motivated by theoretical accounts of reading in English which assume knowledge of word meaning – accessed via a lexical-semantic pathway – inhibits LARC errors produced when reading words that have unpredictable components (see e.g. Patterson & Hodges, 1992). Note that word regularity in English refers to whether a word conforms to grapheme to phoneme correspondence (GPC) rules and, as Chinese does not contain graphemes or GPC rules, then regularity in Chinese is not equivalent to English. It was clear from the results of Weekes and Chen that semantic impairment was associated with poor reading of irregular characters particularly if the characters were low in word imageability and word frequency.

Another type of dyslexia reported in Chinese is called *tonal dyslexia*. This describes the phenomenon of preserved oral reading of a character at the syllable level, but incorrect assignment of tone for that syllable. Some dyslexic individuals produce tonal errors in reading/writing words even though segmental phonology is preserved in their responses (Law & Or, 2001). Others produce tonal errors in addition to errors at the level of the onset (the optional initial consonant or consonant cluster of the syllable) and the rime (the obligatory vowel (the nucleus) and the optional final consonants). Luo and Weekes (2004) reported a Putonghua speaker, ZW, who produced onset errors, rime errors and tonal errors. Among tonal errors, 85% were substitutions of Tone 4 for Tones 1, 2 and 3. Luo and Weekes also found that ZW produced rime errors that included responses with none of the vowel components correct (whole rime substitutions) and errors with one vowel/phoneme wrong, including omission errors (omissions of the coda) and addition errors (additions of the medial and the coda). Of interest, all of the erroneous responses were extant syllables in Chinese, i.e. they were meaningful and no responses were nonextant syllables in Chinese.

The results from these dyslexic individuals suggest important facts about the representation of information in the Chinese speech production system. First, because extant syllables were produced as errors, these are represented at the level of the phonological output lexicon. Second, subsyllabic information might also be represented by components in the Chinese phonological output lexicon because vowel and onset errors were also observed. Third, tonal information can be dissociated from the syllable level.

Models of Reading

Computational models

One goal of cognitive neuropsychological studies of individuals with acquired dyslexia is the development of cognitive models of reading and writing. These models are widely used in the assessment and rehabilitation of reading and writing impairments in English. Coltheart *et al.* (2001) proposed a 'multiroute' model to explain normal oral reading as well as acquired disorders of oral reading in English. The model assumes that a *lexical-semantic* pathway is available for reading known words in addition to a *direct lexical* pathway that reads words aloud without contacting meaning. A third route, called the *non-lexical* pathway, is also assumed and is mandatory for reading nonwords, available for reading regular words, but cannot read irregular words correctly. A radically different theoretical approach is characterised by the connectionist principles of cognitive processing. These models eschew whole-word representations in favour of subword components in onset, vowel and coda positions. Plaut *et al.* (1996) proposed a model of reading based on connectionist principles of subsymbolic processing. Their model assumes bidirectional pathways for reading and for spelling (see Seidenberg & McClelland, 1989). Plaut *et al.* use the terms *semantic* and *phonological* pathways instead of lexical-semantic or non-lexical grapheme to phoneme pathways. The distinction between dual-route and connectionist models is that the former assume independent direct lexical and semantic pathways whereas connectionist models do not. Plaut *et al.* also assume that the reading (and spelling) of nonwords proceeds via the phonological pathway and is performed using a process of analogy with existing subword representations, rather than relying on symbolic letter-to-sound rules.

These models give contrasting accounts of acquired dyslexia in English. According to the multiroute model, surface dyslexia results from damage to the direct lexical and/or the lexical-semantic pathways leading to over-reliance on the non-lexical route for reading aloud. This explains the tendency to regularisation of irregular words using knowledge of letter-to-sound rules in surface dyslexia. Phonological dyslexia results from impairment to the non-lexical pathway with preserved lexical and semantic pathways. This explains the selective inability to read nonwords. Even when the non-lexical pathway is damaged, word reading is possible because the lexical reading route can be used. Deep dyslexia might arise from a loss of the lexical and non-lexical pathways following extensive left hemisphere damage so that reading is exclusively semantic. Surface dysgraphia could result from loss of the lexical-semantic pathway and phonological/deep dysgraphia from a loss of the non-lexical pathway (Houghton & Zorzi, 2003).

According to connectionist models (Plaut *et al.*, 1996), surface dyslexia results from impairment to the semantic pathway due to damaged representations in semantic memory or the bidirectional mappings linking orthographic representations and phonological representations. Similarly, surface dysgraphia could arise from damage to semantic memory or mappings between semantics and orthography (Graham *et al.*, 1997, 2000). This leads to over-reliance on the phonological pathway for reading and spelling. Phonological dyslexia and dysgraphia result from damage to the phonological pathway, which might be abolished in deep dyslexia according to connectionist models (Friedman, 1996). Note that Hillis and Caramazza (1995) also developed a summation account of oral reading (and spelling) that assumes the basic dual-route architecture.

Although multiroute and connectionist models make different assumptions about the cause of impairment in acquired dyslexia, each model assumes that selective damage to independent pathways linking orthography and phonology is possible and damage will lead to different patterns of acquired dyslexia. Thus, all models can explain the patterns of acquired dyslexia seen in English-speaking individuals. These models have also been applied to explaining disorders of reading and writing observed in other Indo–European languages and in bilingual speakers including languages with distinctive orthographies. This is illustrated by a report of a French–Arabic speaker by Beland and Mimouni (2001) who showed characteristics of deep dyslexia when reading in both the Latin (French) and Semitic (Arabic) alphabets (see also Fabbro, 1999; Raman & Weekes, 2005a).

One question of interest is whether different models can explain oral reading in nonalphabetic scripts. For example, the logographic nature of characters makes it likely that lexical knowledge (orthographic or phonological) will be used for reading characters correctly. Because the Plaut *et al.* (1996) model does not contain lexical representations (only subword components), it is not clear how their model would explain oral reading in Chinese even though functional units, such as the rime, may be important for oral reading in both scripts. Similarly, a non-lexical pathway is redundant for oral reading in Chinese because graphemes are orthographic representations of phonemes that are used in an alphabet. By this definition grapheme representations may not exist in Chinese. Moreover, the logographic nature of Chinese characters makes it difficult to test nonword reading in an equivalent way in alphabetic and nonalphabetic scripts. This also means that an equivalent to phonological and deep dyslexia cannot be found in Chinese.

Models of reading in Chinese

Weekes *et al.* (1997a) argued that normal oral reading in Chinese proceeds via two pathways: the lexical-semantic pathway that supports reading for meaning, and a nonsemantic pathway that connects representations of orthography, i.e. strokes, radicals and characters, to phonological representations including syllables, rimes and tones. This framework for oral reading in Chinese is depicted in Figure 11.1. Weekes *et al.* proposed this framework following their report of an anomic individual, YQS, who could not name common objects, but who nevertheless displayed intact reading of high-imageability characters

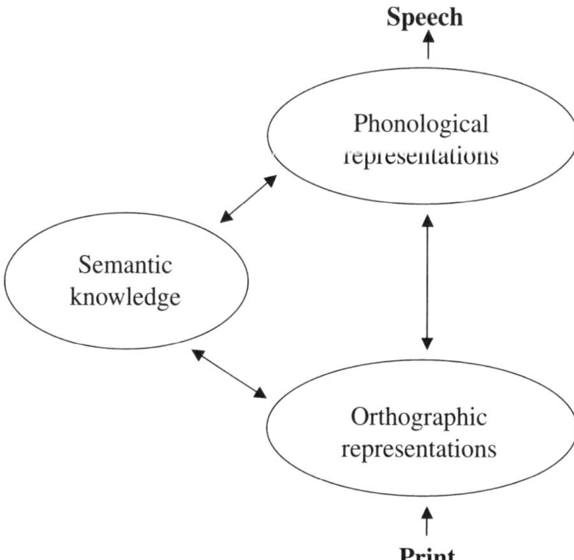

Figure 11.1 Cognitive neuropsychological framework for oral reading and writing in Chinese

(nouns) including the printed names of objects that she could not name from pictures. Weekes *et al.* called this phenomenon *anomia without dyslexia* in Chinese and interpreted this pattern according to the framework depicted in Figure 11.1.

The framework assumes that oral reading can be preserved despite a disconnection between semantic and phonological representations that lead to impaired confrontation naming and category fluency in anomia. The pattern of poor picture naming with superior reading of characters has subsequently been replicated by Weekes and Chen (1999) in another Putonghua-speaking individual (see also Han *et al.*, 2005) and by Law and Or (2001) who reported that CML showed a similar pattern of spared oral reading coincident with impaired naming performance (see also Law, 2004; Law *et al.*, 2005). Note that this framework can explain writing to dictation via direct access from semantics to orthography and a nonsemantic pathway in Chinese (Law & Or, 2000) if bidirectional mappings between orthography and phonology are assumed.

The cognitive neuropsychological framework in Figure 11.1 is not a computational model. A computational model is an advance over frameworks such as these because it requires a more precise set of parameters than those specified in the framework. Different levels of units are assumed in the framework in Figure 11.1, but few details are given. For example, is the phonological representation of the morpheme 糖 *tang2* 'candy' represented twice, once alone as *ang* and once within the syllable *tang2*? When reading 糖, are both *ang* and *tang* activated and how are these eventually selected? These questions require a specific set of parameters to be specified and one advantage of computational models is they require precision. This potentially allows a computational model to explain development of literacy – instantiated in terms of learning mechanisms connecting input (orthography) with output (phonology) – in addition to impairments to skilled reading and writing. We now turn to an evaluation of computational models of word identification and oral reading in Chinese. Although the primary aim of current computational models is to account for skilled word recognition in Chinese, studies of individuals with acquired dyslexia and dysgraphia have influenced the development of computational models of reading and writing in alphabetic languages (Houghton & Zorzi, 2003; Plaut *et al.*, 1996).

Computational models of reading in Chinese

All theorists agree that there are at least two independent pathways for reading and spelling in English: one that proceeds via semantic knowledge and another that makes no contact with meaning, i.e. a nonsemantic pathway. This consensus was reached in part by the requirement to accommodate patterns of preserved and impaired reading and spelling in individuals who have acquired dyslexia and dysgraphia. Although there is still debate about the success of computational models in explaining reading of nonwords and whether a lexical nonsemantic pathway is required, theorists agree that a complete model of reading needs to explain the data from acquired dyslexia.

The computational model proposed by Plaut *et al.* (1996) was not designed to explain reading in Chinese and we have argued that there are problems extending these models to explaining reading in Chinese. However, Perfetti *et al.* (2005) have proposed a general computational framework for reading across writing systems, called the lexical constituency (LC) model, and described in detail an implementation of their model to oral reading in Chinese. This is illustrated in Figure 11.2.

Like the framework in Figure 11.1, the LC model assumes two pathways from orthography to phonology. One pathway links orthography to phonology via semantics comprising connections from orthography to semantics and connections from semantics to phonology (similar to the lexical-semantic pathway in Figure 11.1), and the other links orthography to phonology directly (similar to the nonsemantic pathway in Figure 11.1). However, unlike the framework in Figure 11.1, the LC model assumes a level of representation referred to as radical units. These map directly to an additional level of orthography representing characters. One reason for assuming radicals are necessary is that Chinese script is not systematic enough to support a component approach to reading – unlike letters in an alphabet. It is important to note that (1) separate levels of representation may be redundant in alphabetic scripts because letter representations are input to computational simulations, and in most simulations it is not necessary to assume separate word level representations and (2) contact between radical units and semantic and phonological knowledge is always mediated by character

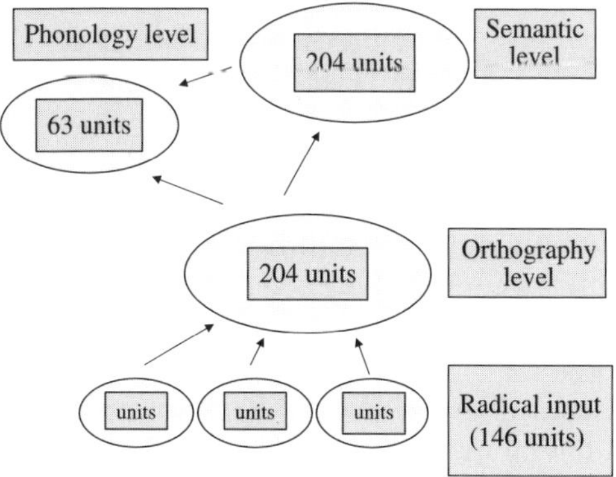

Figure 11.2 The lexical constituency model adapted from Perfetti *et al.* (2005)

knowledge. Another difference is that computational models of oral reading in English assume that subword knowledge is available in normal oral reading – whether it is symbolic, e.g. GPC rules, or subsymbolic (Plaut *et al.*) – whereas Perfetti *et al.* do not.

Perfetti *et al.* (2005) demonstrate that their model can simulate priming of normal word identification in Chinese. However, we are not concerned with the success of their model in explaining these behavioural phenomena. The question we pose here is whether the model can explain known facts about disorders of reading in Chinese. We will begin with cognitive neuropsychological data that we believe the model does explain and then describe data that appears to be a challenge for the model. The LC model needs to explain why some individuals produce semantic reading errors and others produce LARC errors (Weekes & Chen, 1999; Yin & Butterworth, 1992, 1998) and read ambiguous characters out-of-context (Law, 2004). Semantic, LARC and out-of-context errors are revealing because they suggest that oral reading in Chinese involves multiple levels of cognitive processing. Semantic errors show that knowledge about character meaning is activated whereas LARC and out-of-context errors show that the knowledge about the mappings between orthography and phonology in character components is activated during oral reading – albeit at a level that is insufficient to support correct oral reading in individuals with dyslexia. Perfetti *et al.*'s model assumes that character recognition involves lexical identification at semantic and phonological levels. Therefore, the model can accommodate semantic errors as reading via meaning, i.e. without access to the mappings between orthography and phonology, and conversely LARC and out-of-context errors as evidence of oral reading via those same mappings (without support from the semantic system). By assuming two independent pathways, the model also explains anomia without dyslexia as a consequence of reading via the nonsemantic pathway.

Any model of reading in Chinese must explain the effect of tone on literacy. Tone awareness is one predictor of literacy for Chinese-speaking children (Siok & Fletcher, 2001) and is independent of knowledge of syllables and orthographic awareness. Chen *et al.* (2002) observed priming effects on adult reading for syllables but not for tone (and vice versa), suggesting independent representations for syllable and tone. The LC model assumes phonology is a fully distributed representation that is implemented with the Chinese *pinyin* system. The model assumes a set of phonological representations for onset, vowel and tone and represents syllables of Putonghua for which 23 onsets, 34 vowels and five tones are sufficient. There are no within-level linkages in the phonological system. This means that lateral inhibition is not possible in the model in contrast to the representations for orthography (specifically radicals and characters) as well as presumed semantic representations at the level of meaning. There are also no local representations for whole words (monosyllabic or polysyllabic) and no representations of rime level units.

The LC model has the potential to explain the features of tonal dyslexia. The most striking feature of tonal dyslexia is that errors occur with onset and rime intact, suggesting tone is dissociated from the syllable. At present, the LC model can explain tonal dyslexia as a consequence of damage to the tone layer of representation. However, all tones are given equal status in the model and no consideration is given to the weight assigned to each tone. Luo and Weekes (2004) found a tendency for their participant to assign the fourth tone and proposed an economy principle to explain this effect, i.e. if the tonal system is disrupted following brain damage, the Chinese speaker adopts the fourth tone as a default because the fourth tone takes least time to produce in Chinese. This would in principle allow syllables that had no meaning to be produced, although these were not noted in the case of ZW. The LC model would have difficulty accounting for this observation because a model with phonological representations that are fully distributed should produce tonal errors with the same frequency.

Although the LC model can explain some of the characteristics observed in individuals with tonal dyslexia, there are outstanding questions. The first concerns the desirability of a rime level of representation in the phonological system. The LC model assumes a distributed level of representation for onset and vowel in the phonological output system. This assumption is supported by data from Chinese dyslexic individuals who show selective impairment in production of the onset relative to the tone and rime (Shu *et al.*, 2005). However, Luo and Weekes (2004) reported evidence of whole rime substitution errors, suggesting the rime is represented by components in the lexicon and assignment of tone with the syllable intact. Thus, a rime level representation that is independent of tone is needed (see also Law & Or, 2001). The second question concerns how the phonological representations for monosyllabic or polysyllabic words that represent a morpheme, e.g. 玫瑰 *mei2 gui1* 'rose' and 蚯蚓 *qiu1 yin3* 'earthworm', are identified in a fully distributed system. Semantic errors in oral reading show that although whole-word knowledge can be lost, morphemes related to the target are activated. This suggests a level of representation for whole-word forms that can be selectively impaired with brain damage. Law *et al.* (2005) argued that whole-word representations for polysyllabic words in the Chinese lexicon are necessary at the phonological level following testing with two character words. Their claim for whole-word (polysyllabic) representations was based on evidence from an individual who could read aloud but not comprehend polysyllabic words containing phonologically ambiguous characters that must be disambiguated by word context. Assuming a fully distributed phonological system, damage would need to be prephonological, i.e. within the semantic system, or a stage that involves a lemma level of representation to explain the data from these individuals. Although this is possible in theory, no such level of representation is implemented in the LC model.

The LC model simply cannot explain other data from cases of acquired dyslexia. For example, Yin and Butterworth's (1998) report of radical-by-radical reading whereby character components including semantic and phonetic radicals were read instead of the name of the character. The critical result from reports of radical-by-radical reading is that character components can be read aloud without contacting character knowledge. As the model assumes that reading of radicals is mediated by access to characters, it cannot explain this phenomenon. One objection to our claim is that some radicals can act alone as characters (i.e. they represent a morpheme) and hence have a legitimate pronunciation. However, individuals with acquired surface dyslexia produce LARC errors showing that components may be read aloud without contacting character knowledge. The model cannot explain surface dyslexia because it assumes that orthography and phonology are connected at the character level only. Recall also that surface dyslexia in Chinese is impaired in oral reading of irregular characters that have unpredictable correspondences between orthography and phonology, particularly if characters are low frequency and abstract in meaning. Although LARC errors reflect contact with lexical representations (radicals), the target is unavailable. The evidence from surface dyslexia therefore suggests reliance on direct mappings between character components and phonology, and moreover it is possible to read aloud via these mappings even if the mappings between characters and phonology are not available. Taken together, the data from individuals with radical-by-radical reading and surface dyslexia show that access to phonological output from radical representations is not necessarily mediated by character recognition and can bypass the representations of characters containing the radical. This is assumed in all cognitive neuropsychological frameworks as depicted in Figure 11.1 (see also Law and colleagues), but not in the LC model.

The reading errors in surface dyslexia also cast doubt on the assumption of the LC model that radicals and characters are represented at independent levels of processing. There is justification for assuming separate levels of radical and character representations. Although most phonetic radicals are themselves characters, there are phonetic radicals that do not exist alone (nonfree-standing phonetic radicals) (Lee *et al.*, 2005; Peng *et al.*, 1994). Ding *et al.* (2004) propose these phonetic radicals are represented at the radical level and differ from free-standing counterparts because they are not connected to semantic and phonological representations. Perfetti *et al.* (2005) do not assume these units, but argue that pronunciation of such radicals might be attached to the orthographic character level in the LC model. However, the LC model must still explain why radical and character knowledge interact in individuals with surface dyslexia. This is because character components that are consistent pronunciations are read instead of the correct pronunciation of the target character. Also LARC errors typically are syllables with a higher frequency than the target itself (Weekes & Chen, 1999).

A lesion simulation in the model would refute our contention that the model does not account for surface dyslexia (see e.g. Plaut *et al.*, 1996). This can be done via reducing activation in the LC model so that alternative and higher frequency syllables representing a component are produced instead of the target. Reduced activation could occur at several levels in the model, including orthographic input, the mappings between orthography and phonology or the mappings between semantic and phonological levels. Another possibility is to instantiate within-level competition at the character level to prevent whole character reading but allow reading of components. However, it is unclear how this would work as long as radicals are mediated by character units. Note also that this would require within-level competition at the phonological level and it is not clear how the LC model would allow this. For example, if all the phonological representations are activated at once, what criterion would be used to produce a correct response?

One response to the observation of preserved reading of character components that is coincident with impaired character reading might be to assume independent mappings connecting orthography and phonology at the subcharacter level (Han *et al.*, 2005; Luo & Weekes, 2004; Weekes & Chen, 1999). By subcharacter we mean below the character (not word) level. For example, if radical units were connected to phonological output directly, this would allow reading of a component when whole character reading is not possible (see e.g. Taft and colleagues 1995, 1997, 1999 who propose a model that assumes subcharacter representations). This is not equivalent to non-lexical processes assumed for oral reading by Plaut *et al.* (1996). No model of oral reading in Chinese assumes a non-lexical level of representation. All representations are assumed to have lexical content. Some of these representations may be considered 'sublexical', e.g. radical units. As such they may be similar to the subcomponents of words in alphabetic languages, such as the rime. A rime typically depicts an existing syllable in the language, e.g. eat, and may also be a word, i.e. have a meaning although not all rimes are words, e.g. *ong*. Graphemes and phonemes are also considered to be subcomponents in all models of reading including connectionist models. However, these units are non-lexical because they have no meaning. Note that the debate over the status of a non-lexical unit in alphabetic scripts is ongoing and the reader is referred to Plaut *et al.* (1996) for further discussion. Graphemes do not exist in Chinese and, like radical units in non-alphabetic scripts, are language specific. Many radicals have identifiable meaning or pronunciation making them lexical according to accepted definitions of that term. Some radicals have no meaning or pronunciation and cannot stand alone, such as the top component of the character 充 *chong1* 'to fill' (note the latter type of orthographic representation has no equivalent in English). Radical units may be considered subcharacter components and hence sublexical, but this does not make them equivalent to the representations assumed in models of oral reading in English. A non-lexical reading process is assumed in all models of reading in alphabetic scripts. This allows a nonextant syllable to be read aloud when depicted in print, e.g. *zint*. A nonextant syllable cannot be depicted in a nonalphabetic script. This redundancy of non-lexical reading in Chinese is the key difference between reading in alphabetic and nonalphabetic scripts and challenges universal architectures for reading across scripts. The adaptation of the LC model to oral reading in Chinese is an attempt to show that the same computational architecture can be applied universally to oral reading in alphabetic and nonalphabetic scripts. However, we question whether this is viable.

In our view, a key theoretical question that needs to be addressed in computational modeling of reading in Chinese is what are the relevant units for reading? One response might be that the minimal unit of orthographic representation should represent a syllable. However, this definition would not capture non-free-standing phonetic radicals linked to pronunciations via characters; semantic radicals with meaning but no pronunciation; or radicals with no meaning or pronunciation. The LC model assumes independent units of representation at the character and radical levels. However, in our view the inclusion of a radical level representation that is independent of other orthographic representations is an error of commission.

Peripheral Disorders of Reading

There are few reports of peripheral disorders of reading in Chinese. Pure alexia was characterised earlier as a disorder of word recognition. Cognitive neuropsychologists assume that pure alexia reflects damage to a word form system. This is a functional module responsible for parsing letter strings into familiar units and visual categorisation of units into meaningful entities. However, the notion of whole-word recognition impairment has been challenged by data showing that some individuals can access whole-word representations implicitly with no awareness of the presented stimuli. Thus, unlike cases of acquired central dyslexia it may be inappropriate to interpret pure alexia in terms of damage to the normal reading system. This is because the normal reading system in the left hemisphere may not be damaged if individuals recognise written words via oral spelling. A different explanation assumes a disconnection between the left and right occipital cortices and the mechanisms representing visual forms of words in the left hemisphere. This account assumes normal reading of words that are presented to the right visual field is achieved by (1) initial visual processing in the right visual cortex that is followed by (2) transfer of information via the splenium to normal reading centres in the left hemisphere. However, this right-to-left transfer cannot occur when the splenium is damaged. This account of pure alexia is supported by neuropathological data, showing all reported cases of pure alexia have two lesions, one in the left occipital lobe and a lesion to the splenium. Single letters can be transferred from the right occipital lobe reflected in letter-by-letter reading. However, visual input to the normal reading system is unavailable because of splenium damage. This is the pathology reported by Yin and Butterworth (1998) for their radical-by-radical reader.

One issue to emerge from studies of pure alexia is whether the human brain has separate letter processing and word processing systems or whether the word form system is unitary, i.e. made up of letter and word representations that are activated in parallel (Fiset *et al.*, 2006). Data from Chinese are not relevant to this question as letters do not exist. Most models of word recognition assume that recognition occurs in a hierarchical fashion with letter units activated first in a spatially parallel manner, and these are then mapped to the higher level orthographic representations of whole words. An alternative view is that letter activation is functionally different to word activation because words are made up of interdependent letters and are more numerous statistically than single letters. This would explain suboptimal lexical access in pure alexia even if there is a common orthographic mechanism involved in letter and word identification. This mechanism may be defective because competing representations are activated thus precluding word identification. This could account for the observation that some individuals gain access to whole-word representations via a spatially parallel mapping procedure despite letter-by-letter reading (Fiset *et al.*, 2006). It would be of interest theoretically to find a Chinese-speaking individual who showed a pattern of implicit character recognition.

Other peripheral dyslexias include visual, attentional and neglect dyslexia. *Visual dyslexia* refers to reading errors where the response shares letters with the target, e.g. *arrangement* → *argument* and *calm* → *claim* (Lambon Ralph & Ellis, 1997). The same phenomenon is observed when the speaker reads nonwords, e.g. *belm* misread as a visually similar word, e.g. *beam* or *bell*. This error is also called a lexicalisation. When asked to spell aloud the letters of a word, the subject can do this correctly, e.g. *calm* read as 'C''A''L''M' → *calm*. *Attentional dyslexia* refers to letter migration errors, e.g. *window* read as *widnow* together with impaired naming of letters in words (Warrington *et al.*, 1993). Migration errors diminish if the speakers focus their attention on each letter in a word (Davis & Coltheart, 2002).

Neglect dyslexia refers to a pattern of reading whereby the left side of a word, a passage or a whole page is ignored even when print falls within the intact portions of both visual fields (Caramazza & Hillis, 1990). Reading errors arise because letters in a word or nonword are omitted or misidentified. Almost all individuals with neglect dyslexia omit the letters to the left of the stimulus, e.g. *cap* → *tap*. Neglect dyslexia can also be seen on different tasks. For example, the left side of an open book is ignored or the beginning of lines of text may be omitted. Furthermore, the beginning letters of single words may be neglected, leading to substitution errors, e.g. *book* → *hook*; omission errors, e.g. *farm* → *arm*; and addition errors, e.g. *love* → *glove*. Neglect dyslexia usually accompanies the syndrome of unilateral neglect of space where s/he fails to pay attention to the left side of space and may engage in conversation only if the speaker is in the right side of space, may eat only the food on the right side of the plate, may dress only the right side of his or her body and may deny ownership of their left arm and leg.

Visual, attentional and neglect dyslexia all involve difficulties identifying word components such as letters. It is important to note that these disorders are not necessarily the result of a common syndrome. The neglect syndrome follows extensive damage to the right hemisphere. However, neglect dyslexia is a separate disorder because individuals with neglect dyslexia do not always show unilateral neglect of space (Haywood & Coltheart, 2000). For these individuals, processing the left half of space is impaired only if a letter-string is processed. Also, cases of right-sided neglect dyslexia, where errors arise with the rightmost letters of a letter-string, have been reported (Ellis & Young, 1988). Neglect dyslexia can occur when words are presented horizontally or vertically. This suggests that neglect dyslexia results from a problem with attention that is related to the phenomenon of letter migration in reading (Davis & Coltheart, 2002). Neglect dyslexia can be extinguished in some individuals if all the letters of a word are presented in the right visual field, i.e. if s/he fixates to the left of a word that is being read. However, in other individuals, neglect occurs even for words presented entirely in the right visual field, and in others the right-hand side of a word is neglected when it is mirror reversed, e.g. *pac* → *car*. Neglect of printed material has also been dissociated from neglect on line bisection and symbol detection tasks. This shows that neglect of printed material can be stimulus bound rather than result from a general neglect of space (Haywood & Coltheart, 2000, 2001). Also, some neglect individuals show left-sided neglect on reading tasks, but right-sided neglect on visuospatial tasks (Haywood & Coltheart, 2000, 2001). Neglect dyslexia is most likely due to a deficit in visuospatial attention because reading impairments can be minimised by cueing and exacerbated with bilateral simultaneous stimulus presentation (Haywood & Coltheart, 2000, 2001). There are as yet no Chinese individuals reported with attentional, visual or neglect dyslexia. However, identifying such individuals has the potential to add significantly to our knowledge about basic processes in reading Chinese characters.

Conclusion

Studies of cases of acquired dyslexia suggest there are at least two independent pathways available for normal reading in Chinese. If these pathways are labelled lexical semantic and nonsemantic, then differences between nonalphabetic and alphabetic scripts – such as whether reading via non-lexical mechanisms is necessary – can inform the development of cognitive models of reading and writing across scripts. However, the unique properties of a script require modification to this basic framework. We have illustrated similarities between acquired dyslexia in Chinese and alphabetic languages. However, this should not imply that disorders of reading should be viewed as universal (Beland & Mimouni, 2001; Eng & Obler, 2002; Miceli & Caramazza, 1993; Raman & Weekes, 2005a). In fact, patterns of acquired dyslexia and dysgraphia in Chinese *cannot* be identical to patterns observed in alphabetic languages because the properties of Chinese script do not allow direct comparisons between disorders. Thus, it will not be possible to replicate the pattern of preserved nonword processing observed in surface dyslexia and dysgraphia in English and Spanish (Coltheart, 1984). We recommend approaching the problem of acquired dyslexia in Chinese by testing predictions that are derived from a cognitive model developed to explain reading *in Chinese*. The LC model has the potential to do this although the model is in an early stage of development. The simulation reported by Perfetti *et al.* (2005) involved only 204 characters out of a possible 50,000. In our view, the weakest part of the model is a lack of specificity regarding the status of the orthographic units of representation. No doubt further work including simulations of impaired oral reading will refine the explanatory power of the model and hence make a contribution to understanding disorders of reading in Chinese.

Acknowledgements

This paper was supported by grants from the Australian Research Council and the Royal Society.

References

Angelelli, P., Judica, A., Spinelli, D., Zoccolotti, P. and Luzzatti, C. (2004) Characteristics of writing disorders in Italian dyslexic children. *Cognitive and Behavioural Neurology* 17, 18–31.

Ardilla, A. (1991) Errors resembling semantic paralexias in Spanish speaking aphasics. *Brain and Language* 41, 437–445.

Behrmann, M. and Bub, B. (1992) Surface dyslexia and dysgraphia: Dual routes, single lexicon. *Cognitive Neuropsychology* 9, 209–251.

Beland, R. and Mimouni, Z. (2001) Deep dyslexia in the two languages of an Arabic/French bilingual patient. *Cognition* 82, 77–126.

Caramazza, A. and Hillis, A. (1990) Levels of representation, coordinate frames and unilateral neglect. *Cognitive Neuropsychology* 7, 391–445.

Cardebat, D., Puel, M., Demonet, J.F. and Nespoulous, J.L. (1991) Les differentes 'boites' de la repetition: Analyse d'un case de dysphasie profonde. *Revue de Neuropsycholgie* 1, 215–232.

Castles, A. and Coltheart, M. (1993) Varieties of developmental dyslexia. *Cognition* 47, 149–180.

Chen, J.Y., Chen, T.M. and Dell, G.S. (2002) Word-form encoding in Mandarin Chinese as assessed by the implicit priming task. *Journal of Memory and Language* 46, 751–781.

Coltheart, M. (1982) The psycholinguistic analysis of acquired dyslexia: Some illustrations. *Philosophical Transactions of the Royal Society London B* 298, 151–164.

Coltheart, M. (1984) Writing systems and reading disorders. In L. Henderson (ed.) *Orthographies and Reading: Perspectives from Cognitive Psychology, Neuropsychology, and Linguistics* (pp. 81–89). London: Erlbaum.

Coltheart, M., Rastle, K., Perry, C., Langdon, R. and Ziegler, J. (2001) DRC: A dual route cascaded model of visual word recognition and reading aloud. *Psychological Review* 108, 204–256.

Cuetos, F. (1993) Writing processes in a shallow orthography. *Reading and Writing: An Interdisciplinary Journal* 5, 17–28.

Cuetos, F. and Labos, E. (2001) The autonomy of the orthographic pathway in a shallow language: Data from an aphasic patient. *Aphasiology* 15, 333–342.

Cuetos, F., Martinez, T., Martinez, C., Izura, C. and Ellis, A. (2003) Lexical processing in Spanish patients with probable Alzheimer's disease. *Cognitive Brain Research* 17, 549–561.

Cuetos, F., Valle-Arroyo, F. and Suarez, M. (1996) A case of phonological dyslexia in Spanish. *Cognitive Neuropsychology* 13, 1–24.

Davis, C. and Coltheart, M. (2002) Paying attention to reading errors in acquired dyslexia. *Trends in Cognitive Sciences* 6, 359–361.

de Partz, M.P. (1986) Re-education of a deep dyslexic patient: Rationale of the method and results. *Cognitive Neuropsychology* 3, 147–177.

de Partz, M.P., Seron, X. and Van der Linden, M.V. (1992) Re-education of surface dysgraphia with a visual imagery strategy. *Cognitive Neuropsychology* 9, 369–401.

Diesfeldt, H.F.A. (1992) Impaired and preserved semantic memory functions in dementia. In L. Blackman (ed.) *Memory Functioning in Dementia* (pp. 227–263). Amsterdam: Elsevier Science.

Ding, G., Peng, D. and Taft, M. (2004) The nature of the mental representation of radicals in Chinese: A priming study. *Journal of Experimental Psychology: Learning Memory, and Cognition* 30, 530–539.

Ellis, A.W. and Young, A.W. (1988) *Human Cognitive Neuropsychology*. Hove: Psychology Press.

Eng, N. and Obler, L.K. (2002) Acquired dyslexia in a biscript reader following traumatic brain injury: A second case. *Topics in Language Disorders* 22, 5–19.

Fabbro, F. (1999) *The Neurolinguistics of Bilingualism: An Introduction*. Hove: Psychology Press.

Ferreres, A.R. and Miravalles, G. (1995) The production of semantic paralexias in a Spanish speaking aphasic. *Brain and Language* 49, 153–172.

Fiset, D., Arguin, M. and McCabe, E. (2006) The breakdown of parallel letter processing in letter-by-letter dyslexia. *Cognitive Neuropsychology* 23, 240–260.

Friedman, R.B. (1996) Recovery from deep alexia to phonological alexia: Points on a continuum. *Brain and Language* 52, 114–128.

Fushimi, T., Komori, K., Ikeda, M., Patterson, K., Ijuin, M. and Tanabe, H. (2003) Surface dyslexia in a Japanese patient with semantic dementia: Evidence for similarity-based orthography-to-phonology translation. *Neuropsychologia* 41, 1644–1658.

Goldblum, J. (1985) Word comprehension in surface dyslexia. In K. Patterson, J. Marshall and M. Coltheart (eds) *Surface Dyslexia*. London: Lawrence Erlbaum.

Graham, N.L., Patterson, K. and Hodges, J.R. (1997) Progressive dysgraphia: Co-occurrence of central and peripheral impairments. *Cognitive Neuropsychology* 14, 975–1005.

Graham, N.L., Patterson, K. and Hodges, J.R. (2000) The impact of semantic memory impairment on spelling: Evidence from semantic dementia. *Neuropsychologia* 38, 143–163.

Han, B.Z., Bi, Y.C., Shu, H. and Weekes, B.S. (2005) The interaction between semantic and sublexical routes in reading: Converging evidence from Chinese. *Brain and Language* 95, 235–236.

Haywood, M. and Coltheart, M. (2000) Neglect dyslexia and the early stages of visual word recognition. *Neurocase* 6, 33–44.

Haywood, M. and Coltheart, M. (2001) Neglect dyslexia with a stimulus-centred deficit and without visuospatial neglect. *Cognitive Neuropsychology* 18, 577–615.

Hillis, A. and Caramazza, A. (1995) Converging evidence for the interaction of semantic and phonological information in accessing lexical information for spoken output. *Cognitive Neuropsychology* 12, 187–227.

Houghton, G. and Zorzi, M. (2003) Normal and impaired spelling in a connectionist dual-route architecture. *Cognitive Neuropsychology* 20, 115–162.

Iribarren, I.C., Jarema, G. and Lecours, A.R. (2001) Two different dysgraphic syndromes in a regular orthography, Spanish. *Brain and Language* 77, 166–175.

Laine, M., Neimi, P., Neimi, J. and Koivuselkä-Sallinen, P. (1990) Semantic errors in deep dyslexia. *Brain and Language* 38, 207–214.

Lambon Ralph, M.A. and Ellis, A.W. (1997) Patterns of paralexia revisited: Report of a case of visual dyslexia. *Cognitive Neuropsychology* 14, 953–974.

Law, S.P. (2004) A morphological analysis of object naming and reading errors by a Cantonese dyslexic patient. *Language and Cognitive Processes* 19, 473–501.

Law, S.P. and Or, B. (2000) Nonsemantic pathways of reading and writing Chinese: Data from a Cantonese-speaking brain-damaged patient. *Brain and Language* 74, 524–526.

Law, S.P. and Or, B. (2001) A case study of acquired dyslexia and dysgraphia in Cantonese: Evidence for nonsemantic pathways for reading and writing Chinese. *Cognitive Neuropsychology* 18, 729–748.

Law, S.P., Wong, W. and Chiu, K. (2005) Preserved reading aloud with semantic deficits: Evidence for a non-semantic lexical route for reading Chinese. *Neurocase* 11, 167–175.

Lee, C.Y., Tsai, J.L., Su, S.C., Tzeng, O. and Hung, D. (2005) Consistency, regularity and frequency effects in naming Chinese characters. *Language and Linguistics* 6, 175–197.

Luo, Q. and Weekes, B.S. (2004) Tonal dyslexia in Chinese. *Brain and Language* 91, 102–103.

Luzzi, S., Bartolini, M., Coccia, M., Provinciali, L., Piccirilli, M. and Snowden, J.S. (2003) Surface dysgraphia in a regular orthography: Apostrophe use by an Italian writer. *Neurocase* 9, 285–296.

Majerus, S., Leku, F., Van de Linden, M. and Salmon, E. (2001) Deep dysphasia: Further evidence on the relationship between phonological short term memory and language processing impairments. *Cognitive Neuropsychology* 18, 385–410.

Marshall, J.C. and Newcombe, F. (1966) Syntactic and semantic errors in paralexia. *Neuropsychologia* 4, 169–176.

Marshall, J.C. and Newcombe, F. (1973) Patterns of paralexia: A psycholinguistic approach. *Journal of Psycholinguistic Research* 2, 175–200.

Miceli, G. and Caramazza, A. (1993) The assignment of word stress in oral reading: Evidence from a case of acquired dyslexia. *Cognitive Neuropsychology* 10, 273–296.

Miozzo, M. and de Bastiani, P. (2002) The organization of letter-form representations in written spelling: Evidence from acquired dysgraphia. *Brain and Language* 80, 366–392.

Patterson, K. (1990) Basic processes of reading: Do they differ in Japanese and English? Japanese. *Journal of Neuropsychology* 6, 4–14.

Patterson, K. and Hodges, J.R. (1992) Deterioration of word meaning: Implications for reading. *Neuropsychologia* 30, 1025–1040.

Patterson, K. and Lambon Ralph, M.A. (1999) Selective disorders of reading? *Current Opinion in Neurobiology* 9, 235–239.

Patterson, K., Okada, S. and Suzuki, T. (1998) Fragmented words: A case of late-stage progressive aphasia. *Neurocase* 4, 219–230.

Patterson, K., Suzuki, T., Wydell, T. and Sasanuma, S. (1995) Progressive aphasia and surface alexia in Japanese. *Neurocase* 1, 155–165.

Peng, D.L., Yang, H. and Chen, Y. (1994) Consistency and phonetic independency effects in naming task of Chinese phonograms. In Q.C. Jing and H.C. Zhang (eds) *Information Processing of Chinese Language* (pp. 26–41). Beijing: Beijing Normal University Press.

Perfetti, C.A., Liu, Y. and Tan, L.H. (2005) The Lexical Constituency Model: Some implications of research on Chinese for general theories of reading. *Psychological Review* 112, 43–59.

Plaut, D.C., McClelland, J.D., Seidenberg, M.S. and Patterson, K. (1996) Understanding normal and impaired word reading: Computational principles in quasi-regular domains. *Psychological Review* 103, 56–115.

Raman, I. and Weekes, B.S. (2005a) Acquired dyslexia in a Turkish-English speaker. *Annals of Dyslexia* 55, 71–96.

Raman, I. and Weekes, B.S. (2005b) Deep dysgraphia in Turkish. *Behavioural Neurology* 16, 59–69.

Ruiz, A., Ansaldo, A.I. and Lecours, A.R. (1994) Two cases of deep dyslexia in unilingual Hispanophone aphasics. *Brain and Language* 46, 245–256.

Seidenberg, M.S. and McClelland, J.L. (1989) A distributed, developmental model of word recognition and naming. *Psychological Review* 96, 523–568.

Shu, H., Xiong, H.Z., Han, Z.H., Bi, Y.C. and Bai, X.L. (2005) The selective impairment of the phonological output buffer: Evidence from a Chinese patient. *Behavioural Neurology* 16, 179–189.

Siok, W.T. and Fletcher, P. (2001) The role of phonological awareness and visual-orthographic skills in Chinese reading acquisition. *Developmental Psychology* 37, 886–899.

Taft, M., Liu, Y. and Zhu, X. (1999) Morphemic processing in reading Chinese. In J. Wang, A.W. Inhoff and H.C. Chen (eds) *Reading Chinese Script: A Cognitive Analysis* (pp. 91–113). Mahwah, NJ: Lawrence Erlbaum.

Taft, M. and Zhu, X. (1995) The representation of bound morphemes in the lexicon: A Chinese study. In L.B. Feldman (ed.) *Morphological Aspects of Language Processing* (pp. 293–316). Hillsdale, NJ: Lawrence Erlbaum.

Taft, M. and Zhu, X. (1997) Using masked priming to examine lexical storage of Chinese compound words. In H.C. Chen (ed.) *Cognitive Processing of Chinese and Related Asian Languages* (pp. 233–241). Hong Kong: The Chinese University Press.

Valdois, S., Cabonnel, S., David, D., Rouset, S. and Pellat, J. (1995) Confrontation of PDP models and dual route models through the analysis of a case of deep dysphasia. *Cognitive Neuropsychology* 12, 681–724.

Warrington, E.K., Cipolotti, L. and McNeil, J. (1993) Attentional dyslexia: A single case study. *Neuropsychologia* 31, 871–885.

Weekes, B.S. (2005) Acquired disorders of reading and writing: Cross-script comparisons. *Behavioural Neurology* 16, 51–57.

Weekes, B.S. and Chen, H-Q. (1999) Surface dyslexia in Chinese. *Neurocase* 5, 161–172.

Weekes, B.S., Chen, M.J. and Yin, W. (1997a) Anomia without dyslexia in Chinese. *Neurocase* 3, 51–60.

Weekes, B.S. and Coltheart, M. (1996) Surface dyslexia and surface dysgraphia: Treatment studies and their theoretical implications. *Cognitive Neuropsychology* 13, 277–315.

Weekes, B.S., Coltheart, M. and Gordon, E.V. (1997b) Deep dyslexia and right hemisphere reading: A regional cerebral blood-flow study. *Aphasiology* 11, 1139–1158.

Woollams, A., Lambon Ralph, M., Plaut, D. and Patterson, K. (2007) SD-squared: On the association between semantic dementia and surface dyslexia. *Psychological Review* 114, 316–339.

Yin, W.G. and Butterworth, B. (1992) Deep and surface dyslexia in Chinese. In H.C. Chen and O.J.L. Tzeng (eds) *Language Processing in Chinese* (pp. 349–366). Amsterdam: Elsevier Science.

Yin, W.G. and Butterworth, B. (1998) Chinese pure alexia. *Aphasiology* 12, 65–76.

Chapter 12

Age of Acquisition Effects on Picture Naming in Chinese Anomia

SAM-PO LAW, BRENDAN S. WEEKES, OLIVIA YEUNG and KAREN CHIU

Introduction

The age at which an individual acquires a word, i.e. age of acquisition (AoA), has been found to influence lexical processing significantly. AoA effects have been reported in various processing tasks using normal subjects, including word naming, picture naming, lexical decision, object recognition, word-associate generation and semantic categorization (see Ghyselinck *et al.*, 2004; Johnston & Barry, 2006; Juhasz, 2005 for review). Items that are learned early in life generally take less time to retrieve their names, read aloud, decide their lexicality or make semantic judgments.

Given the high correlation between AoA and word frequency, the reality of AoA effects has been questioned by some researchers (Lewis, 1999a, 1999b; Lewis *et al.*, 2001; Zevin & Seidenberg, 2002). In particular, Zevin and Seidenberg argue that the AoA effect is in fact a type of frequency effect, as early-acquired words tend to be encountered more frequently over a person's life span than late-acquired words. In other words, lexical items with early AoA have higher cumulative frequency than those with late AoA. However, the hypothesis meets with great difficulty in accounting for the presence of AoA effects in studies where the cumulative frequencies of stimuli have been controlled (e.g. Bonin *et al.*, 2004; Weekes *et al.*, 2006). Findings of a similar nature were reported in simulation studies (Ellis & Lambon Ralph, 2000). In addition, the hypothesis would predict a diminished impact of AoA in older compared with younger adults, but this was not supported by the word- and picture-naming performance of younger and older subjects in Morrison *et al.* (2002). Equally challenging findings to the hypothesis come from lexical decision of expert vocabularies (Stadthagen-Gonzalez *et al.*, 2004). Comparable decision latencies and error rates were found for late AoA/high frequency and early AoA/low frequency words, even though the cumulative frequency for the former was estimated to be at least 13 times higher than the latter.

Among the various language-processing tasks, AoA effects have been most consistently found in picture naming. In fact, all studies of picture naming that have invesigated the role of AoA have found its effects on naming latencies, often without a corresponding frequency effect. This is the case whether the design is one of regression (e.g. Bonin *et al.*, 2002; Laws *et al.*, 2002; Morrison *et al.*, 1992) or semifactorial (e.g. Barry *et al.*, 2001; Bonin *et al.*, 2001; Ellis & Morrison, 1998). Nevertheless, there are studies reporting both AoA and word frequency effects (e.g. Bonin *et al.*, 2003; Lachman, 1973; Lachman *et al.*, 1974; Snodgrass & Yuditsky, 1996). More importantly, the effects of AoA have been observed cross-linguistically, including English, French (Kremin *et al.*, 2000), Greek (Bogka *et al.*, 2003), Icelandic (Pind & Tryggvadottir, 2002), Italian (Dell'Acqua *et al.*, 2000), Spanish (Cuetos *et al.*, 1999) and more recently Chinese (Weekes *et al.*, 2007).

Not only has the effect of AoA been found in naming latencies of normal subjects, it also affects naming accuracy of other participant populations including those with neurogenic language disorders, such as semantic dementia (Lambon Ralph *et al.*, 1998; Taylor, 1998), Alzheimer's disease (Holmes *et al.*, 2006; Kremin *et al.*, 2000; Silveri *et al.*, 2002) and aphasia (e.g. Cuetos *et al.*, 2005; Hirsh & Ellis, 1994; Hirsh & Funnell, 1995; Nickels & Howard, 1995). Indeed, the first investigation of AoA effects was by Rochford and Williams (1962), who reported a close correspondence in naming accuracy and errors between 32 anomic speakers and 120 children between two and 12 years of age. Subsequently, Feyereisen *et al.* (1988) found that AoA and picture familiarity were significant predictors of naming performance of 18 aphasic subjects in a multiple regression analysis. More recent studies have focused on single case studies. Hirsh and Ellis described the performance of an aphasic speaker (NP) with semantic deficits, on spoken and written naming, reading aloud and repetition. AoA significantly predicted response accuracy in spoken naming, written naming and reading aloud, while there were no effects of imageability or word frequency. NP also made many semantic errors in the naming tasks. Hirsh and Ellis proposed that AoA effects resided at the level of access to phonological forms for output. Hirsh and Funnell reported picture-naming accuracy of two individuals with progressive aphasia, Mary with intact comprehension in the initial stage and EP with disrupted semantic processing. While Mary's performance was affected by AoA, EP's was influenced by object familiarity. On this basis, the researchers suggested that the locus of AoA was at the lexical-phonological level and the effect of familiarity was semantically-based.

Although both group and single case studies have reported significant AoA effects, some researchers have questioned the reliability of grouped data. Nickels and Howard (1995) analyzed the picture-naming accuracy of two groups of aphasic subjects who each named a different set of stimuli. Grouped data of the first aphasic group revealed significant effects of AoA, operativity (defined as the extent to which an object may be manipulated in daily life situations) and number of phonemes (i.e. word length). However, when individual data were analyzed, AoA was a significant predictor in less than half of the subjects (5/12), operativity in 7/12, both AoA and operativity in 2/12 and word length in 2/12 participants. In a second set of stimuli, all of which had at least 90% name agreement and for which frequency and length were orthogonally varied, AoA, imageability and word length were significant predictors for the grouped data. Individually, AoA effects were only found for 3/15 subjects. With frequency and familiarity removed from the regression analysis, three additional participants showed significant AoA effects, and 9/15 subjects exhibited the word length effect. Similarly, Ellis *et al.* (1997) presented response accuracy of six aphasic subjects naming 139 pictured objects three times. The data were analyzed as a group, individually by combining the three naming attempts using simultaneous multiple regression, and individually by each attempt using logistic regression. Highly variable patterns of significant predictors emerged across results of the three analyses. However, the more problematic situation was the failure of the model to reach significance in half of the subjects when scores were combined across naming attempts and in two thirds of the cases when naming accuracy of each test session by each participant was separately analyzed. Great variablity between results of grouped and individual data were also reported of Spanish anomic subjects (Cuetos *et al.*, 2002).

The discrepancies between findings from grouped and individual data may at least be due partly to heterogeneity of subjects in the foregoing studies. In fact, details of the participants in these studies were limited to demographic information, aetiology, aphasia type or severity. It is quite likely that the subjects had different underlying deficits resulting in their naming disorders. The averaging or grouping of patient data in neurolinguistic research has been the center of a debate about the usefulness of grouped data in cognitive neuropsychological investigations (Caramazza, 1984, 1986). In response to this, Cuetos *et al.* (2005) conducted two studies involving 'pure' anomic individuals with preserved comprehension and phonological output. Naming difficulties in these subjects were attributed to disruption to lexical access. The first study employed a semifactorial design manipulating word frequency and AoA in turn, while controlling for other variables including familiarity, imageability and word length. Significant AoA effects, not word frequency, were found for both subjects and items. The second study was a full factorial design with AoA and word frequency being orthogonally manipulated. Again, only AoA was found to exert significant influence on naming accuracy.

The present study took a similar approach to examine the effect of AoA on object naming among language-impaired individuals. The subjects were five Cantonese anomic speakers with dissociation between largely preserved reading aloud and impaired naming abilities. Four of them showed normal performance on non-verbal semantic tests. As mentioned before, Weekes *et al.* (2007) have recently found unique and independent contributions of AoA, name agreement and object familiarity to naming latencies in normal Mandarin Chinese participants. This study represents the first investigation into the role of AoA in naming accuracy of Cantonese Chinese aphasic subjects.

Method

Participants

The background information on the five subjects is given in Table 12.1. They were all right-handed, native speakers of Cantonese and at least eight months post-onset at the beginning of this study.

Initial assessment

The tasks included (1) repetition of 30 single words and phrases of up to four syllables in length, (2) three visuospatial analysis tests from the Birmingham Object Recognition Battery (BORB) (Riddoch & Humphreys, 1993), minimal feature view, foreshortened view and item match, (3) oral naming of selected pictures in Snodgrass and Vanderwart (1980),[1] (4) reading aloud of names of the same pictured objects and (5) two non-verbal semantic tests, including the Pyramid and Palm Trees Test (PPTT) (Howard & Patterson, 1992) and the Associative Match Test in the BORB (Riddoch & Humphreys, 1993). In terms of the order of tasks, the stimuli for oral naming and reading aloud were divided into two blocks, and the two tasks were rotated across the blocks. In other words, half of the items were named before reading aloud, and vice versa for the other half. The whole set of stimuli was tested on these tasks over at least two occasions with test sessions being at least one day apart. The same stimulus was never tested on both oral naming and reading aloud in a single session. The order of the other tasks varied across subjects, depending on the availability of time and the time required for administering a given task within a test session. The subjects' performance is shown in Table 12.2.

Picture naming and predictor variables

Naming accuracy of 217 pictures of each participant was taken from the oral-naming task in initial assessment. For each stimulus item, properties along seven variables were obtained.

Table 12.1 Background information on aphasic subjects

	CKY	*FSY*	*LKH*	*YYW*	*WYL*
Age	45	56	53	60	39
Gender	Male	Female	Male	Male	Male
Education	Secondary 3	Secondary 2	University degree	Secondary 6	Secondary 5
Onset date	May 2004	December 2003	March 2005	May 2004	August 2003
Etiology	Left capsular hemorrhage	Left basal ganglia hemorrhage	Hemorrhagic transformation in left frontal-parietal lobe, corona radiata and left basal ganglia	Left MCA infarct	Hypodense lesion over parietal region suggestive of acute infarction involving left tempero-parietal region and left external capsule
Motor/ sensory impairment	Right hemiparesis, mild dysarthria	Mild right hemiparesis	Right hemiparesis, mild dysarthria	Right hemiparesis, mild dysarthria	Nil
Aphasia type	Anomic	Anomic	Transcortical motor	Anomic	Conduction
Premorbid occupation	Cook	Housewife	Art Teacher	Accountant	Decorator
Period of assessment	April 2006	February 2006	December 2005	December 2004	March 2006

Table 12.2 Results of initial assessment

	CKY	*FSY*	*LKH*	*YYW*	*WYL*
Repetition ($n = 30$)	22 (73.3%)	30 (100%)	24 (80.0%)	29 (96.7%)	25 (83.3%)
Visuo-spatial analysis					
Minimal feature view ($n = 25$)	25 (100%)	23 (92.0%)	25 (100%)	25 (100%)	25 (100%)
Foreshortened view ($n = 25$)	25 (100%)	22 (88.0%)	23 (92.0%)	21 (84.0%)	24 (96.0%)
Item match ($n = 32$)	32 (100%)	31 (96.9%)	32 (100%)	32 (100%)	32 (100%)
Non-verbal semantic tests					
PPTT ($n = 37$)	34 (91.9%)	35 (94.6%)	31 (83.8%)	30 (81.1%)	35 (94.6%)
BORB ($n = 23$)	23 (100%)	22 (95.7%)	22 (95.7%)	15 (65.2%)	22 (95.7%)
Oral naming ($n = 217$)	166 (76.5%)	172 (79.3%)	125 (57.6%)	153 (70.5%)	156 (71.9%)
Reading aloud object names ($n = 217$)	193 (90.3%)	215 (99.1%)	195 (89.9%)	215 (99.1%)	206 (96.8%)
Picture versus word naming (McNemar's Chi-square)	$Z = 13.56$, $p < 0.001$	$Z = 38.52$, $p < 0.0001$	$Z = 55.36$, $p < 0.0001$	$Z = 58.14$, $p < 0.0001$	$Z = 40.02$, $p < 0.0001$

(1) Subjective AoA and object familiarity[2]: a total of 60 native Cantonese speakers (30 males and 30 females) equally distributed across three age groups (young: 20–39 years, middle: 40–59 years and older people: 60 years and over) and two education levels (0–14 years of education and above 14 years of education) were asked to estimate the age at which they learned each item and to rate the degree of their familiarity with each object. AoA was rated using a seven-point scale with a two-year age band for each point on the scale (1: 0–2 years, 2: 3–4 years, 3: 5–6 years, 4: 7–8 years, 5: 9–10 years, 6: 11–12 years, 7: 13 years or above). Object familiarity was rated on a five-point scale from 1: unfamiliar (rarely encountered) to 5: highly familiar (encountered nearly everyday). The participants gave both estimates for each picture, one object at a time.

(2) Image agreement, visual complexity and name agreement: the same group of 60 subjects who provided normative naming data on the Snodgrass and Vanderwart pictures was asked to rate image agreement and visual complexity for each stimulus. The ratings were obtained following the same instructions and procedures described in Snodgrass and Vanderwart (1980). For image agreement, the experimenter would call out an object name, wait for about three seconds, during which the subject would close his/her eyes and try to imagine the named object. This was followed by presentation of the picture, which the subject rated on a five-point scale how closely the pictured object resembled his/her mental image. For visual complexity, the subject rated each picture on a five-point scale in terms of 'the amount of detail or intricacy of line in the picture' (Snodgrass & Vanderwart, 1980: 183). Name agreement was computed based on the oral responses of the normal subjects and using the *H* statistic (Morrison *et al.*, 2003).

(3) Word length: this was measured in terms of the number of syllables in each modal name.

Data analysis

The last response to each item by a participant was scored. It was considered correct if it was recognizable as the modal name or an acceptable alternative. In other words, minor phonological errors in which the target and the response shared at least half of the phonemes, including tone and segmentals, were tolerated. Each erroneous response was classified in terms of its error type. The data were analyzed as a group using simultaneous multiple regression and individually using simultaneous logistic regression. We were not only interested in finding whether AoA and other variables could significantly predict naming performance of Chinese aphasic speakers, but also how consistent the results would be between grouped and individual analyses given a relatively homogeneous subject group.

Results

Table 12.2 shows that all five participants demonstrated significantly better reading aloud than oral-naming performance. They were at least 90% correct on reading the object names, but varied between 57% and 79% accuracy for naming the same items. Three subjects, CKY, LKH and WYL, had phonological output disruption. All participants were by and large able to process visual-spatial information. Finally, all of them except YYW performed normally on the two non-verbal semantic tests. On the basis of these results, the naming difficulties experienced by the subjects were attributed to impairment to access from semantics to phonology, with YYW having additional deficits at the semantic level.

The descriptive statistics of the six predictor variables are given in Table 12.3. The distributions of name agreement and image agreement were relatively skewed. For the former, 60% of the stimuli had complete response agreement among the 60 normal subjects and therefore had a value of 0; for the latter, the subjects' ratings tended to be near the high

Table 12.3 Descriptive statistics of predictor variables

	Minimum	*Maximum*	*Mean*	*Standard deviation*	*Skewness*
Subjective age of acquisition	1.63	5.85	3.46	0.89	0.04
Object familiarity	1.97	4.92	3.66	0.82	– 0.26
Word length	1	4	1.80	0.68	0.45
Name agreement	0.00	1.59	0.34	0.42	0.98
Log (name agreement + 0.1)	– 1.00	0.23	– 0.58	0.45	0.30
Image agreement	3.08	4.67	4.25	0.29	– 1.20
Log (image agreement)	0.49	0.67	0.63	0.03	– 1.39
Visual complexity	1.42	4.62	3.30	0.98	– 0.36

end of the scale. Log transformation was used to reduce skew. While name agreement approximated a normal distribution after transformation, image agreement did not improve.

In subsequent correlation and regression analyses, stimuli to which the anomic subjects provided alternative acceptable names were eliminated, as these responses may differ in AoA and word length from their respective modal name. This resulted in the exclusion of 65 items as a group from the multiple regression analysis. For the logistic regression analysis, elimination of items was done individually. This means 26, 28, 15, 4 and 28 stimuli were removed for CKY, FSY, LKH, YYW and WYL, respectively.

Intercorrelations among the predictors are presented in Table 12.4. Simple correlations between naming accuracy of the group and all predictors were significant. The results of a simultaneous multiple regression reveal that the predictor variables taken together significantly predicted naming performance ($F(6, 145) = 13.86$, $p < 0.001$). The model explained about 36% of the variance. Subjective AoA, word length and image agreement were significant predictors of roughly the same importance as indicated by the standardized coefficients β. The earlier an item is learned, the shorter its name is, or the more a picture resembles a subject's mental image of the object, the more probable is the correct name.

Data from each participant was then analyzed. To ensure that failure to name an item was not likely to be due to the unavailability of the target phonological representation, only those stimuli with object names correctly read by each subject were included in data analysis. Table 12.5 illustrates that the three significant predictors from the simultaneous multiple regression were significantly correlated with naming accuracy of every subject. In addition, object familiarity was significant in four participants and visual complexity in one. None of the subjects' performance was associated with name agreement. The independent variables as a group significantly predicted naming accuracy in every case. Subjective AoA made a significant unique contribution to predicting performance in FSY, LKH and YYW and marginally significant in CKY ($p = 0.065$), word length in CKY, LKH and WYL and image agreement in CKY and FSY. The other three variables were never significant predictors. In other words, subjective AoA was the most robust predictor, followed by word length and then image agreement.

Table 12.6 presents the distribution of subjects' naming errors. The majority of errors for CKY, FSY and YYW, and half of LKH's incorrect responses were semantically related to the targets. On the other hand, omissions were as frequent as semantic errors in the case of WYL.

Table 12.4 Intercorrelation matrix and results of simultaneous multiple regression

	Subjective age of acquisition	*Object familiarity*	*Word length*	*Log name agreement*	*Image agreement*	*Visual complexity*
Subjective age of acquisition		– 0.624 (**)	0.455 (**)	0.150	– 0.394 (**)	0.296 (**)
Object familiarity			– 0.116	– 0.105	0.360 (**)	– 0.364 (**)
Word length				0.065	– 0.137	0.213 (**)
Log of name agreement					– 0.231 (**)	– 0.046
Image agreement						– 0.126
Oral naming						
Correlation						
$r =$	– 0.493	0.273	– 0.445	– 0.177	0.399	– 0.164
$p <$	0.001	0.001	0.001	0.05	0.001	0.05
Multiple regression						
$t =$	– 2.719	– 0.291	– 3.683	– 0.930	3.325	– 0.065
$p <$	0.01	n.s.	0.001	n.s.	0.01	n.s.
Standardized coefficients β	– 0.271	– 0.027	– 0.286	– 0.064	0.247	– 0.005

Note. $^{*}p < 0.05$, $^{**}p < 0.01$. n.s. = nonsignificant

Table 12.5 Correlations and results of simultaneous logistic regressions

	Naming accuracy	*Model Chi-square (df=6)*		*Subjective age of acquisition*	*Word length*	*Image agreement*	*Object familiarity*	*Log name agreement*	*Visual complexity*
CKY	72.9% (124/170)	39.376 (**)	Corr:	− 0.351 (**)	− 0.339 (**)	0.299 (**)	0.180 (*)	− 0.151	− 0.164 (*)
			Wald:	3.412[a]	7.566 (**)	5.446 (*)	0.133	1.314	0.339
			β:	− 0.587	− 0.963	1.740	− 0.115	− 0.523	− 0.139
FSY	75.9% (142/187)	36.498 (**)	Corr:	− 0.354 (**)	− 0.188 (**)	0.314 (**)	0.270 (**)	− 0.099	− 0.074
			Wald:	5.061 (*)	2.514	7.546 (**)	0.922	0.138	0.767
			β:	− 0.701	− 0.499	1.833	0.296	− 0.167	0.196
LKH	56.7% (102/180)	39.054 (**)	Corr:	− 0.317 (**)	− 0.384 (**)	0.164 (*)	0.133	− 0.030	− 0.051
			Wald:	5.202 (*)	12.496 (**)	1.559	0.124	0.032	1.614
			β:	− 0.629	− 1.106	0.781	− 0.097	0.070	0.249
YYW	70.1% (148/211)	30.867 (**)	Corr:	− 0.331 (**)	− 0.208 (**)	0.198 (**)	0.152 (*)	− 0.048	− 0.034
			Wald:	11.165 (**)	1.564	2.819	0.793	0.084	1.130
			β:	− 0.937	− 0.338	1.014	− 0.245	0.110	0.198
WYL	69.1% (123/178)	22.330 (**)	Corr:	− 0.276 (**)	− 0.281 (**)	0.142 (*)	0.203 (**)	− 0.094	− 0.124
			Wald:	0.427	7.387 (**)	0.345	1.505	0.489	0.110
			β:	− 0.186	− 0.824	0.391	0.346	− 0.283	− 0.067

Note. [a]Subjective AoA was marginally significant in CKY at $p = 0.065$. $^*p < 0.05$, $^{**}p < 0.01$. Corr = correlation between naming accuracy and each predictor variable

Table 12.6 Distribution of naming errors

	CKY	*FSY*	*LKH*	*WYL*	*YYW*
No. of errors	51	45	92	61	64
Error type					
Semantic (e.g. 蜜蜂 *mat6fung1* 'bee' → 蝴蝶 *wu4dip2* 'fly')	60.8%	82.2%	48.9%	34.4%	67.2%
Partial (e.g. 青蛙 *cing1waa1* 'frog' → 青 *cing1*)	3.9%	0.0%	1.1%	6.6%	3.1%
Jargon (e.g. 裙 *kwan4* 'skirt' → 套衫 *tou3saam1* CL-clothes)	5.9%	6.7%	12.0%	13.1%	7.8%
Unrelated (e.g. 欄杆 *laan4gon1* 'fence' → 南瓜 *naam4gwaa1* 'pumpkin')	3.9%	4.4%	18.5%	1.6%	9.4%
No response	25.5%	6.7%	17.4%	34.4%	12.5%
Others (e.g. 叉 *caa1* 'fork' → [fork])	0.0%	0.0%	2.2%	9.8%	0.0%

Note. CL = classifier

In summary, in contrast with the observations of previous studies that compared results of grouped and individual analyses (Cuetos *et al.*, 2002; Ellis *et al.*, 1997; Nickels & Howard, 1995), more highly consistent patterns of significant predictors were found in the present study between grouped and individual data.

General Discussion

Our findings of significant effects of subjective AoA on picture naming are compatible with previous observations that this variable routinely affects naming latencies in normal subjects and accuracy in aphasic individuals. It was a robust predictor of our data as it was significant for the group analysis and in four of five participants. The influence of word length has been reported of normal and aphasic speakers (e.g. Cuetos *et al.*, 1999; Laws *et al.*, 2002; Morrison *et al.*, 1992; Nickels & Howard, 1995) and is found in naming performance of three of our subjects. Its effects have been suggested to be related to one's difficulties at the phonological output or articulatory levels (Cuetos *et al.*, 2002). Our data seem to support this view. The subjects with word length effects, CKY, LKH and WYL, are also the ones who showed impaired repetition. In contrast, FSY and YYW, with normal repetition were not affected by this variable. Despite its narrow range of ratings, image agreement significantly predicted performance in CKY and FSY. Barry *et al.* (1997), Cuetos *et al.* (1999) and Ellis *et al.* (1997) observed an effect and proposed that the variable refers to how well a target picture matches the subject's mental imagery of that object, and therefore it exerts its influence at the level of structural representations of objects or object recognition. Unlike the case of word length, we could not discern patterns of performance on the language and cognitive tasks in initial assessment that would distinguish CKY and FSY from other participants to account for the selective effects of image agreement.

The other variables, object familiarity, name agreement and visual complexity, were not important determinants in any of the participants. Among the six predictors, visual complexity was least frequently found to be associated with picture-naming performance (Juhasz, 2005; Nickels & Howard, 1995). Our failure to find significant effects of name agreement despite frequent reports of its influence, including Weekes *et al.* (2007) in which naming latencies of normal Chinese subjects were examined, might be due to the fact that 60% of our stimuli had complete name agreement. A different set of stimuli with a wider range of and more evenly distributed values might reveal stronger effects of this variable. Object familiarity is not commonly found to be a significant predictor in picture-naming studies. Nevertheless, it made a unique contribution to predicting naming latencies of Chinese subjects, along with AoA and name agreement, in Weekes *et al.* The absence of its significance in the present study could be the result of its high correlation with subjective AoA (– 0.606). In Weekes *et al.* the two variables were not nearly as highly correlated (– 0.25).

As the effect of AoA has been quite firmly established in picture naming in a growing number of languages, its locus (or loci) is naturally the focus of interest. Earlier hypotheses attributed the effects to the level of phonological output, i.e. the phonological completeness hypothesis (Brown & Watson, 1987). Late-acquired words are assumed to have more segmented phonological representations compared with early-acquired words. However, the observations of AoA effects in tasks that do not involve verbal responses, such as lexical decision (e.g. Gerhand & Barry, 1999; Morrison & Ellis, 1995, 2000) and face recognition (Lewis, 1999a), are problematic to the hypothesis. The most challenging evidence is the results of a more recent study showing a lack of relationship between one's ability to segment a word and the AoA of the word (Monaghan & Ellis, 2002a). In the present context, findings against an account associating phonological output with the AoA effect come from its significant contribution in subjects with supposedly preserved target phonological representations. Moreover, the only subject, WYL, with naming accuracy not significantly predicted by subjective AoA was the subject who produced the lowest proportion of semantic errors and many omissions (see Table 12.6). Although semantic errors are generally assumed to originate at the semantic level, there have been reports showing that they may also arise from impairment to access from semantics to phonology or the phonological output level (Hillis, 1998; Rapp & Caramazza, 1997). Therefore, WYL's naming disorders might stem from disruption in other components, as a consequence, his naming performance was not affected by AoA. In light of our observation that naming accuracy of participants believed to have preserved semantic processing, i.e. CKY, FSY and LKH, and semantic deficits, namely YYW, is significantly predicted by AoA, and the fact that there is little evidence for AoA effects being localized at the phonological output level, we suggest that the effects reside at the semantic level and access from semantics to phonology.

Our proposal is consistent with the semantic locus hypothesis (Brysbaert *et al.*, 2000a, 2000b) and the arbitrary mapping (AM) hypothesis (Ellis & Lambon Ralph, 2000). The former is based on the idea that concepts acquired later in life are often built on or defined in terms of those learned earlier (Gilhooly & Gilhooly, 1979). As object familiarity was not a significant contributor, our pattern of results can be considered frequency-independent AoA effect (Belke *et al.*, 2005; Brysbaert & Ghyselinck, 2006). According to these researchers, the advantage of early over late AoA words is explained in terms of richness of conceptual representations; that is, early-acquired concepts have more semantic connections, thus facilitating access to them and their associated lemmas (Steyvers & Tenenbaum, 2005). The latter hypothesis suggests that AoA is a property of the development of a learning system which gradually loses its plasticity as training progresses. Within this account, it has been argued that the AoA effect is only evident if the mappings between input and output are arbitrary. The greater the degree of inconsistency of input-to-output mappings is, the larger the AoA effect will be (Monaghan & Ellis, 2002b). Hence, in the case of English, stronger AoA effects are predicted for picture naming than word reading (Lambon Ralph & Ehsan, 2006; Zevin & Seidenberg, 2002). The AM hypothesis, therefore, contends that the locus of AoA resides in the connections between different levels of representation, including access from semantics to phonology. Clearly, our data is inadequate in adjudicating these alternative accounts.

In conclusion, our study is the first to provide confirmation of AoA effects in picture naming of Chinese anomic speakers. In light of the participants' largely preserved phonological level, the influence of the timing at which items are acquired is hypothesized to be located at a prelexical level, that is, semantic and/or access from meaning to phonology.

Acknowledgements

The work reported here was supported by a grant from the Seed Funding Programme for Basic Research at the University of Hong Kong. We are grateful to CKY, LKH, FSY, YYW and WYL for participating in this study.

Notes

1. Only culturally appropriate items were used for oral naming and non-verbal semantic tests. The criteria for selection were based on the performance of 30 female and 30 male Hong Kong Cantonese speakers equally distributed in three age groups: 25–39, 40–59 and more than 60 years of age, and two educational levels, less than 13 years and at least 14 years of schooling. An arbitrary cutoff of 80% correct or higher was used for oral naming, and the criterion of at least 70% correct was adopted for the two non-verbal semantic tests. A total of 217, 23 and 37 items were then chosen from the Snodgrass and Vanderwart picture set, BORB and PPTT, respectively.
2. As only 40% of the stimuli had norms in available frequency counts, subjective frequencies were obtained instead. Twenty students at the Division of Speech and Hearing Sciences of the University of Hong Kong were asked to rate the frequency at which they encountered each target name in different modalities (listening, speaking, reading and writing) on a six-point scale. It was found that subjective AoA, object familiarity and subjective frequency were highly correlated. This was particularly the case between familiarity and subjective frequency ($r = 0.771$). Given that familiarity is often considered a measure of subjective frequency (Feyereisen *et al.*, 1988; Hirsh & Ellis, 1994; Nickels & Howard, 1995), to avoid the problem of collinearity, only one of these variables was entered into regression analyses. Familiarity was chosen as its ratings were collected from a larger group of normal subjects and thus believed to be more reliable. It is worth pointing out that whether object familiarity or subjective frequency was used as a predictor, the statistical results remained the same.

References

Barry, C., Hirsh, K.W., Johnston, R.A. and Williams, C.L. (2001) Age of acquisition, word frequency, and the locus of repetition priming of picture naming. *Journal of Memory and Language* 44, 350–375.

Barry, C., Morrison, C.M. and Ellis, A.W. (1997) Naming the Snodgrass and Vanderwart pictures: Effects of age of acquisition, frequency and name agreement. *Quarterly Journal of Experimental Psychology* 50(A), 560–585.

Belke, E., Brysbaert, M., Meyer, A.S. and Ghyselinck, M. (2005) Age of acquisition effects in picture naming: Evidence for a lexical-semantic competition hypothesis. *Cognition* 96, B45–B54.

Bogka, N., Masterson, J., Druks, J., Fragkioudaki, M., Chatziprokopiou, E-S. and Economou, K. (2003) Object and action picture naming in English and Greek. *European Journal of Cognitive Psychology* 15, 371–403.

Bonin, P., Barry, C., Meot, A. and Chalard, M. (2004) The influence of age of acquisition in word reading and other tasks: A never ending story? *Journal of Memory and Language* 50, 456–476.

Bonin, P., Charlard, M., Meot, A. and Fayol, M. (2002) The determinants of spoken and written picture naming latency. *British Journal of Psychology* 93, 89–114.
Bonin, P., Fayol, M. and Chalard, M. (2001) Age of acquisition and word frequency in written picture naming. *Quarterly Journal of Experimental Psychology* 54(A), 469–489.
Bonin, P., Peereman, R., Malardier, N., Meot, A. and Chalard, M. (2003) A new set of 299 pictures for psycholinguistic studies: French norms for name agreement, image agreement, conceptual familiarity, visual complexity, image variability, age of acquisition and naming latencies. *Behavior Research Methods, Instruments and Computers* 35, 158–167.
Brown, G.D.A. and Watson, F.L. (1987) First in, first out: Word learning age and spoken word frequency as predictors of word familiarity and word naming latency. *Memory and Cognition* 15, 208–216.
Brysbaert, M. and Ghyselinck, M. (2006) The effect of age of acquisition: Partly frequency related, partly frequently independent. *Visual Cognition* 13, 992–1011.
Brysbaert, M., Lange, M. and Van Wijnendaele, I. (2000a) The effects of age-of-acquisition and frequency of occurrence in visual word recognition: Further evidence from the Dutch language. *European Journal of Cognitive Psychology* 12, 65–85.
Brysbaert, M., Van Wijnendaele, I. and de Deyne, S. (2000b) Age-of-acquisition effects in semantic processing tasks. *Acta Psychologica* 104, 215–226.
Caramazza, A. (1984) The logic of neuropsychological research and the problem of patient classification in aphasia. *Brain and Language* 21, 9–20.
Caramazza, A. (1986) On drawing inferences about the structure of normal cognitive systems from the analysis of patterns of impaired performance: The case for single-patient studies. *Brain and Cognition* 5, 41–66.
Cuetos, F., Aguado, G., Izura, C. and Ellis, A.W. (2002) Aphasic naming in Spanish: Predictors and errors. *Brain and Language* 82, 344–365.
Cuetos, F., Ellis, A.Q. and Alverez, B. (1999) Naming times for the Snodgrass and Vanderwart pictures in Spanish. *Behavior Research Methods, Instruments, & Computers* 31, 650–658.
Cuetos, F., Monsalve, A. and Perez, A. (2005) Determinants of lexical access in pure anomia. *Journal of Neurolinguistics* 18, 383–399.
Dell'Acqua, R., Lotto, L. and Job, R (2000) Naming times and standardized norms for the Italian PD/DPSS set of 266 pictures: Direct comparisons with American, English, French, and Spanish published databases. *Behavior Research Methods, Instruments, & Computers* 32, 588–615.
Ellis, A.W. and Lambon Ralph, M.A. (2000) Age of acquisition effects in adult lexical processing reflect loss of plasticity in maturing systems: Insights from connectionist networks. *Journal of Experimental Psychology: Learning, Memory, and Cognition* 26, 1103–1123.
Ellis, A.W., Lum, C. and Lambon Ralph, M.A. (1997) On the use of regression techniques for the analysis of single case aphasic data. *Journal of Neurolinguistics* 6, 165–174.
Ellis, A.W. and Morrison, C.M. (1998) Real age-of-acquisition effects in lexical retrieval. *Journal of Experimental Psychology: Learning, Memory, and Cognition* 24, 515–523.
Feyereisen, P., Van der Borght, F. and Seron, X. (1988) The operativity effect in naming: A re-analysis. *Neuropsycholgia* 26, 401–415.
Gerhand, S. and Barry, C. (1999) Age of acquisition, word frequency and the role of phonology in the lexical decision task. *Memory & Cognition* 27, 592–602.

Ghyselinck, M., Lewis, M.B. and Brysbaert, M. (2004) Age of acquisition and the cumulative frequency hypothesis: A review of the literature and a new multi-task investigation. *Acta Psychologica* 115, 43–67.

Gilhooly, K.J. and Gihooly, M.L. (1979) Age-of-acquisition effects in lexical and episodic memory tasks. *Memory & Cognition* 7, 214–223.

Hillis, A.E. (1998) What's in a name? A model of the cognitive processes underlying object naming. In E.G. Visch-Brink and R. Bastiaanse (eds) *Linguistic Levels in Aphasia* (pp. 35–48). San Diego, CA: Singular.

Hirsh, K.W. and Ellis, E.W. (1994) Age of acquisition and lexical processing in aphasia. *Cognitive Neuropsychology* 11, 435–458.

Hirsh, K.W. and Funnell, E. (1995) Those old, familiar things: Age of acquisition, familiarity and lexical access in progressive aphasia. *Journal of Neurolinguistics* 9, 23–32.

Holmes, S.J., Fitch, F.J. and Ellis, A.W. (2006) Age of acquisition affects object recognition and naming in patients with Alzheimer's disease. *Journal of Clinical and Experimental Psychology* 28, 1010–1022.

Howard, D. and Patterson, K. (1992) *Pyramids and Palm Trees Test*. Edmunds, UK: Thames Valley Test Company.

Johnston, R.A. and Barry, C. (2006) Age of acquisition and lexical processing. *Visual Cognition* 13, 789–845.

Juhasz, B.J. (2005) Age-of-acquisition effects in word and picture identification. *Psychological Bulletin* 131, 684–712.

Kremin, H., Hamerel, M., Dordain, M., de Wilde, M. and Perrier, D. (2000) Age of acquisition and name agreement as predictors of mean response latencies in picture naming of French adults. *Brain and Cognition* 43, 286–291.

Lachman, R. (1973) Uncertainly effects on time to access the internal lexicon. *Journal of Experimental Psychology* 99, 199–208.

Lachman, R., Shaffer, J.P. and Hennrikus, D. (1974) Language and cognition: Effects of stimulus codability, name-word frequency, and age of acquisition on lexical reaction time. *Journal of Verbal Learning and Verbal Behavior* 13, 613–625.

Lambon Ralph, M.A. and Ehsan, S. (2006) Age of acquisition effects depend on the mapping between representations and the frequency of occurrence: Empirical and computational evidence. *Visual Cognition* 13, 928–948.

Lambon Ralph, M.A., Graham, K.S., Ellis, A.W. and Hodges, J.R. (1998) Naming in semantic dementia – What matters? *Neuropsychologia* 36, 775–784.

Laws, K.R., Leeson, V.C. and Gale, T.M. (2002) The effect of 'masking' on picture naming. *Cortex* 38, 137–148.

Lewis, M.B. (1999a) Age of acquisition in face categorization: Is there an instance-based account? *Cognition* 71, B23–B39.

Lewis, M.B. (1999b) Are age-of-acquisition effects cumulative frequency effects in disguise? A reply to Moore, Valentine and Turner (1999) *Cognition* 72, 311–316.

Lewis, M.B., Gerhand, S. and Ellis, H.D. (2001) Re-evaluating age-of-acquisition effects: Are they simply cumulative-frequency effects? *Cognition* 78, 189–205.

Monaghan, J. and Ellis, A.W. (2002a) Age of acquisition and the completeness of phonological representations. *Reading and Writing* 15, 759–788.

Monaghan, J. and Ellis, A.W. (2002b) What exactly interacts with spelling-sound consistency in word naming? *Journal of Experimental Psychology: Learning, Memory, and Cognition* 28, 183–206.

Morrison, C.M. and Ellis, A.W. (1995) Roles of word frequency and age of acquisition in word naming and lexical decision. *Journal of Experimental Psychology: Learning, Memory, and Cognition* 21, 116–133.

Morrison, C.M. and Ellis, A.W. (2000) Real age of acquisition effects in word naming and lexical decision. *British Journal of Psychology* 91, 167–180.

Morrison, C.M., Ellis, A.W. and Quinlan, P.T. (1992) Age of acquisition, not word frequency, affects object naming, not object recognition. *Memory & Cognition* 20, 705–714.

Morrison, C.M., Hirsh, K.W., Chappell, T. and Ellis, A.W. (2002) Age and age of acquisition: An evaluation of the cumulative frequency hypothesis. *European Journal of Cognitive Psychology* 14, 435–459.

Morrison, C.M., Hirsh, K.W. and Duggan, G.B. (2003) Age of acquisition, ageing, and verb production: Normative and experimental data. *The Quarterly Journal of Experimental Psychology* 56A, 705–730.

Nickels, L. and Howard, D. (1995) Aphasic naming: What matters? *Neuropsychologia* 33, 1281–1303.

Pind, J. and Tryggvadottir, H.B. (2002) Determinants of picture naming in Icelandic. *Scandinavian Journal of Psychology* 43, 221–226.

Rapp, B.C. and Caramazza, A. (1997) The modality specific organization of lexical categories: Evidence from impaired spoken and written sentence production. *Brain and Language* 56, 248–286.

Riddoch, M.J. and Humphreys, G.W. (1993) *Birmingham Object Recognition Battery.* Hove, UK: Lawrence Erlbaum.

Rochford, G. and Williams, M. (1962) Studies in the development and breakdown of the use of names. *Journal of Neurology, Neurosurgery & Psychiatry* 25, 222–233.

Silveri, M.C., Cappa, A., Mariotti, P. and Puopolo, M. (2002) Naming in patients with Alzheimer's disease: Influence of age of acquisition and categorical effects. *Journal of Clinical and Experimental Psychology* 24, 755–764.

Snodgrass, J.G. and Vanderwart, M. (1980) A standardised set of 260 pictures: Norms for name agreement, image agreement, familiarity and visual complexity. *Journal of Experimental Psychology: Learning, Memory, and Cognition* 6, 174–215.

Snodgrass, J.G. and Yuditsky, T. (1996) Naming times for the Snodgrass and Vanderwart pictures. *Behavior Research Methods, Instruments, & Computers* 28, 516–536.

Stadthagen-Gonzalez, H., Bowers, J.S. and Damian, M.F. (2004) Age-of-acquisition effects in visual word recognition: Evidence from expert vocabularies. *Cognition* 93, B11–B26.

Steyvers, M. and Tenenbaum, J.B. (2005) The large-scale structure of semantic networks: Statistical analyses and a model of semantic growth. *Cognitive Science* 29, 41–78.

Taylor, R. (1998) Effects of age of acquisition, word frequency, and familiarity on object recognition and naming in dementia. *Perceptual and Motor Skill* 87, 573–574.

Weekes, B.S., Castles, A.E. and Davies, R.A. (2006) Effects of consistency and age of acquisition on reading and spelling among developing readers. *Reading and Writing* 19, 133–169.

Weekes, B.S., Shu, H., Hao, M-L., Liu, Y-Y. and Tan, L.H. (2007) Predictors of timed picture naming in Chinese. *Behavior Research Methods, Instruments, & Computers* 39, 335–342.

Zevin, J.D. and Seidenberg, M.S. (2002) Age of acquisition effects in word reading and other tasks. *Journal of Memory and Language* 47, 1–29.

Chapter 13

The Effect of Semantic Integrity of Words with Preserved Lexico-phonological Representation on Verbal Recall

WINSY WONG and SAM-PO LAW

Introduction

The role of semantics in verbal recall has generated much interest in studies of short-term memory (STM). Some researchers investigate this issue by examining how psycholinguistic factors (e.g. imageability) affect verbal recall in neurologically intact individuals (e.g. Bourassa & Besner, 1994) and aphasic participants (Martin & Saffran, 1997). Other studies have contrasted the performance on immediate serial recall (ISR) of words in individuals with neurological diseases who have degraded semantic knowledge, such as semantic dementia (Knott *et al.*, 1997; McCarthy & Warrington, 1987, 2001; Patterson *et al.*, 1994). However, the involvement of semantics in verbal STM remains inconclusive.

Patterson *et al.* (1994) proposed a semantic-binding hypothesis after studying the ISR performance of subjects with semantic dementia. Their hypothesis was based on results showing that semantically preserved (known) words were better recalled than degraded (unknown) words. Such findings are explained via the differential semantic support of known and unknown words from the feedback-feedforward mechanism between the semantic and phonological levels in the language-processing system. The phonological nodes activated during verbal input spread activation to the associated semantic nodes; the feedback from the semantic nodes then helps to bind the corresponding phonological segments for output. The phonological representations of known words receive more support from the semantic level and are thus better recalled than the unknown counterparts. Subsequent studies adopting the same methodology obtained similar results not only from individuals with semantic dementia (e.g. Jefferies *et al.*, 2005; Knott *et al.*, 1997), but also with other etiologies, including carbon-monoxide poisoning (Forde & Humphreys, 2002) and encephalitis (Caza *et al.*, 2002).

Martin and Saffran (1997) proposed a different model to explain the contribution of semantic memory to verbal recall. By examining the ISR performance of aphasic participants, they found that imageability effects in verbal recall were correlated with semantic-processing abilities, i.e. imageability effects were more pronounced in aphasic participants with more preserved semantic processing. Such findings were explained by the direct interaction between semantic and phonological levels. In patients with severe semantic impairment, the phonological representations for output receive less feedback from the semantic level and are thus more prone to decay. Their framework is similar to Patterson *et al.* (1994) in that performance on verbal recall is dependent on the direct interaction between semantic and phonological levels and neither model assumes a separate semantic buffer. However, these models differ from each other in that an additional lexical level representing word forms is assumed in Martin and Saffran.

Another model, proposed by Martin *et al.* (1994), also recognizes the role of semantics in verbal recall. It differs from the above-mentioned models in the distinction between processing and STM components at both the semantic and phonological levels, and the buffers for holding semantic and phonological information, respectively. In such a framework, one may have intact processing but impaired STM (e.g. cases reported in Martin, 1995; Martin & Breedin, 1992), and vice versa. It is also possible that language impaired individuals may suffer deficits to one of the STM buffers (e.g. Majerus *et al.*, 2005).

Although the aforementioned studies, contrasting known versus unknown word recall, provide evidence for semantic contribution to verbal recall, there are studies that do not find semantic effects (Funnell, 1996; McCarthy & Warrington, 1987, 2001; Warrington, 1975). Jefferies *et al.* (2004) reported that only two of their four participants showed an advantage when recalling known words. McCarthy and Warrington (2001) suggested that preserved lexical-phonological processing and phonological STM are sufficient to support word repetition, which is functionally independent of semantic processing. However, their account seems incompatible with reports of the presence of semantic effects in participants with intact phonology (e.g. Caza *et al.*, 2002; Jefferies *et al.*, 2005).

Attempts have been made to accommodate the mixed findings. Jefferies *et al.* (2004) suggested that the negative findings (e.g. Funnell, 1996) might be attributable to the small set size tested. As a consequence, subjects would be more familiar with the phonological form of items when they appeared repeatedly, and this might reduce the significance of the semantic effect. Caza *et al.* (2002) pointed out that the ceiling performance on recalling unknown words in McCarthy and Warrington (1987) did not allow potential differences to be observed. Nevertheless, these explanations are not able to accommodate all the results. The accounts offered by Jefferies *et al.* and Caza *et al.* are not applicable to the findings of McCarthy and Warrington (2001), because the set size was reasonably large (20 for each of the known and unknown condition) and the accuracy of recalling unknown words was well below ceiling (52.5% accuracy at list length four).

We propose that the mixed findings may be explained in terms of methodological procedures. Research findings of previous work might have been confounded with the lexical status of the stimuli. The lexical-phonological integrity of the stimuli was rarely checked except in Caza *et al.* (2002). This perhaps may be related to the fact that the semantic-binding hypothesis does not assume a lexical level. This potential lexical effect might interact with other language-processing levels, which result in the inconsistent findings reported previously. The interpretation regarding the experimental findings therefore becomes questionable.

The present study examined the role of semantics in verbal recall by taking into consideration the lexical-phonological integrity of test stimuli. This was evaluated using an auditory lexical decision test administered to each participant. Only stimuli with preserved lexical-phonological representations were used in known and unknown word sets. By doing this, we could assess the effect of semantic integrity on verbal recall by effectively removing a potential confounding variable characteristic of previous studies. In addition, it should be noted that in studies contrasting known versus unknown word recall, the significance of the semantic STM buffer has not been considered. By adopting some of the STM tasks developed by Martin and colleagues (e.g. Freedman & Martin, 2001; Martin *et al.*, 1994), our aim was to give a more comprehensive psycholinguistic profile of the participants and explore if and how semantic STM has an influence on verbal recall of words with varying semantic integrity.

Method

Background information on participants

Two native Cantonese-speaking aphasic individuals, CSW and FWL, took part. They had no hearing or motor speech impairments. Six age and education-matched controls were tested on various phonological and semantic processing and STM tasks. Two more females who were age matched to FWL were also administered the task of ISR with known and unknown words. Semantic tasks included verbal and non-verbal tests. Non-verbal tests included selected items from the associative match tasks of the Birmingham Object Recognition Battery (Riddoch & Humphreys, 1993) and the Pyramids and Palm Trees Test (PPTT; Howard & Patterson, 1992). Verbal semantic tests comprised word-picture matching and attribute judgment of object names, and synonym judgment of disyllabic nouns. The object names were selected from Snodgrass and Vanderwart (1980). Yes/no questions concerning the attributes of each target object (e.g. category, functions and properties) were probed in the attribute judgment task. Disyllabic nouns, which were used to examine the extent of semantic effect in verbal recall, were assessed by synonym judgment and auditory lexical decision tasks so as to evaluate their semantic and lexico-phonological integrities, respectively. In addition, the imageability of the nouns was rated by five graduates of the Speech and Hearing Sciences program of the University of Hong Kong following the procedures reported in Chiarello *et al.* (1999). Phonological processing was assessed via the immediate auditory discrimination and rhyme judgment tasks. Normative data for the synonym judgment, auditory lexical decision, immediate auditory discrimination and rhyme judgment tasks was based on the performance of controls subjects, while control performance on the non-verbal semantic tasks was taken from Law *et al.* (2005).

Background information and the performance of aphasic and normal participants on the phonological- and semantic-processing tasks are reported in Table 13.1. Both participants had intact phonological-processing abilities, but different degrees of semantic deficit. CSW's semantic impairment was relatively mild; she showed normal performance on all tasks except synonym judgment. On the other hand, FWL performed below the normal range on all tasks except PPTT, indicating a moderate-to-severe semantic impairment. Finally, both subjects scored below normal in the lexical decision task.

Tasks and procedures

Semantic STM tasks

Category probe task. We adopted the procedure used by Martin *et al.* (1994). Disyllabic object names known to each of the participants, i.e. those items that were scored correct in the spoken word-picture matching and attribute judgment tasks were used. Sequences containing two to seven items from different semantic categories were presented auditorily, and the target object was presented after two seconds. Subjects had to decide if the target name was in the same category as any of the items in the list. Ten lists were prepared for each of the 'same' and 'different' category conditions for each list length. Each serial position was probed equally frequently. The probe span was determined by taking the longest list length in which the participant could obtain an accuracy of at least 50% in both conditions.

ISR of semantically related versus unrelated words. Normal subjects are better at recalling word lists comprised of items of the same semantic category compared to those from unrelated categories (Channon & Daum, 2000; Poirier & Saint-Aubin, 1995). Object names known to both CSW and FWL were selected. In the semantically related condition, items in each word list belonged to one or two semantic categories, whereas in the unrelated condition, none of the items were semantically related. As

Table 13.1 Background information and performances on phonological and semantic processing tasks of aphasic and control participants

	CSW	*FWL*	*Control mean (range)*
Age/gender	44/F	49/F	46 (43–48)
Years of education	14	14	14
Etiology	CVA	TBI (due to traffic accident)	NA
Lesion site	Left frontoparietal region	Left temporal region	
No. of onset years	5	1	NA
Aphasia type	Transcortical motor	Anomia	NA
Semantic processing			
Non-verbal semantic tasks			
BORB ($n = 23$)	23	19[a]	22.3 (20–23)
PPTT ($n = 37$)	36	32	31.9 (16–37)
Verbal semantic tasks			
Spoken word-picture matching ($n = 74$)	74	66[a]	
Attribute judgment ($n = 74$)	74	55[a]	
Synonym judgment ($n = 84$)	57[a]	50[a]	80.7 (74–84)
Auditory lexical decision ($n = 84$)	82[a]	79[a]	83.7 (83–84)
Phonological processing			
Immediate auditory discrimination ($n = 80$)	80	80	78.7 (77–80)
Rhyme judgment ($n = 40$)	38	39	37.7 (36–39)

Note. [a]Denotes below normal performance. BORB = associative match tasks of the Birmingham Object Recognition Battery (Riddoch & Humphreys, 1993). PPTT = Pyramid and Palm Trees Test (Howard & Patterson, 1992)

frequency counts of many object names in Cantonese are not available, familiarity ratings were used, similar to Shibahara *et al.* (2003). The stimuli were matched for familiarity in both conditions, with ratings collected from 20 age- and education-matched controls using the same procedures as in Snodgrass and Vanderwart (1980). The recall task started at list length two and the longest list length with at least 50% accuracy was considered the maximum span for that list condition for each participant.

Synonym selection task. This task was considered a semantic STM test as the participants had to hold several pieces of semantic information at one time for comparison. Stimuli scored correct in the synonym judgment task were included (57 for CSW and 50 for FWL). Two versions of the tasks, three-choice and four-choice, were given. In the three-choice version, three stimuli were presented serially on a trial and the participants had to select which two out of the three stimuli were synonymous. In the four-choice version, the subject was asked to select two stimuli that shared similar meaning from an array of four. Stimuli were presented in auditory and written modalities in the three-choice version, while the four-choice version was tested in the written modality only. In the auditory mode, a piece of paper with printed numbers (depending on the number of choices) was prepared. The experimenter pointed to each number and a stimulus was presented verbally. The participant responded by either pointing to the two numbers representing the synonymous pair or by producing the answers verbally. In the written mode, the participants responded by pointing to the two choices they considered to be synonymous.

Phonological STM tasks

Filled delayed auditory discrimination (n = 80). The stimuli were identical to those in the immediate auditory discrimination task. On each trial, the first item of a pair was aurally presented and the participant was asked to count from one to five verbally together with the experimenter before the presentation of the second item.

Rhyme probe. Existing Cantonese monosyllables with CV or CVC structures served as stimuli. There were 10 trials in both the rhyming and nonrhyming conditions for all list lengths. The scoring criterion was identical to that of the category probe task.

ISR of phonologically similar versus dissimilar syllables. Twenty existing syllables with a CV structure where the vowel might be a monophthong or diphthong were chosen as stimuli. Based on the corpus of spoken Cantonese of Leung *et al.* (2004), the selected vowels had frequency counts higher than 700 (mean = 5024.4; SD = 3585.9). Fifteen lists were created in both the phonologically similar and dissimilar conditions for each list length. Stimuli of the same lists in the former condition shared the same vowels. The procedures were similar to that of the ISR with semantically related versus unrelated words.

Digit span. The span was determined by taking the longest list length in which all the items were recalled in the correct order in at least one out of two trials.

ISR of known versus unknown words

Two word sets were compiled according to the accuracy of the items in the synonym judgment and lexical decision tasks. The known word set included items that were scored correct in both lexical decision and synonym judgment. Unknown words were those from failed trials in synonym judgment but with preserved lexical status according to the results of the lexical decision task. The disyllabic words used for the known and unknown word sets for each participant were matched on frequency, imageability and number of phonemes. The characteristics of the stimuli are summarized in Table 13.2.

Fifteen lists were generated for each list length (from one to six) for each condition by random selection of items from the respective stimulus set. Items in the same list did not rhyme with their neighboring items. ISR started at list length one and lists of both conditions were presented in an ABBA manner. The experimenter presented the list auditorily at the rate of one item per second and the participant was asked to repeat the list verbally in the order of presentation. One point was given if the item was recalled in its correct serial position. The ISR of either list type was terminated if the participant scored lower than 50% accuracy for a given length.

The Chi-square test and semantic effect scores were used to contrast performance between known and unknown word recall. The former has

Table 13.2 The characteristics of known and unknown word stimuli for CSW and FWL

	Frequency	*Imageability*	*Numbero. of phonemes*	*Set size*
CSW				
Known	20.57 (21.47)	2.15 (0.52)	5.0 (0.71)	21
Unknown	20.09 (20.10)	2.23 (0.52)	5.10 (0.70)	21
FWL				
Known	14.71 (15.93)	2.21 (0.54)	5.0 (0.66)	24
Unknown	15.29 (16.50)	2.19 (0.55)	5.0 (0.75)	24

Note. Word frequency values were obtained from Wu and Liu (1987). Figures in parentheses represent standard deviations

been employed to compare verbal recall of lexical items of different degrees of semantic integrity (Forde & Humphreys, 2002; Hodges *et al.*, 1994; Patterson *et al.*, 1994). In our study, the test was administered for every list length. A semantic effect score was calculated according to the formula proposed by Caza *et al.* (2002) and gave an index that was equal to (the number of known words recalled–the number of unknown words recalled)/number of known words recalled. However, we calculated the scores for each participant in all list lengths tested, and then the highest semantic effect score of each control participant was selected to represent the semantic effect manifested by that individual. The scores of the normal participants were then pooled in order to compute *z*-scores for the aphasic participants.

The aforementioned tasks were administered to the aphasic participants over four 90-minute sessions with phonological STM tasks preceding the semantic STM tasks, which were followed by the ISR tasks. The tests were carried out with the control participants in two to three separate sessions with the same test sequence and procedures used with the aphasic participants.

Results

The results in Table 13.3 reveal that the aphasic participants were impaired in both STM components, but the patterns of impairment were different. CSW had severe impairments in semantic STM, while her phonological STM was mildly impaired. She performed poorly on all semantic STM tasks, far below the normal range. The semantic relatedness effect was absent, as shown by comparable performance on recalling semantically related and unrelated items at list length two (14/15 versus 15/15) and three (5/15 versus 5/15). On the other hand, she performed within the normal range on all phonological STM tasks except the ISR of phonologically similar and dissimilar syllables. Nevertheless, a phonological similarity effect was observed, as the span of dissimilar syllables was longer than the span with similar syllables.

FWL showed normal performance on the category probe and written version of three-choice synonym selection tasks, but the scores she obtained in the auditory three-choice and written four-choice selection were below normal. While the control participants demonstrated the semantic relatedness effect by recalling more related items than unrelated items, the spans for both conditions were the same in FWL. Nonetheless, she recalled more items in the related condition than the unrelated condition at list length five (55/75 versus 43/75, $\chi^2(1) = 4.24$; $p = 0.04$), indicating the presence of an effect. We therefore suggest that although her semantic STM was not unimpaired, her deficit is less severe than CSW's. Her phonological STM disruption was considered to be

Table 13.3 Performance on phonological and semantic STM tasks

	CSW	*FWL*	*Control mean (range)*
Semantic STM			
Category probe span	3[a]	6	6.8 (6–8)
Span of semantically related lists	2[a]	4[a]	5.6 (5–6)
Span of semantically unrelated lists	2[a]	4	4.6 (4–5)
Synonym selection ($n = 57$ for CSW; $n = 50$ for FWL)			
Auditory three-choice	43[a]	43[a]	CSW controls: 56 (55–57); FWL controls: 48.7 (48–49)
Written three-choice	49[a]	49	CSW controls: 57; FWL controls: 49.6 (49–50)
Written four-choice	43[a]	43[a]	CSW controls: 57; FWL controls: 50
Phonological STM			
Filled-delayed auditory discrimination ($n = 80$)	77	75[a]	77.1 (77–79)
Rhyme probe span	6	5	6.5 (5–7)
Span of phonologically similar syllables	2[a]	5	5.5 (5–6)
Span of phonologically dissimilar syllables	4[a]	5	6.3 (5–7)
Digit span	7	8	8.2 (7–11)

Note. [a]Denotes below normal performance

mild. She performed below the normal range in the filled-delayed auditory discrimination task, whereas performance on the other tasks was normal. Phonological similarity effects were exhibited in terms of a significant difference in the number of items correctly recalled in phonologically similar versus dissimilar conditions at list length four

(58/60 versus 51/60; $\chi^2(1) = 4.90$; $p = 0.03$). A comparison between the performances of the two participants on the STM tasks reveals that FWL had better preserved semantic STM than CSW, while their phonological STM capacities were highly comparable.

The results of ISR for known versus unknown words are illustrated in Table 13.4. The scores at list length six for the control group are not reported, as one of the control subjects did not reach the passing criterion at list length five. The highest semantic effect scores from the control subjects were obtained from list lengths four to six, except for two control participants who had a zero effect score at list length three, but negative scores from list lengths four to six. Therefore, their performances on list length three were selected to calculate the mean semantic effect score of the control group. As a result, a mean semantic effect score of 0.061 (SD = 0.084; range = 0–0.205) was obtained.

For the two aphasic participants, CSW in general performed poorly on the ISR task. She had a span of two items in recalling both known and unknown items. Although known words were better recalled than unknown ones at both list length one and two, the greater semantic effect score of 0.111 selected at list length two gave a *z*-score of 0.595, indicating the absence of semantic effect. FWL had a span of five in both the known and unknown conditions. This was similar to the control group. Her performance at list length four rendered the highest semantic score of 0.216 giving a *z*-score of 1.84, which was higher than that of CSW. Similar findings were obtained in the Chi-square tests. No significant differences were found for CSW and the control participants between known versus unknown item recall in all list lengths tested. On the other hand, FWL recalled more known words than unknown ones at list length four ($\chi^2(1) = 5.50$; $p = 0.02$).

Discussion

A full examination of the issue of semantic contribution to verbal recall needs to consider the status of lexical-phonological knowledge of the stimuli. The present study compared the ISR performances of two Cantonese aphasic speakers, CSW and FWL. Their language profiles indicate that they had comparable phonological processing and STM abilities, but with different semantic STM abilities: FWL had relatively better semantic STM than CSW.

These two aphasic participants took part in the task of ISR with words of varying semantic integrity. As all the stimuli chosen in the ISR tasks had preserved lexical-phonological representations as assessed by the auditory lexical decision task, this potentially confounding effect was eliminated. Furthermore, the stimuli in the known and unknown word sets were matched on various linguistic variables, including frequency,

Table 13.4 ISR of known and unknown words

	List length					
	***1* (n =*15*)**	***2* (n =*30*)**	***3* (n =*45*)**	***4* (n =*60*)**	***5* (n =*75*)**	***6* (n =*90*)**
	No. of items correctly recalled (%)					
CSW						
Known	15 (100)	18 (60)	5 (11.1)	NT	NT	NT
Unknown	14 (93.3)	16 (53.3)	11 (24.4)	NT	NT	NT
FWL						
Known	15 (100)	30 (100)	43 (95.6)	51* (85)	44 (58.7)	28 (31.1)
Unknown	15 (100)	30 (100)	42 (93.3)	40 (66.7)	47 (62.7)	20 (22.2)
Control mean [(range])						
Known	15 (100)	30 (100)	45 (100)	55.6 (92.7) [52–59]	52.5 (70.0) [39–67]	NR
Unknown	15 (100)	30 (100)	44.9 (99.8)	54.8 (91.3) [54–60]	54.8 (73.1) [31–66]	NR

Note. NT = not tested, NR = not reported. Figure marked with an asterisk (*) denote significantly better recall of known than unknown words at $p < 0.05$

imageability and the number of phonemes. As a result, better recall of known words must be due to their semantic integrity. We used both Chi-square test and a semantic effect score to measure the extent of semantic effect on known versus unknown word recall. As the normal control subjects knew both the two word sets, the semantic effect scores obtained from them should be close to zero. The use of z-score served as a reliable means to compare the degrees of deviation manifested by the aphasic participants with respect to the control group. CSW showed minimal (if any) semantic effects in the ISR task. FWL seemed to exhibit a somewhat stronger semantic effect, as measured by both statistical measures. In short, after controlling for the lexical-phonological status of the stimuli, no semantic effects were seen in one of the aphasic participants ($z = 0.595$), while a weak effect was observed in the other ($z = 1.84$).

The tentative finding of a difference in the semantic effect, albeit small, between CSW and FWL deserves further attention, especially in light of their different degrees of semantic STM deficits. As they had similar phonological processing and STM abilities, their performances on verbal recall could not be attributed to these factors. We suggest that the rough correlation between the extent of semantic effect and their semantic STM abilities could be understood in models that assume the existence of semantic STM, e.g. Martin *et al.* (1994).

As the semantic STM is responsible for temporary retention of lexico-semantic information via interactive activation at the lexico-semantic processing level, known words elicit stronger activation at the semantic level and the associated information will be stored in the semantic STM component, which then feeds backward to the associated lexico-semantic nodes. The reverberation between semantic processing and STM in turn activates the corresponding phonological nodes, and thus stabilizes the phonological representations for output. On the other hand, recall of unknown words receives little or no support from semantic processing, and the involvement of semantic STM in the maintenance of lexico-semantic activation becomes minimal. In the case of CSW, her semantic buffer was severely impaired; as a result, she was less able to maintain lexico-semantic information. The different levels of activation for known and unknown words at the lexico-semantic processing level might not be sufficient to manifest a known versus unknown recall discrepancy due to rapid decay. Consequently, the integrity of the semantic representation of a stimulus had little effect in ISR tasks, leading to similar performances on recalling known and unknown words. On the other hand, FWL showed a weak semantic effect in the ISR task. It is plausible that the differential semantic support of known words over unknown ones was partially maintained by FWL's mildly impaired semantic STM. We suggest that stronger evidence for our hypothesis may be sought by recruiting participants with more preserved semantic STM abilities and examine if their semantic effect size is larger.

Another possible way to test our hypothesis would be to include a series of participants with a gradation of semantic STM deficits. If the semantic effects observed in the ISR task pattern with their semantic STM capacities, i.e. a negative relationship between the magnitude of semantic effects and the degree of semantic STM disruption, our suggestion about the role of semantic STM in verbal recall would be strengthened.

Our hypothesis about the role of semantic STM in verbal recall may give a clue to the absence of semantic effects reported previously. More specifically, it is possible that the participants in Funnell (1996) and McCarthy and Warrington (1987) had disruption in semantic STM. In McCarthy and Warrington (2001), the lack of semantic relatedness effect found in the participant MNA might be taken as additional support for her compromised semantic STM, although the semantic integrity of the stimuli used in the task was not tested.

Given the very poor verbal recall of CSW, one may question whether her performance might be attributed to other underlying deficits, such as executive dysfunctions. Unfortunately, we were unable to compare the executive functioning of the two aphasic participants. CSW was not able to perform the Chinese version of the Stroop Color-Word Test (Regard, 1981) due to her inability to name colors. She refused to complete the Wisconsin Card Sorting Test (Grant & Berg, 1993) after 21 trials. Nevertheless, executive function impairments may be reflected by error patterns of ISR tasks in terms of source errors (i.e. intrusion of interlist items) and repetitions due to inability to inhibit nontarget items. Therefore, we analyzed the error patterns of the two participants at their supraspan (three for CSW and six for FWL), as more errors were observed at these list lengths. We did not find CSW making excessive repetition or source errors. There were no repetition errors in recalling either known or unknown items, and source errors accounted for only 5% and 9.7% in the known and unknown conditions, respectively. On the contrary, FWL's repetition errors in the corresponding conditions constituted 11.7% and 8% of the total number of errors. Moreover, she made more source errors than CSW (33.3% in the known condition and 14% in the unknown condition). In other words, there is no strong evidence for the claim that CSW's poor verbal recall was associated with executive dysfunctions.

In conclusion, by controlling for the lexico-phonological status of the known and unknown words in an ISR task administered to two aphasic participants, we found no semantic effect in an individual with severe semantic STM impairment, and a small effect in another individual with relatively better semantic STM. These results raise questions about the possible role of semantic STM in verbal recall. Furthermore, our hypothesis may provide a new perspective on understanding the mixed findings in the literature.

References

Bourassa, D.C. and Besner, D. (1994) Beyond the articulatory loop: A semantic contribution to serial order recall of subspan lists. *Psychonomic Bulletin and Review* 1, 122–125.

Caza, N., Belleville, S. and Gilbert, B. (2002) How loss of meaning with preservation of phonological word form affects immediate serial recall performance: A linguistic account. *Neurocase* 8, 255–273.

Channon, S. and Daum, I. (2000) The effect of semantic categorization on recall memory in amnesia. *Behavioral Neurology* 12, 107–117.

Chiarello, C., Shears, C. and Lund, K. (1999) Imageability and distributional typicality measures of nouns and verbs in contemporary English. *Behavior Research Methods, Instruments, & Computers* 31, 603–637.

Forde, E.M.E. and Humphreys, G.W. (2002) The role of semantic knowledge in short-term memory. *Neurocase* 8, 13–27.

Freedman, M.L. and Martin, R.C. (2001) Dissociable components of short-term memory and their relation to long-term learning. *Cognitive Neuropsychology* 18, 193–226.

Funnell, E. (1996) Response bases in oral reading: An account of the co-occurrence of surface dyslexia and semantic dementia. *The Quarterly Journal of Experimental Psychology* 49A, 417–446.

Grant, D.A. and Berg, E.A. (1993) *Wisconsin Card Sorting Test*. Tampa, FL: Psychological Assessment Resources.

Hodges, J.R., Patterson, K. and Tyler, L.K. (1994) Loss of semantic memory: Implications for the modularity of mind. *Cognitive Neuropsychology* 11, 505–542.

Howard, D. and Patterson, K. (1992) *Pyramids and Palm Trees Test*. Edmunds, UK: Thames Valley Test Company.

Jefferies, E., Jones, R., Bateman, D. and Lambon-Ralph, M.A. (2004) When does word meaning affect immediate serial recall in semantic dementia? *Cognitive, Affective, & Behavioral Neuroscience* 4, 20–42.

Jefferies, E., Jones, R., Bateman, D. and Lambon Ralph, M.A. (2005) A semantic contribution to nonword recall? Evidence for intact phonological processes in semantic dementia. *Cognitive Neuropsychology* 22, 183–212.

Knott, R., Patterson, K. and Hodges, J.R. (1997) Lexical and semantic binding effects in short-term memory: Evidence from semantic dementia. *Cognitive Neuropsychology* 14, 1165–1216.

Law, S-P., Yeung, O., Wong, W. and Chiu, K.M-Y. (2005) Processing of semantic radicals in writing Chinese characters: Data from a Chinese dysgraphic patient. *Cognitive Neuropsychology* 22, 885–903.

Leung, M-T., Law, S-P. and Fung, S-Y. (2004) Type and token frequencies of phonological units in Hong Kong Cantonese. *Behavior Research Methods, Instruments, & Computers* 36, 500–505.

Majerus, S., Van der Linden, M., Poncelet, M. and Metz-Lutz, M-N. (2005) Can phonological and semantic short-term memory be dissociated? Further evidence from Landau-Kleffner syndrome. *Cognitive Neuropsychology* 21, 491–512.

Martin, N. and Saffran, E.M. (1997) Language and auditory-verbal short-term memory impairments: Evidence for common underlying processes. *Cognitive Neuropsychology* 14, 641–682.

Martin, R.C. (1995) A multiple capacities view of working memory in language. Paper presented at the Annual Meeting of the Psychonomic Society, Los Angeles, CA, November.

Martin, R.C. and Breedin, S.D. (1992) Dissociations between speech perception and phonological short-term memory deficits. *Cognitive Neuropsychology* 9, 509–534.

Martin, R.C., Shelton, J.R. and Yaffee, L.S. (1994) Language processing and working memory: Neuropsychological evidence for separate phonological and semantic capacities. *Journal of Memory and Language* 33, 83–111.

McCarthy, R.A. and Warrington, E.K. (1987) The double dissociation of short-term memory for lists and sentences: Evidence from aphasia. *Brain* 110, 1545–1563.

McCarthy, R.A. and Warrington, E.K. (2001) Repeating without semantics: Surface dysphasia? *Neurocase* 7, 77–87.

Patterson, K., Graham, N. and Hodges, J.R. (1994) The impact of semantic memory loss on phonological representations. *Journal of Cognitive Neuroscience* 6, 57–69.

Poirier, M. and Saint-Aubin, J. (1995) Memory for related and unrelated words: Further evidence on the influence of semantic factors in immediate serial recall. *Quarterly Journal of Experimental Psychology* 48, 384–404.

Regard, M. (1981) Cognitive rigidity and flexibility: A neuropsychological study. Unpublished doctoral dissertation, University of Victoria, BC.

Riddoch, M.J. and Humphreys, G.W. (1993) *Birmingham Object Recognition Battery*. Hove: Lawrence Erlbaum.

Romani, C. and Martin, R.C. (1999) A deficit in the short-term retention of lexical-semantic information: Forgetting words, but remembering a story. *Journal of Experimental Psychology: General* 128, 56–77.

Shibahara, N., Zorzi, M., Hill, M.P., Wydell, T. and Butterworth, B. (2003) Semantic effects in word naming: Evidence from English and Japanese kanji. *Quarterly Journal of Experimental Psychology* 56A, 1–24.

Snodgrass, J.G. and Vandervart, M. (1980) A standardized set of 260 pictures: Norms for name agreement, image agreement, familiarity and visual complexity. *Journal of Experimental Psychology: Learning, Memory, and Cognition* 6, 174–215.

Warrington, E.K. (1975) The selective impairment of semantic memory. *Quarterly Journal of Experimental Psychology* 27, 635–657.

Wong, W. and Law, S-P. (2006) The relationship between semantic integrity and recall of known and unknown words and nonwords: Preliminary data from Chinese aphasic individuals. *Brain and Language* 99, 98–99.

Wu, R-T. and Liu, I-M. (1987) 中文字詞語音，語意屬性的研究 [*A Study of the Phonological and Semantic Properties of Chinese Lexical Items*]. Taipei, Taiwan: National University of Taiwan.

Chapter 14

Cantonese Linguistic Communication Measure (CLCM): A Clinical Tool for Assessing Aphasic Narrative Production

ANTHONY PAK-HIN KONG and SAM-PO LAW

Introduction

Objective measurement of discourse production as part of a comprehensive assessment has recently been promoted and become more popular in Western countries (e.g. American Speech-Language-Hearing Association, 2004; Armstrong *et al.*, 2006; Capilouto *et al.*, 2006; Royal College of Speech & Language Therapists, 2005). In this chapter, we describe the first clinically oriented assessment tool for Cantonese aphasic narratives, the Cantonese linguistic communication measure (CLCM). In addition, we present findings demonstrating how well the tool can discriminate fluent and non-fluent aphasic speakers from normal speakers using multivariate analysis of variance (MANOVA) and discriminant function analysis (DFA).

An overview of analytic tools for English aphasic narratives

One of the most influential quantitative systems for analyzing aphasic production in English is the Quantitative Production Analysis (QPA; Saffran *et al.*, 1989), which has a detailed procedure for extracting propositional speech and segmenting the extracted samples into utterances, as well as a system for evaluating performances on lexical content and sentence structure. This system was found to be able to distinguish agrammatic output from normal speech as well as from nonagrammatic aphasic speech. In addition, the scores of variables reflecting sentence complexity in nonagrammatic aphasia speakers were found to be significantly lower than those of their normal counterparts. However, as the system involves time-consuming data collection and transcription, as well as complex index computation and result interpretation by linguistically trained researchers, it has not been widely used in clinical settings.

A number of clinically oriented tools have been developed for a quick evaluation of aphasic narratives. Yorkston and Beukelman (1980) introduced a scoring method for analyzing the description of the Cookie

Theft picture of the Boston Diagnostic Aphasia Examination (BDAE; Goodglass & Kaplan, 1993). The procedure focuses on the amount and efficiency of information conveyed. The former is measured by comparing target words produced by an individual with a list of content units, defined as information expressed to describe a key element of the picture. The efficiency of communication is indicated by speaking rate (syllables per minute) and the rate at which content units are uttered per minute. These indices were reported to be able to differentiate between low-moderate and mild aphasic speakers as well as high-moderate aphasic speakers and normal individuals. Another quantitative system was introduced in Shewan (1988a), namely the Shewan Spontaneous Language Analysis (SSLA). Language samples were elicited through the description of the picture stimulus from the standardized version of the Western Aphasia Battery (WAB; Shewan & Kertesz, 1980). They were then analyzed using 12 SSLA variables that are meant to evaluate the semantic (e.g. content units, errors and paraphasic productions), phonological (e.g. melody and articulation) and syntactic (e.g. length of utterances and complex sentences) aspects of the samples. Ten of the variables were reported to reveal significant differences between aphasic and normal speakers, with the content units, speech rate and the number of utterances being the three most discriminating variables. The SSLA was also used to monitor changes in expressive language during recovery as a function of severity (Shewan, 1988b). Eight of the variables were found to be useful in tracing the recovery of language function as they showed positive changes towards the level of the older normal subjects from Shewan's (1988a) study. More recently, Menn *et al.* (1994) presented a simple method of analyzing aphasic narratives, referred to as the Linguistic Communication Measure (LCM). This tool was designed to supplement standard tests. Using the Cookie Theft picture as the stimulus, its aim was to reflect patient progress or deterioration in oral narratives over time. It contained three indices, including the number of content units, Index of Lexical Efficiency (ILE) and Index of Grammatical Support (IGS), the computation of which required minimal clinical experience and linguistic training. Although these performance indices were not intended to differentiate between aphasia types, it was argued that they reflected clinically important differences among aphasic individuals that were missing in the Yorkston and Beukelman scoring method (i.e. the use of correct grammatical morphemes). Similar to the SSLA, the LCM was examined in terms of its ability to monitor changes in aphasic individuals over time. It was found that speakers' performances either approached the normal means or became more stable by the end of the recovery period.

An overview of analytic tools for Cantonese aphasic narratives

Compared with the English literature, investigations of Cantonese aphasic narratives have only appeared in the last decade, using the QPA as the basis for analysis. Yiu (1995) was the first to apply the QPA to perform quantitative analysis of sentence production in 30 Cantonese aphasic subjects and 10 normal controls. Modifications were made to adapt to the characteristics of the Chinese grammar. This involved the inclusion of classifiers and sentence final particles as part of the lexical contents and the adoption of the descriptive system of predicate-argument structure from Byng and Black (1989) for structural analysis. Law (2001) put forth a modified QPA for Cantonese by describing more appropriate procedures to extract narrative words, to classify words into parts-of-speech, to perform structural analysis of compound words and to quantify embedding. There are 33 indices in the system that reflect the amount, fluency, efficiency of speech production, use of grammatical morphemes, distribution of lexical items of different form classes, sentence structure, and sentence complexity and elaboration of narratives. The results indicated that the system could reflect different patterns of language performance in one Broca's aphasic subject, one anomic aphasic subject and their control speakers. Due to similar practical issues regarding data transcription and analyses as the original QPA in English, both Yiu's and Law's systems have rarely been used in general clinical settings in Hong Kong.

In light of this, Kong (2006) has devised a clinically oriented analytic system for quantifying aphasic narratives in Cantonese based on the LCM (Menn *et al.*, 1994), referred to as the Cantonese Linguistic Communication Measure (CLCM). The tool is designed to be quick and simple, requiring little linguistic background of the user and straightforward computation of the indices. As such, it ensures a short rater training period and good intra-rater and inter-rater reliabilities. In the preliminary version of the CLCM (Kong & Law, 2004), four new pictures containing local characteristics were developed, including revised pictures from the BDAE (Goodglass & Kaplan, 1993), the WAB (Kertesz, 1982) and its Cantonese version (CAB; Yiu, 1992) and a picture depicting a Chinese restaurant. Each participant is required to describe the picture set and orthographic transcriptions of the language samples are analyzed in the following eight indices (an example illustrating the computation of these indices is shown in the Appendix):

(1) The total number of words (NW): all the words a speaker produced, except for hesitation noises, interjections, intranscribable mumbles, false starts and direct responses to questions or probes, are included.

(2) The number of informative words (IW): an informative word, or i-word in short, is similar to the 'content unit' mentioned earlier and are counted only when they are used correctly.

(3) The ILE: it is the ratio of NW to IW, reflecting the efficiency of information conveyed.
(4) The Index of Communication Efficiency (ICE): it is computed by dividing the IW by the duration of the recording in minutes, reflecting the rate of information conveyed.
(5) The IGS: it is computed by dividing the total number of correctly used functors by the NW.
(6) The Index of Elaboration (IEl): it is the ratio of correctly used stem morphemes to i-word.
(7) The Index of Error (IEr): it is obtained by dividing the total number of errors produced by the IW.
(8) The Index of Lexical Richness (ILR): language sample elicited from each picture is trimmed to 40 words. The type-token ratio for the total 160 words is then computed.

In the following sections, we present the major findings of Kong (2006). In that study, a MANOVA and a DFA were carried out to demonstrate the ability of the CLCM in discriminating fluent and non-fluent individuals from normal speakers. More importantly, the most discriminating indices were identified. These statistical analyses have been used in previous studies to describe major differences among speaker groups and/or to classify subjects into groups based on their language output. For example, Yiu *et al.* (1998) have conducted a DFA to determine whether the criterion and subtest scores in the CAB (Yiu, 1992) are able to classify various aphasia types in Cantonese. More recently, Coelho *et al.* (2003) have attempted to distinguish individuals with closed head injuries from normal speakers based on their story narratives and conversational discourse.

Method

Subjects

Sixty aphasic subjects with unilateral cerebrovascular accidents or traumatic brain injuries participated in the study. They were recruited through an internal clinic and the Aphasia, Dyslexia, and Dysgraphia Laboratory in the Division of Speech and Hearing Sciences at The University of Hong Kong, the Community Rehabilitation Network and the Yan Chai Hospital in Hong Kong. The background information on the aphasic participants and their control subjects is provided in Table 14.1. Sixty normal speakers matched for gender, age (± 4 years), and education level (± 3 years of education) with the aphasic individuals were recruited as controls. Those with a history of neurological disease(s), a head injury(ies) or other medical condition(s) that might affect their oral performance were excluded.

Table 14.1 Background information on aphasic subjects

Subject group	*No. of subjects*[a]	*Mean age*	*Mean years of education*	*Aphasia quotient*[b]	*Etiology*	*Mean length of post-onset time (month)*
Fluent aphasic	34 (20M + 14F)	60.29	7.74	77.75 (35.2–99.0)	–	32.88
Anomic	21 (13M + 8F)	58.38	8.81	88.89 (78.2–99.0)	1 AVM + 1 BT + 18 CVA + 1 TBI	40.86
Transcortical sensory	3 (2M + 1F)	57.33	8.00	65.43 (57.0–75.6)	3 CVA	6.67
Conduction	4 (1M + 3F)	66.00	3.75	64.53 (57.0–70.8)	4 CVA	22.00
Wernicke's	6 (4M + 2F)	64.17	6.50	53.77 (35.2–76.0)	5 CVA + 1 TBI	25.33
Non-fluent aphasic	26 (16M + 10F)	58.19	7.12	60.69 (23.3–80.5)	–	44.42
Broca's	8 (6M + 2F)	59.88	5.13	51.58 (23.3–59.5)	8 CVA	58.75
Isolation	2 (1M + 1F)	67.00	2.50	49.90 (45.6–54.2)	2 CVA	7.00
Transcortical motor	15 (9M + 6F)	55.07	9.13	65.84 (46.7–80.5)	1 AVM + 13 CVA + 1 TBI	44.67
Global	1 (0M + 1F)	74.00	2.00	32.8 (32.8–32.8)	1 CVA	1.00
Control	60 (36M + 24F)	58.48	7.57	–	–	–

Note. [a]The gender distribution of subjects is given in parenthesis. [b]The AQ values are listed in the order 'mean (range)'. M = male, F = female, AVM = arteriovenous malformation, BT = brain tumor, CVA = cerebrovascular accident, TBI = traumatic brain injury

Data collection and analysis

All the subjects were asked to describe each of the four CLCM pictures. The sequence of picture presentation was counterbalanced across subjects. Speech samples were recorded, orthographically transcribed and subsequently analyzed using the eight CLCM indices.

Statistical analysis

Logarithmic transformation of raw scores was applied to the NW, ILE, ICE, IEl and ILR. According to Griffith *et al.* (1998), the transformation can optimize the distribution of variable frequency, such that the distribution would be more symmetrical and approximate more closely a normal distribution. Empirically, the transformation could also lead to more similar variances among the three groups (Fokianos, 2003). As for the IEr, for which most controls scored zero, and the IGS and IEl, for which some of the non-fluent aphasic subjects had a score of zero, a Box-Cox transformation (Box & Cox, 1964) was performed. The transformation was computed by the formula: $\log[(N + 0.5)/D]$, where N and D represent the numerator and denominator of the original index, respectively.

There were 120 cases and nine variables, a factor differentiating among the speaker groups (fluent aphasic, non-fluent aphasic and control) and eight dependent variables (the eight CLCM indices). A one-way MANOVA was employed to test for significant differences in the CLCM indices among the three groups of speakers. It was used to test the hypothesis that the population means for the dependent variables are the same across all groups. The analysis of variance (ANOVA) was then run to examine any group differences for each of the indices. To reduce Type I errors, the Bonferroni method was employed (Silva & Stam, 1995). Each ANOVA was tested at the 0.00625 level of significance, which was obtained based on 0.05 divided by eight (the number of ANOVAs). A direct DFA was conducted to classify speaker groups and to predict group membership for individual subjects. All eight indices (predictors) were entered together without a predetermined order.

Results

MANOVA

The Wilks' Lambda of 0.072 was significant ($F(14, 222) = 43.43$, $p < 0.0001$). The hypothesis that population means of the dependent variables are the same for the three speaker groups could therefore be rejected. The multivariate effect size index of η^2 was found to be 0.73, suggesting that 73% of variance of the dependent variables was associated with the group factor. For the IW, ILE, ICE, IGS, IEr and ILR, *post-hoc* comparisons revealed that both aphasic groups differed significantly from the controls ($p < 0.05$). In addition, the fluent and non-fluent groups were significantly different from each other. Regarding the IEl, there was significant difference only between the two aphasic and control groups. As for the NW, only the non-fluent group was significantly different from the control speakers.

Univariate ANOVAs were conducted as follow-up tests to the MANOVA. It was found that all indices were significant at the 0.000 level. Table 14.2 lists the means and standard deviations of all indices in raw scores. As the four picture stimuli were found to be comparable in terms of their abilities to elicit i-words as well as other index scores from normal and aphasic speakers (Kong, 2006), the values shown were obtained based on the average of the four pictures. The results of the univariate ANOVAs are also given in Table 14.2. Note that the η^2 values of the ICE, IGS and IEr are much higher than the other indices; in contrast, the NW has a very low value despite showing a significant p-level.

Direct DFA predicting fluent and non-fluent aphasic and control groups

The overall Wilks' lambda of 0.07 was significant ($\chi^2(14, 120) = 300.68$, $p < 0.0001$). This indicated that the eight CLCM indices differentiated among the three speaker groups. In addition, the residual Wilks' lambda of 0.51 was also significant ($\chi^2(6, 120) = 76.39$, $p < 0.0001$), showing that the indices also differentiated significantly among the three speaker groups after partialling out the effects of the first discriminant function. The first (F1) and second function (F2) accounted for 86.57% and 13.43% of the variance, respectively. The eigenvalues of F1 and F2, 6.15 versus 0.95, show that F1 is more powerful than F2 in classifying subjects. As these tests were significant at 0.000 level, both discriminant functions were interpreted.

Figure 14.1 displays the centroids and the dispersion of the scores for each speaker group. The scores of the members in a speaker group generally clustered together. While there was a relatively clear distinction between the normal and aphasic speakers, there was some overlap between the two aphasic groups. Moreover, the scores of the control subjects generally clustered around the centroid. In contrast, the scores of fluent and non-fluent aphasic speakers scattered loosely to a similar extent. Concerning the means of canonical variables of the two discriminant functions, the control group had a higher value (2.30) on F1 than the fluent (−1.24) and non-fluent (−3.67) aphasic groups. The canonical mean for the normal group is quite different from the two

Table 14.2 Descriptive results and statistical results of univariate ANOVAs

	Means and standard deviations of indices[a]			*Univariate ANOVAs*		
CLCM index	*Fluent aphasia*	*Non-fluent aphasia*	*Control*	*F(2, 117)*	*p-Level*	η^2
NW	64.21 (29.11)	54.20 (21.38)	69.09 (23.52)	6.01	0.003	0.09
IW	8.07 (3.69)	4.43 (3.01)	14.29 (3.61)	87.18	0.000	0.60
ILE	12.01 (16.26)	19.13 (15.09)	4.91 (1.39)	52.71	0.000	0.47
ICE	8.46 (5.05)	3.06 (2.30)	25.54 (7.96)	202.09	0.000	0.78
IGS	0.13 (0.07)	0.03 (0.04)	0.24 (0.07)	174.49	0.000	0.75
IEl	0.26 (0.26)	0.14 (0.25)	0.57 (0.30)	40.30	0.000	0.41
IEr	0.77 (1.94)	0.75 (0.76)	0.00 (0.01)	202.71	0.000	0.78
ILR	0.45 (0.08)	0.33 (0.11)	0.55 (0.06)	66.76	0.000	0.53

Note. [a]The values are obtained based on the averages of the four-picture stimuli and are listed in the order 'mean (standard deviation)'

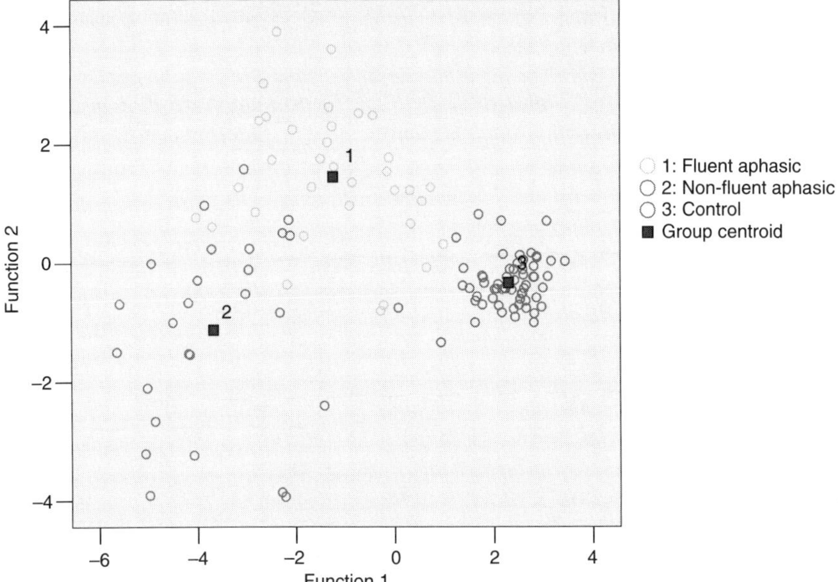

Figure 14.1 Discriminant function scores of (1) fluent aphasic, (2) non-fluent aphasic and (3) control speaker groups with respective group centroids.

aphasic groups. Regarding F2, the fluent group had the highest value (1.45), followed by the control (−0.34) and non-fluent group (−1.13). F1 was therefore able to distinguish well between aphasic and normal speakers, especially between the non-fluent aphasic and normal groups. F2, on the other hand, distinguished between the two aphasic groups more efficiently.

A rotation of the correlation matrix was carried out to facilitate the interpretation of the two functions. A Varimax rotation, a procedure to maximize variance (Tabachnick & Fidell, 2001) was performed to maximize high correlations and minimize low ones. Table 14.3 shows the index correlations after rotation and the rotated standardized coefficients for both functions. According to Stevens (2002), the values of within-groups correlations are used for substantive interpretation of the discriminant functions. It was found that while the IEr was strongly related to F1, the IGS and ICE were associated with F2. The next step was to examine the standardized discriminant function coefficients for each function to determine which of the highly correlated variables were redundant. The standardized discriminant function coefficients of the IEr for F1 as well as the IGS and ICE for F2 were also comparatively high, suggesting that they were not redundant.

Table 14.3 Correlations between CLCM indices and the discriminant functions after Varimax rotation

	Correlation with discriminant functions		*Standardized discriminant function coefficients*	
CLCM index	*F1*	*F2*	*F1*	*F2*
IEr	− 0.76	− 0.27	− 4.80	2.26
ICE	0.47	0.59	2.10	3.41
IEl	0.36	0.10	0.19	0.53
IW	0.26	0.43	− 5.84	− 2.02
ILE	− 0.22	− 0.32	–	–
IGS	0.20	0.77	− 2.08	5.39
ILR	0.14	0.46	3.14	0.28
NW	0.04	0.14	1.25	2.66

When predicting the speaker group membership, the DFA was able to correctly classify 92.5% (111/120) of the individuals in the overall sample. The function correctly identified all normal (specificity = 100%) and 51 out of 60 aphasic speakers (sensitivity = 85.0%). Sensitivity for the non-fluent group (84.6%; 22/26) and that for the fluent group (85.3%; 29/34) were almost the same. For the pattern of misclassification, two anomic aphasic subjects were misclassified as normal, one with transcortical sensory and two with Wernicke's aphasia were misclassified as non-fluent. For the non-fluent subjects, three with transcortical motor aphasia and one with Broca's aphasia were misclassified as fluent aphasic; none were classified as normal. To assess the accuracy of the prediction of group membership, a κ coefficient was computed. A value of 0.88 was obtained, indicating a high level of accuracy in prediction.

To assess how well the classification procedure would predict in a new sample, the percentage of speakers accurately classified using the leave-one-out technique was estimated. With this technique, classification functions were derived based on all cases except one and then the left out case was classified. This was done 120 times until all cases had been left out once and classified based on classification functions for the 119 cases. It was found that the functions correctly classified 88.3% (106/120) of the cases.

Discussion

The overall results indicate that three measures were particularly informative in discriminating subjects, including the production of errors (IEr) in distinguishing between aphasic and normal speakers, the grammatical form of speech output (IGS) and rate and agility of producing key contents (ICE) between fluent and non-fluent aphasic individuals. The IEr is not a detailed quantifying index as the error index in the SSLA (Shewan, 1988a) or the frequency analysis of error production in Ardila and Rosselli (1993) in that it does not specify patterns or types of errors exhibited by fluent and non-fluent aphasia, it was still found to be a powerful index for discriminating the normal and aphasic groups. The separation was clear as more than 95% of the control subjects had not made any errors during the picture description task. This contrasted with only one aphasic subject (with Broca's aphasia) who made no error at all. The IGS was highly correlated with F2. This is consistent with previous studies in English (Basso, 2003) and Chinese (Chu *et al.*, 1986; Packard, 1990; Yiu, 1995; Yiu & Worrall, 1996a, 1996b), in which the use of grammatical morphemes or closed-class elements served as a fundamental standard to make clinical diagnoses of agrammatical and fluent aphasic individuals.

With regard to the classification of speaker groups, the overall accuracy, sensitivity and specificity are somewhat higher than the aphasia studies mentioned previously (ranging between 72.1% and 88.4%). The distinction between normal and aphasic speakers was clearer than that between the two aphasic groups. Moreover, the assignment of aphasic speakers followed the 'normal-fluent-non-fluent' continuum. In particular, for the fluent aphasic group, only individuals with anomic aphasia, who are generally considered to be the least impaired among various types of fluent aphasias, were misclassified as normal. A few other fluent aphasic cases were misclassified into the non-fluent group. None of the normal speakers were classified as non-fluent aphasic or vice versa.

Compared with the other existing objective systems in Cantonese, i.e. Law (2001) and Yiu (1995), the CLCM is undoubtedly a more clinician-friendly evaluation tool. Apart from its good reliability and validity as reported in Kong (2006) and Kong and Law (2004), the analytic procedures are relatively easy to carry out. The CLCM, therefore, fills the gap of clinical tools available for analyzing aphasic narrative output. More importantly, as the population of Hong Kong is aging, it is estimated that 24.0% of the population will reach the age of 65 or above by 2031 (Department of Health, 2006). Given that the prevalence of CVA is higher among older individuals (Woo *et al.*, 1998), it is foreseeable that the incidence of aphasia will increase greatly in future. Having an objective, easily administrable and reliable tool for clinical assessment among aphasic speakers will definitely offer clinicians important diagnostic information (Gao & Benson, 1990), which can be used for devising intervention. Furthermore, communication about patient progress across different clinical settings or among professionals can also be greatly enhanced.

Finally, Yiu *et al.* (1998) showed that the criterion scores of fluency, auditory comprehension and repetition sections in the CAB (Yiu, 1992) were useful in classifying their subjects into various aphasia types. The CLCM at present does not provide clinicians with a diagnosis of aphasia syndrome as in the CAB. More research is needed to evaluate whether the CLCM indices are capable of classifying patients into various types. Future investigation may recruit a much larger number of aphasic subjects to see if it would be possible to establish specific CLCM profiles for different aphasia types.

Acknowledgements

We are very grateful to all of the subjects for their participation in the study. Special thanks to Ms Lorinda Kwan, Dr Man-Tak Leung, Dr Diana Ho, Ms Man-Yu Chi, Ms Joan Ma and Ms Joyce Chun, Division of Speech and Hearing Sciences at The University of Hong Kong, Ms Doris Cho, Speech Therapist of the Yan Chai Hospital, Mr. Siu-Lam Yuen, Chairman of the Self-Help Group for the Brain Damaged, Mr. Tat-Nin Leung, Vice-chairman of the Neuro United, Ms Fook, social worker of the Hong Kong Stroke Association, Ms. Edith Mok, founder of BrainCare Link and Ms Pui-Yuk Iu, Unit-in-charge of Pok Oi Hospital Chan Ping Memorial Neighbourhood Elderly Center, for their help in subject recruitment. Many thanks to Dr Valter Ciocca, Associate Professor in the Division of Speech and Hearing Sciences, and Dr John Bacon-Shone, Director of Social Sciences Research Center, for their statistical advice.

References

American Speech-Language-Hearing Association, Ad Hoc Committee on Admission/Discharge Criteria in Speech-Language Pathology (2004) Guildelines: Admission/discharge criteria in speech-language pathology. *ASHA* 24, 65–70.

Ardila, A. and Rosselli, M. (1993) Language deviations in aphasia: A frequency analysis. *Brain and Language* 44, 165–180.

Armstrong, L., Brady, M. and Norrie, J. (2006) Evaluating a transcription-less approach to the analysis of aphasic discourse. Paper presented at a meeting of the Clinical Aphasiology Conference, Ghent, Belgium, May.

Basso, A. (2003) *Aphasia and its Therapy.* New York: Oxford University Press.

Box, G.E.P. and Cox, D.R. (1964) An analysis of transformation. *Journal of Royal Statistical Society (Series B)* 26, 211–246.

Byng, S. and Black, M. (1989) Some aspects of sentence production in aphasia. *Aphasiology* 3, 241–263.

Capilouto, G.J., Wright, H.H. and Wagovich, S.A. (2006) Reliability of main event measurement in the discourse of individuals with aphasia. *Aphasiology* 20, 205–216.

Chu, Y.W., Peng, F.C.C. and Yiu, H.K. (1986) Agrammatism and conduction aphasia: A Chinese case. *Journal of Neurolinguistics* 2, 209–231.

Coelho, C., Youse, K., Le, K. and Feinn, R. (2003) Narrative and conversational discourse of adults with closed head injuries and non-brain-injured adults: A discriminant analysis. *Aphasiology* 17, 499–510.

Department of Health, Hong Kong Special Administrative Region of the People's Republic of China (2006) *Health Facts* (31 March). On WWW at http://www.info.gov.hk/dh/diseases/index.htm/. Accessed 19.4.06.

Fokianos, K. (2003) Box-Cox transformation for semiparametric comparison of two samples. In Y. Haitovsky, H.R. Lerche and Y. Ritov (eds) *Foundations of Statistical Inference: Proceedings of the Shoresh Conference 2000* (pp. 131–139). Heidelberg/New York: Physica-Verlag.

Gao, S.R. and Benson, D.F. (1990) Aphasia after stroke in native Chinese speakers. *Aphasiology* 4, 31–43.

Goodglass, H. and Kaplan, E. (1993) *The Boston Diagnostic Aphasia Examination.* Philadelphia, PA: Lee & Feliger.

Griffith, D.A., Paelinck, J.H.P. and van Gastel, R.A. (1998) The Box-Cox transformation: New computation and interpretation features of the parameters. In D.A. Griffith, C.G. Amrhein, J.M. Huriot, L.J. Gibson, A. Bailly and N.L. Law (eds) *Econometric Advances in Spatial Modelling and Methodology: Essays in Honour of Jean Paelinck* (pp. 45–56). Dordrecht: Kluwer Academic.

Kertesz, A. (1982) *The Western Aphasia Battery.* New York: Grune & Stratton.

Kong, A.P.H. (2006) A Cantonese linguistic communication measure for evaluating aphasic narrative production. Unpublished doctoral dissertation, The University of Hong Kong, Hong Kong SAR, China.

Kong, A.P.H. and Law, S.P. (2004) A Cantonese linguistic communication measure for evaluating aphasic narrative production: Normative and preliminary aphasic data. *Journal of Multilingual Communication Disorders* 2, 124–146.

Law, S.P. (2001) A quantitative analysis of Cantonese aphasic production. *Journal of Psychology in Chinese Society* 2, 211–237.

Menn, L., Ramsberger, G. and Helm-Estabrooks, N. (1994) A linguistic communication measures for aphasic narratives. *Aphasiology* 8, 343–359.

Packard, J.L. (1990) Agrammatism in Chinese: A case study. In L. Menn, L.K. Obler, G. Miceli and M. O'Connor (eds) *Agrammatic Aphasia: A Cross-language Narrative Sourcebook* (pp. 1191–1223). Amsterdam: J. Benjamins.

Royal College of Speech & Language Therapists (2005) *RCSLT Clinical Guidelines.* Bicester, Oxon: Speechmark.

Saffran, E.M., Berndt, R.S. and Schwartz, M.F. (1989) The quantitative analysis of agrammatic production: Procedure and data. *Brain and Language* 37, 440–479.

Shewan, C.M. (1988a) The Shewan spontaneous language analysis (SSLA) system for aphasic adults: Description, reliability and validity. *Journal of Communication Disorder* 21, 103–138.

Shewan, C.M. (1988b) Expressive language recovery in aphasia using the Shewan spontaneous language analysis (SSLA) system. *Journal of Communication Disorder* 21, 155–169.

Shewan, C.M. and Kertesz, A. (1980) Reliability and validity characteristics of the Western Aphasia Battery (WAB). *Journal of Speech and Hearing Disorder* 45, 308–324.

Silva, A.P.D. and Stam, A. (1995) Discriminant analysis. In L.G. Grimm and P.R. Yarnold (eds) *Reading and Understanding Multivariate Statistics* (pp. 277–318). Washington, DC: American Psychological Association.

Stevens, J. (2002) *Applied Multivariate Statistics for the Social Sciences*. Mahwah, NJ: L. Erlbaum.

Tabachnick, B.G. and Fidell, L.S. (2001) *Using Multivariate Statistics*. Boston, MA: Allyn and Bacon.

Woo, J., Ho, S.C., Yuen, Y.K., Yu, L.M. and Lau, J. (1998) Cardiovascular risk factors and 18-month mortality and morbidity in an elderly Chinese population aged 70 years and over. *Gerontology* 44, 51–55.

Yiu, E.M.L. (1992) Linguistic assessment of Chinese-speaking aphasics: Development of a Cantonese aphasia battery. *Journal of Neurolinguistic* 7, 379–424.

Yiu, E.M.L. (1995) Sentence production in aphasic subjects: A cross-language comparison. Unpublished doctoral dissertation, The University of Queensland, Brisbane.

Yiu, E.M.L. and Worrall, L.E. (1996a) Sentence production ability of a bilingual Cantonese/English agrammatic speaker. *Aphasiology* 10, 505–552.

Yiu, E.M.L. and Worrall, L.E. (1996b) Agrammatic production: A cross-linguistic comparison of English and Cantonese. *Aphasiology* 10, 623–647.

Yiu, E., Worrall, L. and Baglioni, T. (1998) Classification of aphasic Chinese speakers: Cluster and discriminant function analyses. *Aphasiology* 12, 37–48.

Yorkston, K.M. and Beukelman, D.R. (1980) An analysis of connected speech samples of aphasic and normal speakers. *Journal of Speech and Hearing Disorders* 45, 27–36.

Appendix

An example illustrating the computation of the CLCM indices

Original transcription of a language sample describing the revised pictures from the CAB (Yiu, 1992)

哩個圖畫裏面呢有媽媽啦哥哥啦妹妹啦 /e/ 總共三個人... 噉呀 /e/
媽媽呢響個睡廚房嗰度 /e/ ... 洗乾碗就 ... 嗰個水池呀漏晒流晒 ...
噉呀噉呀哥哥呢 /e/ ... 擔張凳走向去 ... 攞嗰啲物件糖果糖果食呀 ...
/dap_1//dap_1/幾佢/dap_1/ 彈咗落嚟嘞 ... 噉嗰個妹妹喇 /ha_2/
響度哈哈笑喇...
(Clinician's probe: 仲有冇其他嘢呀?) ... /m/ / 冇 / 呀...
啊 /e/ 窗外嗰啲 ... 窗外呀嘛 ... /e//m/ 冇呀 (Time = 3:50)

Step 1: Identification of total number of words
1a: Exclusion of unwanted words
1b: Segment utterances into separate words and count the total number of words

Step 2: Identification of i-word (underlined words)

No. of words	***Language sample***	***Remarks***
6	哩/ 個/ 圖畫/ 裏面/ 呢/ 有	
6	媽媽/ 啦/ 哥哥/ 啦/ 妹妹/ 啦	Informative words 媽媽, 哥哥 and 妹妹 are underlined
4	~~/e/~~ / 總共/ 三/ 個/ 人	Hesitation noise /e/ is excluded
1	嗷呀/ ~~/e/~~	Frame or habitual statement 嗷呀 is included
7	媽媽/ 呢/ 響/ 個/ 睡房/ 廚房/ 嗰度/ ~~/e/~~	Self-correction 睡房 for 廚房 is included
4	洗/ 乾/ 碗/ 就	
6	*睡房*	Semantic paraphasia 水池 for 水盤 is included
1	嗷呀	
3	嗷呀/ 哥哥/ 呢/ ~~/e/~~	
6	擔/ 張/ 凳/ 走/ 向/ 去	
8	攞/ 嗰/ 啲/ 物件/ *糖果* / *糖果* / 食/ 呀	

No. of words	*Language sample*	*Remarks*
5	/dap$_1$//dap$_1$/幾佢/dap$_1$// 彈咗/ 落/ 嚟/ 嘞	Neologistic jargon / dap$_1$ dap$_1$ 幾佢 dap$_1$/ is included
8	嗷/ 嘓/ 個/ 妹妹/ 喇/ ~~ha$_2$~~/ 嚮度/ 哈哈笑/ 喇	False start of /ha/ in 嚮度 is excluded
–	~~(仲有有其他嘢呀?)~~	Leading questions or probes from examiner are excluded
0	~~/m// 冇 / 呀~~	Words in response to probes are excluded
1	啊/ ~~/e/~~	
4	窗/ 外/ 嘓/ 啲	
3	窗/ 外/ 呀嘛	Repetition of the word units 窗 and 外 are included
2	~~/e//m/~~ / 冇/ 呀	

Step 3: Identification of i-word units: 13 i-word units in total

Step 4: Calculation of time in minute: 3:50 (= 3.83 minutes)

Step 5: Identification of errors (*italic* text): four errors including *睡房, 水池, 糖果, 糖果*

Step 6: Identification of grammatical morphemes in i-word units (squared text)

Step 7: Identification of stem morphemes in i-word units (shaded text)

A. *i-word unit*	B. *No. of closed-class words in i-word unit* □	C. *No of morphemes in open-class words in i-word unit*
媽媽	0	0
哥哥	0	0
妹妹	0	0
媽媽	0	0
響 / 個 / 廚房 / 嗰度	3	0
洗	0	0
碗	0	0
流 晒	1	0
哥哥	0	0
擔	0	0
張 / 凳	1	0
走 / 去 /攞	0	2
嗰 / 個 / 妹妹 / 喇	3	0
Total: 13	8	2

Step 8: Extraction of 40 words from the text for calculation of the ILR.

The sample size of each speaker is fixed at 160 words for describing the four-picture stimuli. The speech sample elicited from each picture should be trimmed to 40 words and counted toward the final text. We used a method that will consider the entire speech sample and each picture would contribute equally toward the final type-token ratio (TTR) score. To do so, we divide the text into 40 chunks, with the size of each unit equal to NW/40 words, and the first word from each chunk will be selected. For example, in an 80-word text, every other word was counted; in a 120-word text, every third word was selected.

In cases where the word number is not a multiple of 40, we will pool chunks of words such that the combined string would approach a whole number. Then we will select the same number of words as chunks from the word string that are equally spread out. For example, in a 130-word text, each word chunk is supposed to contain 3.25 words. The way of selecting words will be by combining four chunks together and picking the first, fourth, seventh and tenth words.

For a sample of 75 words, as in this example, the sample is first divided into five 15-word chunks. The first, third, fifth, seventh, ninth, eleventh, thirteenth and last word in each chunk are included. The **bolded and squared** words shown next are therefore selected:

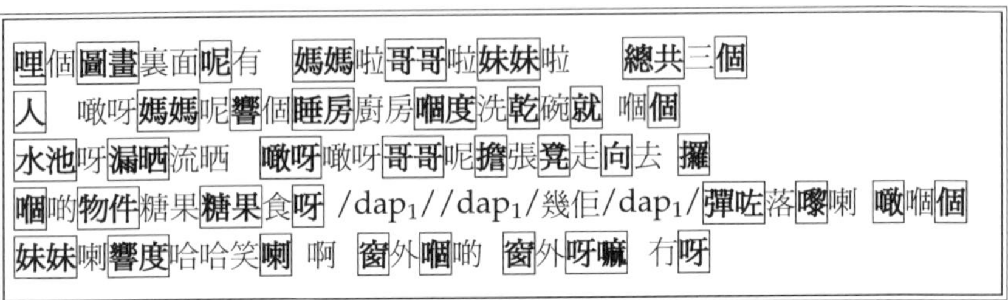
哩個**圖畫**裏面**呢**有 **媽媽**啦**哥哥**啦**妹妹**啦 **總共**三**個**
人 噉呀**媽媽**呢**響**個**睡房**廚房**嗰度**洗**乾**碗**就** 嗰**個**
水池呀**漏晒**流晒 **噉呀**噉呀**哥哥**呢**擔**張**凳**走**向**去 **攞**
嗰啲**物件**糖果**糖果**食**呀** /dap$_1$//dap$_1$/幾佢/dap$_1$/**彈咗**落**嚟**喇 **噉**嗰**個**
妹妹喇**響度**哈哈笑**喇** 啊 **窗**外**嗰**啲 **窗**外**呀嘛** 冇**呀**

Step 9: Computation of CLCM indices

1. Total number of words (NW) = 75
2. Number of informative words (IW) = 13
3. Index of Lexical Efficiency (ILE) = 75/13 = 5.77
4. Index of Communication Efficiency (ICE) = 13/3.83 = 3.39
5. Index of Grammatical Support (IGS) = 8/75 = 0.11
6. Index of Elaboration (IE) = 2/13 = 0.15
7. Index of Error (IEr) = 4/13 = 0.31
8. Index of Lexical Richness (ILR): computed by obtaining the TTR of the four trimmed samples (160 words)

Chapter 15

A Semantic Treatment for Cantonese Anomic Patients: Implications for the Relationship Between Impairment and Therapy

SAM-PO LAW, WINSY WONG and ELVA WONG

Introduction

Evidence-based treatment studies of acquired language disorders have been a vibrant research area for the past several decades. This is particularly the case for anomia therapies. In psycholinguistic models, the failure to retrieve a word for production can be the result of damage to semantic processing, access from semantics to phonology, phonological encoding or any combination of these. Perhaps because of the pervasiveness and persistence of word-finding disorders experienced by aphasic individuals, there is an increasingly large body of work investigating the efficacy of anomia treatments taking different approaches, semantically oriented, phonologically-based or a combination of both, and using various techniques (see Nickels, 2002 for a comprehensive review). Semantic tasks may include discussing semantic properties of the object to be named (e.g. Boyle, 2004; Boyle & Coelho, 1995; Coelho *et al.*, 2000; Hillis, 1998), 'talking around' the target item or circumlocuting as a way to facilitate word retrieval (Francis *et al.*, 2002), word-picture matching (e.g. Byng, 1988; Marshall *et al.*, 1990), categorizing or sorting objects (e.g. Grayson *et al.*, 1997; Kiran & Thompson, 2001), generating or matching synonyms (e.g. Hough, 1993) or making judgments about functions, semantic features or relatedness of objects (e.g. Drew & Thompson, 1999; Nickels & Best, 1996). Phonological tasks include repetition, the most common form of treatment either as a key component or part of the protocol when the patient fails to provide the target name after cueing, reading aloud (e.g. Eales & Pring, 1998; Howard, 1994; Nickels & Best, 1996), phonological cueing (e.g. Hillis & Caramazza, 1994; Raymer & Ellsworth, 2002) or making judgments to promote phonological awareness, such as rhyme judgment, counting syllables or phonemes and segmentation of words into phonemes (e.g. Biedermann *et al.*, 2002; Robson *et al.*, 1998). Although the tasks can often be characterized as semantic- or phonologic-based, most treatment protocols are composed of elements that involve both semantic and phonological processes (Howard, 1994; Nickels, 2002). For instance, in semantic feature analysis (SFA) (Boyle & Coelho, 1995; Coelho *et al.*, 2000; Conley & Coelho, 2003), if the patient is unable to retrieve the correct name after describing the various semantic properties of the stimulus object, she/he will be given the target for repetition.

Nickels' (2002) critical review of anomia treatment reports over the last 15 years shows that, while most therapies improve patients' naming accuracy, our understanding of the relationship between therapy and impairment remains poor. This is because different therapeutic approaches have been shown to be successful for similar deficits, the same treatment may benefit anomic patients with different underlying impairment and positive treatment outcomes may vary in terms of generalization to untrained items or maintenance of treatment gains. To remedy the situation, at least two proposals have been made. Howard (2000) suggests that the same treatment be applied to patients with different deficits, followed by an examination of how they respond to the intervention. Alternatively, Nickels proposes a comparison of the outcomes of different therapies with the same patient. In addition, therapies with the simplest procedures should precede ones that are more complicated. The former approach is exemplified in Fink *et al.* (2002). As for the latter, while there are studies that meet the first criterion (e.g. Raymer & Ellsworth, 2002; Rose *et al.*, 2002), they tend to contrast treatments that are either different in nature or comparable in terms of the number of components involved.

A recent study that has adopted the approach advocated in Howard (2000) is an application of the same semantic-based intervention to three Cantonese-speaking anomic patients who differ in terms of the degree of semantic, phonological, memory and cognitive deficits (Law *et al.*, 2006). The therapy combined SFA (Boyle & Coelho, 1995; Coelho *et al.*, 2000; Conley & Coelho, 2003) and semantic priming. Objects belonging to the same category were trained consecutively, i.e. semantic priming, and the clinician would discuss with the patient the semantic features of each target object, including category, function, usage, properties, location and any semantic associations of the target item the patient could generate. The results showed that the two patients with mild semantic deficits benefited from the therapy, and treatment effects generalized to untrained items that were semantically related as well as those that were unrelated to the trained stimuli. In contrast, no change was observed in the patient with severe disruption to semantic processing. Evidence for specific treatment effects is demonstrated by the patients' long post-onset period, ranging from three to 10 years, minimizing the likelihood of spontaneous recovery, stability in performance during baseline, the co-occurrence in timing of clear progress in naming performance and the introduction of intervention, and significantly greater improvement in naming treated items than other probes. The findings of treatment generalization to related and unrelated untrained items are compatible with the view that SFA is a facilitative or strategic technique that an anomic patient may learn to internalize in naming. The researchers attribute the different outcomes of the three patients to the facilitative nature of SFA and the severity of semantic impairments.

The present study continued the work of Law *et al.* (2006). It replicated their treatment protocol on two additional Cantonese anomic patients, both with moderate semantic deficits but differing in other language aspects. Two questions were asked through comparing the results of the two studies. Law *et al.* concluded that the extent of semantic impairment could predict how well a patient would respond to the combination of SFA and semantic priming; the present study extended the examination of this relationship to patients with moderate semantic disruption. In other words, would anomic patients with moderate degrees of semantic deficit respond positively to the therapy? Furthermore, would the extent of semantic impairment remain the key factor in determining treatment success? Several predictions were made.

(1) If the degree of semantic impairment was the determining factor for treatment outcomes, then treatment progress of the two patients was expected to be similar.

(2) Alternatively, as oral naming involves both semantics and phonological output among other things, the status of postsemantic processes including access from semantics to phonology and the phonological output level may also affect treatment results. In other words, two patients with similar degrees of semantic deficits but differing in the functioning of postsemantic processes may benefit from the same intervention to different extents. More specifically, the patient with better-preserved access from semantics to phonology and/or phonological output was more likely to show treatment gains.

(3) Because SFA is believed to increase the activation of the semantic network surrounding the target word, as naming accuracy improved, the frequency of semantic errors would increase while other error types would decrease.

For ease of reference and comparison, in reporting the findings of the two patients in this study, we also include information on the three patients in Law *et al.* (2006), MTK, YSH and YKM, wherever it is appropriate.

Method

Participants

Two Cantonese brain-injured individuals, YYW and TWT, with naming difficulties were invited to participate in this treatment study. They were native speakers of Cantonese, right-handed, and at least eight months post-onset at the start of the study. Their background information, along with that of the three patients in Law *et al.* (2006), is given in Table 15.1.

Initial assessments and hypothesized nature of impairment

A series of language, memory and cognitive tests as in Law *et al.* (2006) were carried out on YYW and TWT before treatment began. They included (1) an auditory discrimination task consisting of 40 trials with half involving two identical syllables. All stimuli were existing Cantonese syllables with a CVC structure. For those trials where two different items were presented, they were equally likely to differ in the onset, nucleus, coda or tone. (2) Repetition of 30 single words and phrases of up to four syllables in length – there were 10 monosyllabic, 14 disyllabic, five trisyllabic, and one four-syllable items. (3) Oral naming of selected pictures in Snodgrass and Vanderwart (1980). (4) Reading aloud of names of the same items in confrontation naming. (5) Verbal semantic tests, including spoken word-picture matching in which the subject had to match a word with one of three pictures taken from Snodgrass and Vanderwart, i.e. the target, a semantic distractor and an unrelated foil, and a synonym judgment task where the subject had to decide whether two words were similar in meaning or not. The test consisted of 60 trials, on half of which the written words presented were synonymous. (6) Non-verbal semantic tests, including the Pyramid and Palm Trees Test (PPT) (Howard & Patterson, 1992) and the Associative Match Test in the Birmingham Object Recognition Battery (BORB) (Riddoch & Humphreys, 1993). (7) Digit forward sequence task. (8) The Test of Non-verbal Intelligence (TONI-3) (Brown *et al.*, 1997).

The performance of age-matched control subjects on most of the tasks and the results of the anomic patients are shown in Table 15.2 and Table 15.3, respectively. Accuracy rates of auditory discrimination and repetition are assumed to be 100%.

Table 15.3 shows that YYW and TWT performed at comparable levels on most of the tasks except oral naming and reading aloud. YYW named pictured objects (70% correct) much better than TWT (40%); in addition, YYW was able to read aloud almost all the object names (99%), whereas TWT was clearly dyslexic (57%). As for the other tasks, YYW repeated words and phrases somewhat better than TWT. Their performance on the three semantic tests was below the normal range. TWT recalled more

Table 15.1 Background information on YYW and TWT in this study and the patients MTK, YSH and YKM in Law *et al.* (2006)

	MTK	*YSH*	*YYW*	*TWT*	*YKM*
Age	40	71	60	46	61
Gender	Male	Female	Male	Male	Male
Education	9 years	9 years	12 years	11 years	University degree
Onset date	September 1994	August 2000	May 2004	April 1999	First stroke: 1992; second stroke: January 2002
Etiology	Traumatic brain injury with left parietal epidural hematoma	Ischaemic stroke with huge left parietal frontal infarct involving Broca's and Wernicke's areas	Left MCA infarct	Left putaminal hemorrhage without ventricular extension	First stroke: subarachnoid hemorrhage; second stroke: left basal ganglion hemorrhage
Motor/ sensory impairment	Right hemianopia, left hemiparesis, apraxia of speech	Nil	Right hemiparesis, mild dysarthria	Right hemiparesis, mild dysarthria	Right hemiparesis, mild dysarthria
Premorbid occupation	Worker in a photo shop	Accounting	Accounting	Businessman	Broker

Table 15.2 Control subjects' performance on language and memory tests

Task	*Normal performance*		
Control group: Three subjects with ages ranging from 40 to 68 years and at least 9 years education			
Spoken word-picture matching ($n = 126$)	Range: 124–126		
Synonym judgment ($n = 60$)	Range: 54–58		
Control groups of 10 subjects each matched in age and education with each of the anomic patients			
	YKM and YYW	***YSH***	***MTK and TWT***
Oral picture naming ($n = 217$)	212.60 (SD = 2.76; 208–216)	200.50 (SD = 5.68; 188–209)	216.50 (SD = 0.53; 216–217)
PPT ($n = 37$)	33.90 (SD = 5.07; 20–37)	33.20 (SD = 5.49; 19–37)	31.90 (SD = 5.40; 21–37)
Associative Match Test in BORB ($n = 23$)	22.10 (SD = 0.74; 21–23)	21.20 (SD = 2.04; 16–23)	21.90 (SD = 1.20; 20–23)
Data from Lee *et al.* (2002) with control groups most closely matched in age and education with the anomic patients			
	YKM and YYW	***YSH***	***MTK and TWT***
Digit forward sequence	9.12 (SD = 1.16)	8.92 (SD = 1.21)	

Table 15.3 Results of initial assessments

	MTK	*YSH*	*YYW*	*TWT*	*YKM*
Auditory discrimination ($n = 40$)	40 (100%)	39 (97.5%)	39 (97.5%)	40 (100%)	37 (92.5%)
Repetition ($n = 30$)	16 (53.3%)	12 (40.0%)	29 (96.7%)	25 (83.3%)	28 (93.3%)
Oral naming ($n = 217$)	80 (36.9%)	28 (12.9%)	153 (70.5%)	86 (39.6%)	71 (32.7%)
Reading aloud object names ($n = 217$)	51 (23.5%)	42 (19.4%)	215 (99.1%)	124 (57.1%)	206 (94.9%)
Verbal semantic tests					
Spoken word-picture matching ($n = 126$)	120 (95.2%)	120 (95.2%)	117 (92.9%)	112 (88.9%)	102 (81.0%)
Synonym judgment ($n = 60$)	55 (93.2%)	48 (80%)	50 (83.3%)	51 (85%)	43 (71.7%)
Non-verbal semantic tests					
PPT ($n = 37$)	35 (94.6%)	31 (83.8%)	30 (81.1%)	31 (83.3%)	22 (56.5%)
BORB ($n = 23$)	22 (95.7%)	21 (91.3%)	15 (65.2%)	18 (78.3%)	15 (65.2%)
Memory test					
Digit forward sequence	5	2	6	7	8
Cognitive test					
TONI-3: Raw score (percentile)	38 (81)	9 (10)	12 (6)	15 (6)	14 (9)

Note. YSH was unable to carry out the verbal learning test (Law *et al*., 2006) digits than YYW. Both patients scored at the 6th percentile on TONI-3, showing very poor cognitive abilities.

The nature of the patients' language and cognitive impairments is characterized in five areas: phonological input based on auditory discrimination; phonological output based on repetition; semantic processing according to word-picture matching; synonym judgment; and non-verbal semantic tests, phonological memory on the basis of digit span and non-verbal cognitive abilities based on TONI-3. The degree of semantic deficits is determined by the number of semantic tasks on which a patient performs below the normal range. For instance, it is suggested that MTK suffered very mild disruption to semantic processing as he performed below normal on word-picture matching only. YSH scored worse than normal controls on two semantic tests, word-picture matching and synonym judgment; hence, she was classified to have mild semantic impairment. YYW and TWT performed below normal controls on all semantic tasks except for the PPT; they were then considered to have moderate semantic deficits. Finally, YKM was said to have severe semantic processing impairment because his performance was very poor on all four semantic tasks. The hypothesized underlying deficits are summarized in Table 15.4. Taking all the patients together, with the exception of phonological input in which the patients were at most

Table 15.4 Hypothesized nature of impairment in YYW, TWT and patients in Law *et al.* (2006)

	MTK	*YSH*	*YYW*	*TWT*	*YKM*
Phonological input	Preserved	Largely preserved	Largely preserved	Preserved	Mildly impaired
Phonological output	Severe	Severe	Largely preserved	Moderate	Mildly impaired
Semantic processing	Very mild	Mild	Moderate	Moderate	Severe
Phonological memory	Severe	Severe	Moderate	Mild	Preserved
Cognitive abilities	Normal	Severe	Severe	Severe	Severe

Note. For phonological input and phonological output, 'mild impairment' roughly corresponds to a performance level of around 90%, 'moderate impairment' to around 80% and 'severe' impairment to an accuracy rate below 80%. For phonological memory, the degree of impairment is related to the number of standard deviations (SD) below mean performance; 'severe' refers to a span of 3 or more SDs below mean or more, 'moderate' 2 SDs below mean and 'mild' 1 SD below mean mildly impaired, they exhibited various degrees of disruption in the other aspects.

Note that the results of reading accuracy are not interpreted in hypothesizing underlying impairment of the patients. Current models of word production based on data from Chinese aphasic speakers (Law & Or, 2001; Weekes *et al.*, 1997) consist of a semantic level and two levels of form representations, orthographic and phonological, with units corresponding to individual characters and syllables, respectively. There are bidirectional connections among these three levels. Reading characters can proceed along two pathways, from orthography to phonology via semantics, i.e. the semantic reading route, and from orthography to phonology directly, i.e. the nonsemantic reading pathway. This means that reading aloud may or may not involve the semantic system. The relevance of reading performance is discussed when we account for different patterns of treatment outcome in the Discussion.

Materials

A total of 256 black-and-white line drawings of objects belonging to 18 different categories were selected from various sources, including the picture set of Snodgrass and Vanderwart (1980) ($n = 158$), Aphasia Rehabilitation: a clinical and home therapy program outcome (Jipson, 1987) ($n = 39$), British Picture Vocabulary Scale (Dunn, 1982) ($n = 36$), Boston Naming Test (Kaplan *et al.*, 1983) ($n = 12$), and Picture Please! A Language Supplement (Abbate & Lachappelle, 1984) ($n = 11$). Objects of monosyllabic names were excluded so as to avoid ambiguity in accuracy judgment induced by the patient's phonological impairment.

Normative data on naming agreement, familiarity and visual complexity were collected following the procedures in Snodgrass and Vanderwart (1980). For each patient, five normal control subjects, matched for age, education and gender, were asked to orally name the pictures and rate the familiarity and the visual complexity of each picture. Pictures with 60% naming agreement or above in the respective control groups were used in the baseline phase. In other words, the picture sets for YYW and TWT were different.

Treatment design

A multiple baseline treatment design consisting of a baseline, two treatment phases and a maintenance phase was adopted.

Baseline phase

Three sessions were carried out within two weeks during this phase. In each session, the patients were asked to name their selected picture set and were given a time limit of 20 seconds for each picture. Those pictures that individual patients failed to name on two out of three occasions were then chosen. They were subject to the same procedure for assignment to treated, untreated generalization and control items. The mean familiarity rating of each category of objects was calculated. The same category contributed equally to treatment and generalization probe types. Control probes were selected from categories unrelated to those of the treatment and generalization items. Detailed information on the stimuli for YYW and TWT is given in Table 15.5. For both YYW and TWT, the Student's *t*-test found comparable familiarity values across treatment, generalization and control probes of high and low familiarity objects. At the

Table 15.5 Information on treatment, generalization and control probes for YYW and TWT

	YYW	*TWT*
Treatment items		
Phase 1	High familiarity: 3.1 Household items, kitchenware, furniture, toiletries, fruits and vegetables, food ($n = 15$)	High familiarity: 4.4 Household items, clothing, stationery ($n = 14$)
Phase 2	Low familiarity: 1.5 Recreational items, stationery, transportation, musical instruments, birds, four-legged animals, insects ($n = 15$)	Low familiarity: 3.6 Recreational items, transportation means, animals and birds ($n = 16$)
Generalization items		
	High familiarity: 3.1 Household items, kitchenware, furniture, toiletries, fruits and vegetables, food ($n = 15$)	High familiarity: 4.3 Household items, clothing, stationery ($n = 14$)
	Low familiarity: 1.5 Recreational items, stationery, transportation, musical instruments, birds, four-legged animals, insects ($n = 15$)	Low familiarity: 3.6 Recreational items, transportation means, animals and birds ($n = 16$)
Control items		
	High familiarity: 2.7 Tools and clothing ($n = 6$)	High familiarity: 4.6 Furniture and electrical appliances ($n = 8$)
	Low familiarity: 1.7 Electrical appliances and personal items ($n = 6$)	Low familiarity: 3.6 Kitchenware and insects ($n = 8$)

same time, the high and low familiarity items differed significantly for each probe type ($p < 0.05$).

Treatment phases

At the beginning of every treatment session, the patients were asked to name all probe items presented in random order without feedback in order to monitor progress over time.

There were two treatment phases; high familiarity items were introduced in Phase 1, followed by low familiarity items in Phase 2. A treatment phase was considered completed when the patient scored at least 85% correct on naming treated items during probing at the beginning of a treatment session over three consecutive sessions. The treatment protocol was identical for both treatment phases. The training followed exactly the SFA procedure described in Boyle and Coelho (1995). The technique of semantic priming was incorporated through simultaneous presentation of line drawings of the same category. The combined treatment of SFA and semantic priming was possible for TWT, but not so for YYW. As his pretreatment naming performance was relatively high (70%), there were not enough eligible items in any of the semantic categories to be divided into two groups of reasonable sizes for treatment and generalization probes, respectively. In other words, the therapy that YYW received was strictly SFA.

A treatment session would end when all the treatment items of the corresponding phase were presented. The duration of a treatment session averaged about 1.5 hours. The order of presentation of the categories was randomized across sessions to even out the possible effects of fatigue and/or level of attention over the course of a session.

Home practice was not compulsory and depended on the patient's motivation and the extent of family support. The feature analysis charts used in the treatment sessions were given to the patients. They contained written semantic information on each treated item provided by the patient during the treatment. The patients were encouraged to name the pictures in their free time by reviewing all the corresponding semantic features.

Maintenance phase

Patients who successfully completed both treatment phases would proceed to the maintenance phase, during which their naming accuracy of all probe items was measured on three separate occasions in the second, third and fourth week after the last treatment session.

Statistical analyses

To find out whether significant improvement was made in naming treatment, generalization and control probes, and whether greater

Table 15.6 Statistical analyses of naming accuracy of different probe types

Items	*Comparison between*		*Test*
Treatment	Highest accuracy in a session during baseline	Best performance in a treatment session of the corresponding phase	McNemar's test
Generalization	Highest accuracy in a session during baseline	Best performance in a session after baseline	McNemar's test
Control	Highest accuracy in a session during baseline	Best performance in a session after baseline	McNemar's test
Treatment versus control	Best performances in the entire treatment period		Chi-square test
Generalization versus control	Best performances in the entire treatment period		Chi-square test
Treatment versus generalization	Best performances in the entire treatment period		Chi-square test

progress was seen in naming one probe type over another, the McNemar's test and the Chi-square test were used, respectively. Table 15.6 illustrates how comparisons were made.

Results

The performance of YYW and TWT in terms of the number of correctly named stimuli of different probe types across sessions is depicted in Figure 15.1. Results of statistical analyses demonstrating whether there were significant improvement in naming different types of items over the course of therapy and significant differences in accuracy between probe types are given in Table 15.7. Changes in error distribution between baseline and the last three therapy sessions are presented in Table 15.8.

YYW completed both treatment phases and maintained the treatment gains for at least one month. There was no generalization to untrained items. Specific treatment effects in YYW were evidenced by the occurrence of a significant increase in naming accuracy of treated items only, greater improvement in trained than untrained stimuli, and the fact that the timing of noticeable change in performance level coincided with that of introduction of therapy, both high and low familiarity items. On the other hand, TWT did not complete the first treatment phase. Therapy

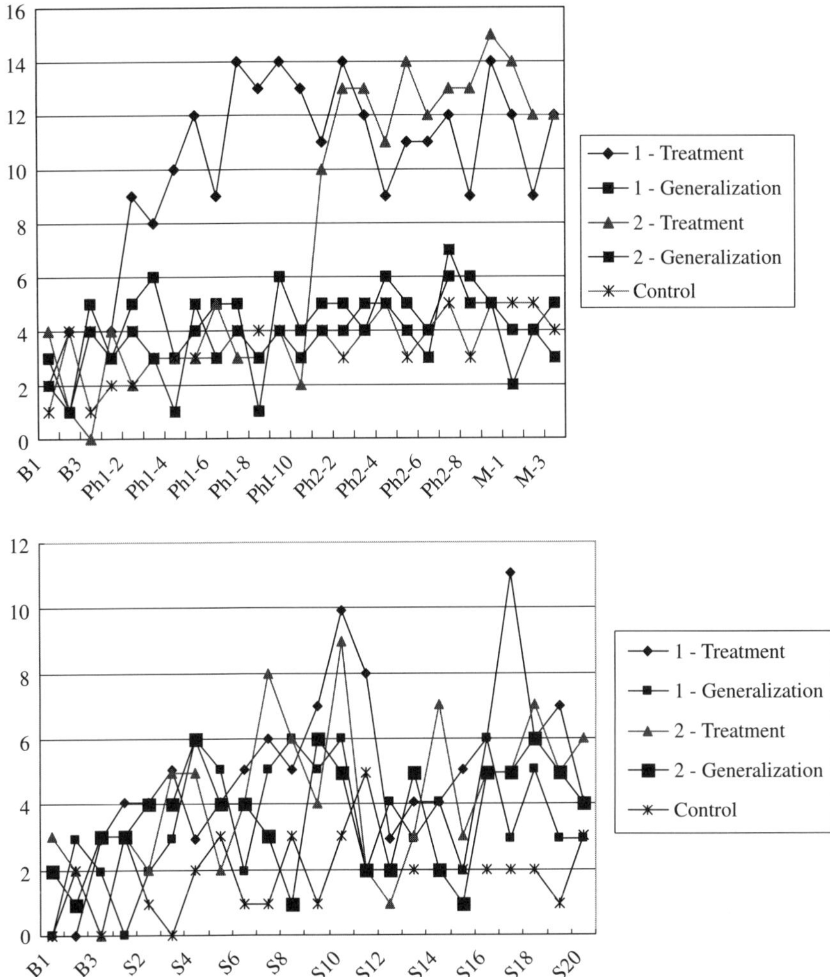

Figure 15.1 Performance of YYW (top panel) and TWT (bottom panel) in terms of number of items correct on different probe types across sessions. B = baseline phase, Ph1 = treatment phase 1, Ph2 = treatment phase 2, M = maintenance phase, S = session.

was withdrawn after 20 sessions. However, the difference was significant between the best performances during baseline and treatment phases, respectively, in naming Phase 1 high familiarity items. No other comparisons reached statistical significance.

As for the distribution of errors before and after therapy, YYW showed a slightly higher rate of semantic errors, but made many more omission responses. In contrast, TWT's responses subsequent to therapy were more likely to be semantically related to the targets. Moreover, omissions

Table 15.7 Results of statistical analyses of YYW and TWT

YYW		
	Phase 1 (High familiarity items)	*Phase 2 (Low familiarity items)*
Treatment items	26.7% (B2) versus 100% (T7)[a]	26.7% (B1) versus 100% (T19)[a]
Generalization items	33.3% (B3) versus 40% (T3)	26.7% (B3) versus 33.3% (T14)
Control items	33.3% (B2) versus 41.7% (T14)	
Treatment versus generalization	100% (T7) versus 40% (T3)[a]	100% (T19) versus 33.3% (T14)[a]
Treatment versus control	100% (T7) versus 41.7% (T14)[a]	100% (T19) versus 41.7% (T14)[a]
Generalization versus control	40% (T3) versus 41.7% (T14)	33.3% (T14) versus 41.7% (T14)
TWT		
	Phase 1 (High familiarity items)	*Phase 2 (Low familiarity items)*
Treatment items	21% (B3) versus 79% (T17)[b]	10% (B1) versus 56% (T10)
Generalization items	21% (B2) versus 43% (T4, T8, T10, T16)	10% (B1) versus 38% (T9, T18)
Control items	12.5% (B2) versus 31% (T11)	
Treatment versus generalization	79% (T17) versus 43% (T4, T8, T10, T16)	56% (T10) versus 38% (T9, T18)
Treatment versus control	79% (T17) versus 31% (T11)	56% (T10) versus 31% (T11)
Generalization versus control	43% (T4, T8, T10, T16) versus 31% (T11)	38% (T9, T18) versus 31% (T11)

Note. [a]$p < 0.005$, [b]$p < 0.05$. B = baseline, T = treatment

during the last three treatment sessions were reduced by more than half of the number of occurrences during the baseline period.

In summary, a positive treatment outcome was found in one of the two patients with moderate semantic deficits. Treatment effects did not

Table 15.8 Error distribution before and after treatment

	YYW		*TWT*	
	B1-B3	***M1-M3***	***B1-B3***	***T18-T20***
No. of errors	167	108	207	161
Error types				
Semantic	59.9%	63.9%	37.5%	68.1%
Unrelated	5.4%	2.8%	3.4%	3.8%
Jargon	6.6%	1.9%	0.4%	
No response	16.8%	26.9%	54.9%	26.4%
Others	8.4%	4.7%	3.6%	1.6%

Note. B = baseline, M = maintenance

generalize to untrained items. Only one patient demonstrated the change in pattern of error distribution expected for SFA.

Discussion

Law *et al.* (2006) have argued that a therapy combining SFA and semantic priming is effective for patients with mild semantic deficits but not for those with severe impairment at that level, on the basis of treatment outcomes of three Chinese anomic patients. The finding is compatible with the view that SFA is facilitative rather than remedial in nature (Coelho *et al.*, 2000; Lowell *et al.*, 1995). It works by strengthening existing connections within the semantic system and those between semantics and phonology. Furthermore, if an anomic patient learns to internalize the technique or strategy of analyzing semantic features, his or her naming of untrained stimuli may also improve.

The results of the present study seem to challenge the conclusions in Law *et al.* (2006). Table 15.9 summarizes the treatment outcomes of patients in these two studies for ease of reference. Although YYW and TWT both suffered moderate degrees of semantic disruption, only YYW benefited from the treatment. This raises the question whether semantic processing alone can predict success of the semantic treatment. Second, there was no treatment generalization to untreated items for YYW. In other words, it is plausible that YYW had not acquired the strategy of SFA. If so, how would one explain his progress in naming treated stimuli? An examination of their performance on the tasks in pretreatment assessment (see Table 15.3) reveals that YYW and TWT differ in two tasks that may be of particular relevance to their different responses to

Table 15.9 Summary of treatment outcomes of YYW, TWT and patients in Law *et al.* (2006)

	MTK	*YSH*	*YYW*	*TWT*	*YKM*
Phase 1 treatment	Completed	Completed	Completed	No	No
Phase 2 treatment	Completed	Completed	Completed	No	No
Generalization to semantically related probes	Yes	Yes	No	NA	NA
Generalization to control items	Yes	Yes	No	NA	NA
Maintenance of treatment gains	Yes	No	Yes	NA	NA

Note. NA = not applicable

the treatment. First, YYW's naming disorder was less severe than TWT's (70.5% versus 39.6%); furthermore, YYW's reading aloud ability was within normal range (99.1%), whereas TWT was clearly dyslexic (57.1%). These observations suggest that although semantic processing was comparably impaired in YYW and TWT, at postsemantic levels including access from semantics to phonology and phonological output, YYW was in better condition than TWT. Near-normal functioning at these levels may enable YYW to take advantage of the phonological component of the treatment protocol, i.e. repetition, which trains him to associate specific concepts with their phonological representation. If this is the case, it explains why his naming performance on untreated items remained low. Nevertheless, it is arguable that the lack of generalization effects can alternatively be attributed to the therapy received by YYW being strictly SFA rather than a combination of SFA and semantic priming, as in the case of TWT and the patients in Law *et al.* While it is difficult to rule out this possibility, previous treatment studies using SFA show improvement in naming untrained items (Boyle, 2004; Boyle & Coelho, 1995; Coelho *et al.*, 2000; Conley & Coelho, 2003; Hillis, 1998; Renvall *et al.*, 2003), suggesting that the technique of semantic priming alone cannot account for the presence of generalization in MTK and YSH in Law *et al.* and its absence in YYW. Future studies could shed light on the issue through administering the combined semantic treatment to anomic patients with moderate semantic deficits but various degrees of impairment to postsemantic components.

In accounting for the different treatment outcomes of YYW and TWT, we have suggested that proper functioning at the phonological output level, which may be taken to indicate largely preserved phonological representations of target names as evidenced by normal reading aloud, may be crucial to YYW's treatment success. It is important to note that the mere presence of target phonological forms may not be sufficient. YKM in Law *et al.* (2006), who did not benefit from the treatment, could also read object names with 95% accuracy. In short, taking into consideration the factors discussed thus far and the treatment outcomes of five anomic patients summarized in Table 15.9, the level of semantic impairment remains an important element for predicting treatment effectiveness and patterns of outcomes with respect to generalization.

Even though TWT never reached a satisfactory level of naming accuracy after intensive training, his improvement with high familiarity items was significant. This is reminiscent of the results of YKM (Law *et al.*, 2006), although YKM at most achieved 40% correct. In addition, similar to YKM, TWT produced more semantic errors and fewer omissions subsequent to semantic treatment. He also made small progress in naming untrained items. Therefore, it is not entirely correct to say that he did not respond to the intervention. Perhaps given more training sessions, he would have been able to maintain a more stable and achieve a higher level of performance.

In contrast with TWT, the rate of semantic errors by YYW was virtually unchanged. More unexpectedly, he made more omissions at the end of the treatment study. One plausible reason for the increase in 'no response' might be his better self-monitoring skills. That is, if he knew that the only name he could retrieve was not the target, he would choose not to produce it. This line of reasoning is based on recent findings that self-rating of monitoring skills is positively correlated with treatment efficacy and maintenance (Fillingham *et al.*, 2005b). These researchers also demonstrate that executive/problem-solving skills of a patient, not performances on language tasks, can predict both short-term and long-term treatment progress (Fillingham *et al.*, 2005a, 2005b). Law *et al.* (2006) hinted at this when accounting for the difference between MTK and YSH with regard to treatment duration and maintenance. However, our speculation about YYW's higher frequency of omission errors after intervention contradicts the observation in both studies by Fillingham *et al.* that self-monitoring skills tend to be positively related to non-verbal problem-solving skills, and YYW's poor performance on TONI-3 (6th percentile). As the Chinese patients in this study and in Law *et al.* did very poorly on the test of cognitive ability, except for MTK, the new data shed no further light on the issue. Nonetheless, we recognize the potential contribution of cognitive abilities to how aphasic patients may react to an intervention, and that future studies should properly address their role(s) in predicting patterns of treatment outcomes.

Conclusion

Through comparing the treatment outcomes and the language deficits of the patients in the present study and Law *et al.* (2006), we demonstrate the soundness of the approach advocated in Howard (2000). Further insights are gained into the relation between word retrieval difficulties and a treatment aimed at activating the semantic network associated with target words. In addition to semantic disruption, the conditions of postsemantic processes, in particular the phonological output level, also has an impact on the effectiveness of the treatment.

Acknowledgements

This study was supported by a grant from the Simon K.Y. Lee Research Fund. We are grateful to YYW and TWT for their participation.

References

Abbate, M.S. and Lachapelle, N.B. (1984) *Pictures Please! A Language Supplement.* Tucson, AZ: Communication Skill Builders.

Biedermann, B., Blanken, G. and Nickels, L. (2002) The representation of homophones: Evidence from remediation. *Aphasiology* 16, 1115–1136.

Boyle, M. (2004) Semantic feature analysis treatment for anomia in two fluent aphasia syndromes. *American Journal of Speech-Language Pathology* 13, 236–249.

Boyle, M. and Coelho, C.A. (1995) Application of semantic feature analysis as a treatment for aphasic dysnomia. *American Journal of Speech-Language Pathology* 4, 94–98.

Brown, L., Sherbenou, R.J. and Johnsen, S.K. (1997) *Test of Nonverbal Intelligence: A Language-free Measure of Cognitive Ability* (3rd edn). Austin, TX: Pro-Ed.

Byng, S. (1988) Sentence processing deficits: Theory and therapy. *Cognitive Neuropsychology* 5, 629–676.

Coelho, C.A., McHugh, R.E. and Boyle, M. (2000) Semantic feature analysis as a treatment for aphasic dysnomia: A replication. *Aphasiology* 14, 133–142.

Conley, A. and Coelho, C.A. (2003) Treatment of word retrieval impairment in chronic Broca's aphasia. *Aphasiology* 17, 203–211.

Drew, R.L. and Thompson, C.K. (1999) Model based semantic treatment for naming deficits in aphasia. *Journal of Speech, Language, and Hearing Research* 42, 972–989.

Dunn, L.M. (1982) *British Picture Vocabulary Scale.* Windsor: Nfer-Nelson.

Eales, C. and Pring, T. (1998) Using individual and group therapy to remediate word finding difficulties. *Aphasiology* 12, 913–918.

Fillingham, J.K., Sage, K. and Lambon Ralph, M.A. (2005a) Further explorations and an overview of errorless and errorful therapy for aphasic word-finding difficulties: The number of naming attempts during therapy affects outcome. *Aphasiology* 19, 597–614.

Fillingham, J.K., Sage, K. and Lambon Ralph, M.A. (2005b) Treatment of anomia using errorless versus errorful learning: Are frontal executive skills and feedback important? *International Journal of Language and Communication Disorders* 40, 505–523.

Fink, R.B., Brecher, A., Schwartz, M.F. and Robey, R. (2002) A computer-implemented protocol for treatment of naming disorders: Evaluation of clinician-guided and partially self-guided instruction. *Aphasiology* 16, 1061–1086.

Francis, D.R., Clark, N. and Humphreys, G.W. (2002) Circumlocution-induced naming (CIN): A treatment for effecting generalization in anomia? *Aphasiology* 16, 243–259.

Grayson, E., Hilton, R. and Franklin, S. (1997) Early intervention in a case of jargon aphasia: Efficacy of language comprehension therapy. *European Journal of Disorders of Communication* 32, 257–276.

Hillis, A. and Caramazza, A. (1994) Theories of lexical processing and rehabilitation of lexical deficits. In M.J. Riddoch and G.W. Humphreys (eds) *Cognitive Neuropsychology and Cognitive Rehabilitation* (pp. 449–484). Hove: Lawrence Erlbaum.

Hillis, A.E. (1998) Treatment of naming disorders: New issues regarding old therapies. *Journal of the International Neuropsychological Society* 4, 648–660.

Hough, M.S. (1993) Treatment of Wernicke's aphasia with jargon: A case study. *Journal of Communication Disorders* 26, 101–111.

Howard, D. (1994) The treatment of acquired aphasia. *Philosophical Transactions of the Royal Society London, B* 346, 113–120.

Howard, D. (2000) Cognitive neuropsychology and aphasia therapy: The case of word retrieval. In I. Papathanasiou (ed.) *Acquired Neurogenic Communication Disorders: A Clinical Perspective* (pp. 76–100). London: Whurr.

Howard, D. and Patterson, K. (1992) *Pyramids and Palm Trees Test*. Edmunds: Thames Valley Test Company.

Jipson, T.W. (1987) *Aphasia Rehabilitation: A Clinical and Home Therapy Program.* Tulsa, OK: Modern Education Corporation.

Kaplan, E., Goodglass, H. and Weintraub, S. (1983) *Boston Naming Test*. Philadelphia, PA: Lea & Fabiger.

Kiran, S. and Thompson, C.K. (2001) Typicality of category exemplars in aphasia: Evidence from reaction time and treatment data. *Brain and Language* 79, 27–31.

Law, S-P. and Or, B. (2001) A case study of acquired dyslexia and dysgraphia in Cantonese: Evidence for nonsemantic pathways for reading and writing Chinese. *Cognitive Neuropsychology* 18, 729–748.

Law, S-P., Wong, W., Sung, F. and Hon, J. (2006) A study of semantic treatment of three Chinese anomic patients. *Neuropsychological Rehabilitation* 16, 601–609.

Lee, T.M.C., Yuen, K.S.L. and Chan, C.C.H. (2002) Normative data for neuropsychological measures of fluency, attention, and memory measures for Hong Kong Chinese. *Journal of Clinical and Experimental Neuropsychology* 24, 615–632.

Lowell, S., Beeson, P. and Holland, A. (1995) The efficacy of a semantic cueing procedure on naming performance of adults with aphasia. *American Journal of Speech-Language Pathology* 4, 109–114.

Marshall, J., Pound, C., White-Thomson, M. and Pring, T. (1990) The use of picture/word matching tasks to assist word retrieval in aphasic patients. *Aphasiology* 4, 167–184.

Nickels, L. (2002) Therapy for naming disorders: Revisiting, revising, and reviewing. *Aphasiology* 16, 935–979.

Nickels, L. and Best, W. (1996) Therapy for naming deficits (part II): Specifics, surprises and suggestions. *Aphasiology* 10, 109–136.

Raymer, A.M. and Ellsworth, T. (2002) Response to contrasting verbal retrieval treatments: A case study. *Aphasiology* 16, 1031–1045.

Renvall, K., Laine, M., Laakso, M. and Martin, N. (2003) Anomia treatment with contextual priming: A case study. *Aphasiology* 17, 305–328.

Riddoch, M.J. and Humphreys, G.W. (1993) *Birmingham Object Recognition Battery.* Hove: Lawrence Erlbaum.

Robson, J., Marshall, J., Pring, T. and Chiat, S. (1998) Phonological naming therapy in jargon aphasia: Positive but paradoxical effects. *Journal of the International Neuropsychological Society* 4, 675–686.

Rose, M., Douglas, J. and Matyas, T. (2002) The comparative effectiveness of gesture and verbal treatments for a specific phonologic naming impairment. *Aphasiology* 16, 1001–1030.

Snodgrass, J.G. and Vanderwart, M. (1980) A standarised set of 260 pictures: Norms for name agreement, image agreement, familiarity and visual complexity. *Journal of Experimental Psychology: Learning, Memory, and Cognition* 6, 174–215.

Weekes, B., Chen, M-J. and Yin, W.G. (1997) Anomia without dyslexia in Chinese. *Neurocase* 3, 51–60.

Chapter 16

Acquired Dyslexia in Mongolian and Chinese

BRENDAN S. WEEKES, I FAN SU and WENGANG YIN

Introduction

How does the brain process more than one language? This question can be addressed by investigating whether language processing in the first acquired language (L1) uses the same or different brain regions to the second language (L2) with brain imaging techniques such as fMRI, EEG and MEG studies of bilingual speakers (Vaid & Hull, 2002). However, a more traditional method is to study bilingual speakers with acquired language problems following brain damage (aphasia). Although studies of bilingual aphasia date back to the late 19th century (Fabbro, 1999), today this method forms a part of the cognitive neuropsychological approach to studying brain mechanisms in bilingual language processing (Gollan & Kroll, 2001; Paradis, 1977, 1995).

Studies of bilingual aphasia suggest that brain damage produces dissociations in language processing, i.e. one language more impaired than the other (Paradis, 1977). These patterns suggest that L1 and L2 may be processed in different brain regions (Albert & Obler, 1978; Lebrun, 1971). For example, some participants display a pattern of *differential recovery* from stroke whereby L2 is recovered only after recovery in L1. Another pattern is *selective recovery* whereby L2 is not recovered at all. Two further patterns are *alternating antagonism*, i.e. participants access only one language in spontaneous speech for alternating periods of time (Nilipour & Ashayeri, 1989; Paradis *et al.*, 1982), and *selective aphasia*, i.e. impairment to one language with no deficits to the other (Paradis & Goldblum, 1989). An alternative explanation of these phenomena is that dissociations in language processing result from extraneous factors, including the age of acquisition, premorbid proficiency and familiarity with each language (Paradis, 2001), or from the linguistic properties of L1 and L2 that constrain manifestations of aphasia (Nilipour & Paradis, 1995; Yiu & Worrall, 1996). Yet another possibility is that these patterns of differential recovery result from damage to the brain regions that regulate inhibition and control over language use, e.g. the cingulate gyrus (Green, 2006).

Most studies of bilingual aphasia focus on production and comprehension of single words in L1 and L2. One claim to emerge from this research is that knowledge about word meaning (semantic representations) is shared across languages, whereas representations for word forms are stored in separate lexica. This is assumed in most cognitive models of bilingual language processing (e.g. Potter *et al.*, 1984; Smith, 1997), including the Revised Hierarchical (RH) model of Kroll and Stewart (1994) (see Figure 16.1), which assumes that access to word meanings from the most familiar word forms (typically L1) is more efficient than access from less familiar forms. Although this is the most

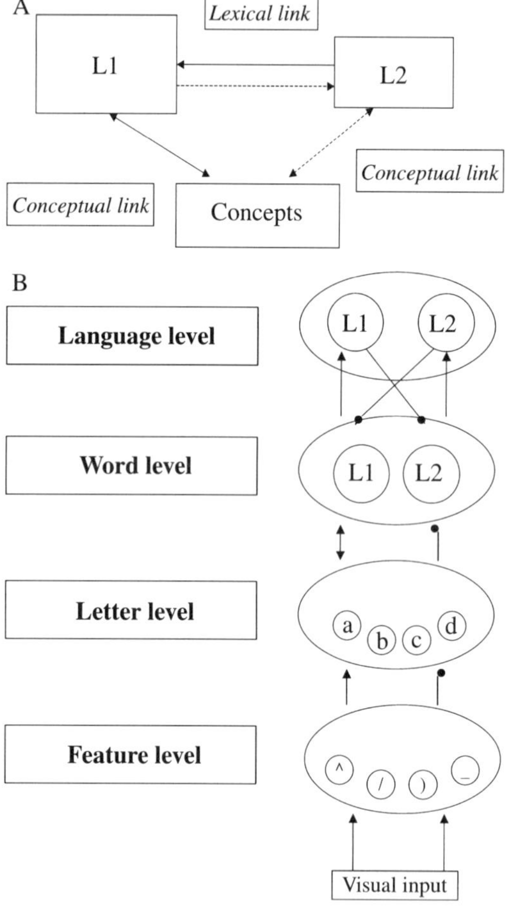

Figure 16.1 Models of bilingual language processing (A) the revised Hierarchical model and (B) the computational BIA model (adapted from Dijkstra & Van Heuven, 1998).

typical pattern observed in bilingual aphasia (Edmonds & Kiran, 2004; Ferrand & Humphreys, 1996), there are exceptional cases. For example, Aglioti and Fabbro (1993) report participant EM who showed paradoxical selective aphasia where L2 (Italian) was better than L1 (Venetian). The RH model can explain selective effects of brain damage in bilingual aphasia because the store of word forms in one language can be damaged without damage to the other. Moreover, the model can generate predictions about dissociations in bilingual aphasia, i.e. brain damage will impact more on the premorbidly less familiar language (L1 or L2). Although the assumption of common conceptual representations in L1 and L2 is not controversial (see Francis, 1999), not all models assume independent lexica. For example, the computational model, the Bilingual Interactive Activation (BIA) model developed by Dijkstra and Van Heuven (2002) (see Figure 16.1), assumes the abstract orthographic representations of word forms in each language are stored at the same level of processing. The BIA model could simulate selective effects of brain damage by instantiating differences in the familiarity of word forms in L1 and L2. This is done using weight adjustment within the network, i.e. less familiar words have a weaker set of connections between representations.

The BIA model is an adaptation of McClelland and Rummelhart's (1981) Interactive Activation model to written word recognition in bilinguals. Different layers of nodes represent the features of printed words as in the monolingual model. However, bottom-up activation that starts from feature nodes results in activation of word nodes in both languages in the BIA model. There is also a layer of language nodes in the BIA model, allowing top-down inhibition of words in the nontarget language. This model accounts for selective effects of language on performance, not by assuming independent abstract orthographic representations for word forms in L1 and L2, but by assuming that word nodes in the dominant language have a higher average resting level than less dominant language nodes. Note the term dominant refers to the more familiar language, which may or may not be the first acquired language. The BIA model predicts that brain damage will lead to differential effects on written word recognition because of differences in familiarity with words, leading to stronger residual activation in the more dominant language. The model also allows brain damage to have a greater effect on lexical processing in one language, because of more top-down inhibition of that language following brain damage (see also Green, 2006).

Extant evidence for the BIA model comes from studies of unimpaired speakers showing that the statistical properties of an L1 script have an impact on reading performance in L2 (and vice versa). For example, Jared and Kroll (2001) showed that the statistical properties of French had an impact on English language processing (see also Bijeljac-Babic *et al.*, 1997; Van Hueven *et al.*, 1998) compatible with the BIA assumption of shared orthographic representations in L1 and L2. Note, however, that cross-script effects on oral reading depend on language proficiency. For speakers who are proficient in both languages, the evidence is that representations of both languages become active. However, for less proficient speakers, the representations in L1 may be more active than the representations in L2 (Jared & Kroll, 2001).

It is perhaps not surprising to find activation in both languages during biscriptal reading if the languages share a script. Almost all studies of biscriptal reading tests in languages that share an alphabetic script – Dutch–English (Van Heuven *et al.*, 1998), Spanish–English (Scarbarough *et al.*, 1984), French–English (Beauvillain & Grainger, 1987), Italian–English (Caramazza & Brones, 1979), English–Afrikaans (Doctor & Klein, 1992) and trilingual Dutch–English–French (Dijkstra & Van Hell, 2003) (also Brysbaert *et al.*, 1999). This is also true in studies of participants with bilingual aphasia who typically read better in L1 than L2 (Caramelli *et al.*, 1994; Masterson *et al.*, 1985; Raman & Weekes, 2005). For example, Masterson *et al.* reported a Spanish–English speaker who produced more reading errors in English (L2) than Spanish (L1). Raman and Weekes reported a similar pattern in a Turkish–English speaker. However, one factor that may impact on acquired reading problems (dyslexia) in biscriptal participants is the type of script. This is particularly true for languages that share an alphabet. For example, Spanish is a relatively transparent script when compared to English and French, and the Turkish script has no ambiguities in spelling at all. This means that surface dyslexia, which refers to impaired reading of irregular words, e.g. yacht in English, is impossible in Turkish (see Raman & Weekes, 2005). Some studies have asked if written word representations are active in both languages during biscriptal oral reading by making cross-script comparisons, e.g. Hebrew–English (Gollan *et al.*, 1997), or else by testing languages with two different scripts, e.g. Serbo–Croatian (Havelka & Rastle, 2005). However, it is an open question whether or not differences in script across the two languages of a biscriptal reader have any impact on language processing and, more specifically, on oral reading in either normal or impaired (aphasic) speakers.

Some studies of biscriptal aphasic participants suggest that differences in script may have an impact on reading of participants with bilingual aphasia (Byng *et al.*, 1984; Karanth, 2002). Beland and Mimouni (2001) reported better reading of nonwords in French (L2) than Arabic (L1), and Eng and Obler (2002) reported more semantic reading errors in Chinese (L1) than English (L2). Caramelli *et al.* (1994) reported more reading and writing errors in Japanese than Portuguese in a Brazilian 'Nesei' participant even though the participant had acquired both languages at an early age and was a scribe in Japanese premorbidly. Also, the participant showed a dissociation when reading in Japanese. The Japanese language uses two different scripts, Kana and Kanji. Both scripts are acquired at around the same age when learning to read. Caramelli *et al.*'s participant was more impaired at oral reading and writing in Kana than Kanji (and in Portuguese) compatible with reports of Japanese aphasic participants who show dyslexia in one script but no impairment in the other (Iwata, 1984; Sasanuma, 1975; Sasanuma & Monoi, 1975; though see Sugishita *et al.*, 1992). Although these participants are biscriptal rather than bilingual, the data suggest that different scripts have separate functional anatomy, compatible with the view that L1 and L2 are processed in different parts of the brain (Albert & Obler, 1978; Benson, 1985; Cremaschi & Dujovny, 1996; Lebrun, 1971). The results are in agreement with some evidence from brain imaging suggesting that different scripts might activate separate brain regions (Chen *et al.*, 2002; Paulesu *et al.*, 2000; Sakurai *et al.*, 2000; though see Chee *et al.*, 1999, 2000 who found no effect of script in brain activation). In our view, an effect of script on oral reading in bilingual aphasia is a challenge for the BIA model, because the model assumes that damage to the lexical network will have a similar impact on written word processing in L1 and L2, given that words presented in either script access the same orthographic representation.

Extant reports of oral reading in bilingual aphasia compare performance within alphabetic scripts that are characterized by a finite number of symbols that when combined can produce an infinite number of words. Nonalphabetic scripts such as Chinese use a relatively arbitrary system for mapping orthographic units to phonology to represent words. The great majority of Chinese characters are composed of strokes formed into components that are written together into a square shape to form a character. Ancient characters were pictographic because the written character portrayed the form of the object that it symbolized. These scripts are often defined as logographic because the basic unit of writing is associated with a unit of meaning (morpheme), unlike alphabetic scripts, which use letters as the basic unit of writing. This means that each written form is associated with a morpheme in spoken language whereas in alphabetic scripts, each unit of writing represents a component (phoneme) of a spoken word. The script is therefore *morphographic*, meaning that the smallest pronounceable unit in a character is associated with a monosyllable. This contrasts with the symbols in an alphabet that do not represent meaning. Instead, Chinese scripts use a large number of symbols called characters, which either alone or in combination with other characters form the words of the language. Other differences between alphabetic and nonalphabetic scripts are that the mappings between orthography and phonology in nonalphabetic scripts are relatively opaque (although some phonetic and semantic radicals may denote a common pronunciation across characters or semantic relatedness across characters [Zhou, 1978]), and that the relationship between orthography and meaning is relatively transparent in many characters, whereas the mappings between orthography and meaning are almost always opaque in alphabetic scripts. Given these differences, one interesting question is whether acquired dyslexia manifests differently across scripts in bilingual participants who speak languages with different orthography. We investigated this question by examining Mongolian–Chinese speakers.

Written Mongolian is called the Uighur script and was invented by Genghis Khan in the 13th century. It is considered an alphabetic script that was derived from Aramaic and it shares a common source with Indo-European and Semitic alphabets (Poppe, 1970). Although Uighur was replaced by Cyrillic in the Republic of Mongolia, the traditional script has remained in use in Chinese-controlled Inner Mongolia where it is taught with Chinese characters to all children. Letters and words are written from left to right in a vertical orientation from top to bottom and all letters in a word are connected by a continuous pen stroke. There are few word boundaries and words are written in a continuous line that runs vertically with lines and loops written to the left as the word progresses downward. Examples of Mongolian script, including the word *bolon* (and), are shown in Figure 16.2 and explained in Table 16.1. Although Mongolian is considered an alphabetic script, understanding the word context may be necessary to read aloud correctly. Grapheme to phoneme relationships will be determined by the position of vowels. For example, one letter is used when a vowel is in the first syllable of a word, and another for subsequent occurrences of the vowel in a word. Thus, the word *bolon* could be read as different words (letter combinations) thereby requiring knowledge of the language to be read correctly (Poppe, 1970). Similar to Hebrew, it is difficult to identify ambiguous printed symbols of Uighur script without some contextual knowledge. This is different from other alphabetic scripts such as Turkish where the mappings between print and sound always generate a correct response. It is interesting to note for the present purposes that although Uighur symbols do not represent morpheme units in the same way as Chinese, access to the meaning of whole words from print may be necessary for skilled processing of written words. Further information is provided in Table 16.1.

Extant studies reporting evidence of an effect of script on written language processing in bilingual aphasia have several methodological problems. For example, test stimuli are rarely controlled for variables such as age of acquisition, premorbid proficiency and word familiarity that all impact on performance (Paradis, 2001). Other factors that have an effect on performance include the word frequency and imageability of word forms, i.e. low imageability words, such as *justice*, are more

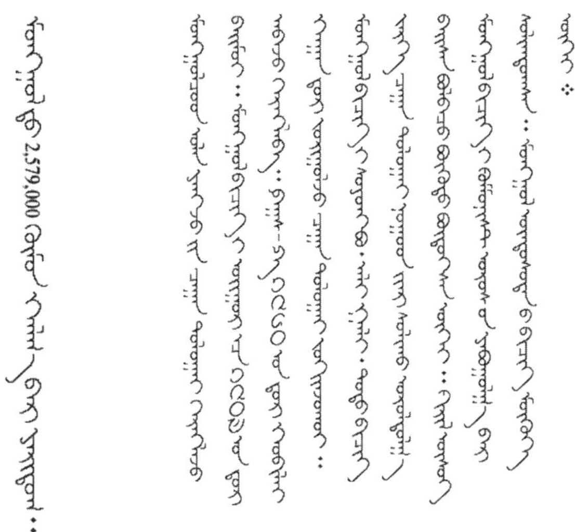

Figure 16.2 Examples of Mongolian script (Kapaj, 2001). The word *bolon* is depicted on the left.

impaired than high imageability words, such as *house* (Kiran & Tuchtenhagen, 2005). We controlled these variables in this study by recruiting participants who had acquired written Mongolian and Chinese at approximately the same (young) age, to minimize the effects of age of acquisition and we compared performance on tasks in both languages using common nouns, e.g. *star, cat, eye* that are high in word frequency, to minimize the effects of premorbid proficiency and word familiarity.

Our primary aim was to examine if type of script has an impact on lexical processing in bilingual aphasia. However, effects of script on lexical processing in Chinese–Mongolian-speaking participants would be of particular interest because the BIA model does not assume independent orthographic representations (unlike the RH model), and therefore would not expect any effect of script when the familiarity of words is controlled. An effect of script would also be informative to the more controversial claim that different brain regions are necessary for written word identification in L1 and L2 (Chen *et al.*, 2002; Paulesu *et al.*, 2000; Sakurai *et al.*, 2000).

Case Reports

Four bilingual Mongolian–Chinese stroke participants were recruited from Tongliao People's Hospital in Inner-Mongolia Autonomous District.

Table 16.1 Explanation of the Mongolian script

The Mongolian script is regular, i.e. most written spellings converge on the same written symbol. However, homophonic heterographs are seen as in English (*there, their*) and Chinese. For example, the word *khana*, which means both 'wall' and 'bleed', is written in different ways:

Sounds may also be written differently according to their position within a word (initial, middle or final). For example, the sound /a/ must be written in three different ways according to position:

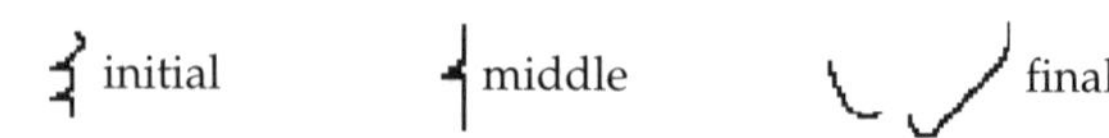

There is also some phonological ambiguity in printed symbols. For example, the sound /i/ has a different printed form to /a/ in the initial position, but not in middle and final positions of a word:

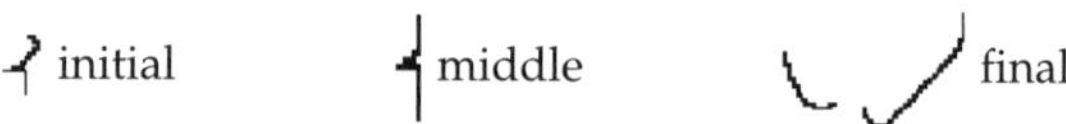

The consonants H and G have the same written form and both change according to position:

Ambiguity in written word pronunciation and writing of sounds suggests that some knowledge of word context may be necessary to read and write in Mongolian as in Chinese and English.

Biographical details of each case including results from CT scans are shown in Table 16.2. Lesion location was not a criterion for selection in order to maximize the number of participants. All participants were native speakers of Mongolian (L1) who learned to read Chinese (L2) at elementary school age. Participants were recruited into the study according to several criteria, including formal instruction in reading and writing Chinese during elementary school, at least average pre-morbid IQ based on education and work history and a preserved ability to comprehend task instructions. The Chinese Aphasia Examination Scale (Wang *et al.*, 1988) and a translation of that scale in Mongolian was used to screen all participants for language problems in Mongolian and Chinese. The purpose of screening was to ensure that participants were capable of comprehending task instructions in both languages. Participants were excluded from the study if they could not perform

Table 16.2 Biographical details of each participant

Case	*Sex*	*Age*	*Handedness*	*Education*	*CT/pathology/test date*
TGX	Male	47	Left-handed	Middle school	Right temporal lobe and basal ganglia infarction
WT	Male	58	Right-handed	Polytechnic	Left basal ganglia infarction
SL	Male	56	Right-handed	Middle school	Left putamen hemorrhage
LH	Male	38	Right-handed	Middle school	Left temporal infarction

above 90% correct on spoken word picture-matching tasks in both languages. It is important to note that screening excluded a large number of participants. Therefore, the present results will be limited to understanding lexical processing of participants with relatively preserved word comprehension in Mongolian and Chinese.

All participants were given four lexical-processing tasks: oral reading, lexical decision, written word-picture matching and spoken word-picture matching. Each task was presented on two different occasions separated by at least a week and items were presented in either Chinese or Mongolian with order counterbalanced across participants to minimize effects of expectation of a bilingual environment (Grosjean, 1998, 2001). Words were selected according to several criteria: concrete words that are early acquired, high imageability and high frequency. Stimuli were thus highly familiar to all participants in both languages premorbidly. Each task contained the same lexical items ($n = 14$) (see Appendix). Performance is summarized in Table 16.3.

McNemar's test (1947) compared performance across the same lexical items in both languages for all tasks by estimating the significance of the difference between correlated proportions following a Chi-squared distribution (Ferguson, 1966). For participant TGX, reading was impaired in both languages and there was also a significant effect of task on performance. Lexical decision in Chinese was significantly better than in Mongolian ($\chi^2(1) = 4.0$, $p < 0.05$). TGX produced semantic errors in oral reading of written words in Mongolian, e.g. woman read as teacher, and in Chinese, e.g. ox read as horse. For participant WT, there was a significant effect of script on written word comprehension which was worse in Chinese than Mongolian ($\chi^2(1) = 4.1$, $p < 0.05$), but no effect of script on other tasks. There were also effects of task, i.e. written word

Table 16.3 Results of experimental investigations in Mongolian and Chinese (% correct)

	TGX	*WT*	*SL*	*LH*
Mongolian				
Oral reading	64	100	57	28
Lexical decision	71	100	100	50
Written-picture matching	85	85	92	78
Spoken-picture matching	71	92	100	78
Chinese				
Oral reading	71	92	14	0
Lexical decision	100	100	100	71
Written-picture matching	85	57	50	78
Spoken-picture matching	85	71	57	78

comprehension in Chinese was worse than oral reading ($\chi^2(1) = 5.0$, $p < 0.05$) and lexical decision ($\chi^2(1) = 6.0$, $p < 0.05$). However, there were no significant effects of task on lexical processing in Mongolian. For participant SL, there were effects of script on performance in written word comprehension ($\chi^2(1) = 6.0$, $p < 0.05$), spoken word comprehension ($\chi^2(1) = 6.0$, $p < 0.05$) and oral reading ($\chi^2(1) = 5.0$, $p < 0.05$). However, lexical decision was preserved in both languages. Similarly for participant SL there were significant effects of task in both languages. In Mongolian, oral reading was more impaired than lexical decision ($\chi^2(1) = 6.0$, $p < 0.05$) and written word comprehension ($\chi^2(1) = 5.0$, $p < 0.05$). In Chinese, spoken word comprehension ($\chi^2(1) = 6.0$, $p < 0.05$) and oral reading were more impaired than lexical decision ($\chi^2(1) = 11.0$, $p < 0.05$), written word comprehension ($\chi^2(1) = 4.1$, $p < 0.05$) and spoken word comprehension ($\chi^2(1) = 5.0$, $p < 0.05$). SL produced semantic errors in Mongolian and Chinese and 'translation errors', i.e. reading aloud a Mongolian word with a Chinese syllable. There was also an effect of script on performance for participant LH, but in oral reading only ($\chi^2(1) = 4.0$, $p < 0.05$). There were significant effects of task for LH in both languages. In Mongolian, oral reading was worse than written word comprehension ($\chi^2(1) = 7.0$, $p < 0.05$) and spoken word comprehension ($\chi^2(1) = 7.0$, $p < 0.05$). In Chinese, oral reading was worse than lexical decision ($\chi^2(1) = 13.0$, $p < 0.05$), written word comprehension ($\chi^2(1) = 11.0$, $p < 0.05$) and spoken word comprehension ($\chi^2(1) = 11.00$, $p < 0.05$). LH produced semantic errors in Mongolian, e.g. table read as stool, but not in Chinese. To summarize, there was an effect of script on written word comprehension for WT and SL with worse performance in Chinese (L2) than Mongolian (L1), and for two participants – SL and LH – type of script had an effect on oral reading which was more impaired for both in L2 than L1.

General Discussion

Performance on tests of written word processing was more impaired in L2 (Chinese) than L1 (Mongolian). These results are compatible with evidence showing brain damage produces dissociations in language processing that affects L2 more than L1 (Fabbro, 1999; Gollan & Kroll, 2001; Paradis, 1977). Of interest was the finding that lexical decision was more impaired in L1 than L2 for participant TGX. Therefore, although brain damage appears to have more impact on language processing in L1 than L2, the reverse pattern can be observed, i.e. brain damage can have more impact on written word recognition in L2 than L1.

Implications for models of bilingual language processing

All models of bilingual language processing assume that lexical processing will be faster and more efficient in L1 than L2. Moreover, the RH model predicts that access to word meaning from L1 will be more efficient than from L2 (Kroll & De Groot, 1997). As brain damage reduces the efficiency of language processing in bilingual aphasia, performance on tests of word comprehension (spoken and written) are expected to be more impaired in L2 than L1 according to this model. The BIA model could explain more efficient access to word meaning from L1 than from L2 as a result of stronger residual activation in the more dominant language or greater top-down inhibition of one language following brain damage. However, the models differ in terms of how differences in oral reading and lexical decision performance across scripts can be explained. The BIA model assumes that lexical processing of written word forms in L1 and L2 address the same orthographic representation. Therefore, the BIA model would expect impaired processing of written word forms in one script to be accompanied by impaired processing in the other script. Consistent performance with the same lexical item across scripts and tasks is compatible with the view that orthographic representations are shared (preserved or lost after brain damage). The RH model makes no differential predictions, but can explain dissociations across both script and task.

Oral reading was more impaired in L2 than L1 for two participants. This is comparable to previous reports of an effect of script on biscriptal reading (Beland & Mimouni, 2001; Caramelli *et al.*, 1994; Eng & Obler, 2002; Masterson *et al.*, 1985; Raman & Weekes, 2005). Moreover, there was evidence of selection impairment from cross-linguistic errors in oral reading, i.e. responses could not be produced in the target language (typically L2). These errors are reported in other biscriptal participants (e.g. Beland & Mimouni, 2001; Eng & Obler, 2002; Masterson *et al.*, 1985; Raman & Weekes, 2005). The RH model accounts for selective reading problems as the result of damage to the Chinese written word lexicon with a spared lexicon for Mongolian. A different possibility is that a mechanism used to switch between written words in each language during reading was impaired after brain damage. However, we can reject a switching hypothesis because all participants could switch between languages when producing oral reading responses.

The pattern of better oral reading in L1 than L2 could be explained by the BIA model if it is assumed that spoken word production in either language can be selectively inhibited. Selective inhibition of spoken word forms is necessary in accounts of bilingual spoken word production to explain the ability of bilingual speakers to ignore properties of one language while processing the other. Selective inhibition of spoken word forms is also necessary to account for 'pathological' inhibition of word forms in L2 in bilingual aphasia (Fabbro, 2001). Inhibition of spoken word forms in the BIA model can be implemented at the level of language nodes that bias the network towards processing in one language only. The temporary nature of word recognition impairments in L2 can also be explained by the model as a result of reduced activation in the network as a whole, thus leading to more impairment in L2 than L1. Reduced activation in the network as a whole would have more impact on language processing in L2 if the representations of L2 word forms have a lower resting state than L1 word forms (Dijkstra & Van Heuven, 1998). One question for the modelers is whether this effect could be simulated by lesioning the BIA model.

The BIA model cannot easily explain why performance on lexical decision was better in Chinese than Mongolian for participant TGX when there was no difference between the two languages on any other task. The model predicts impaired processing of written word forms in one script to be accompanied by impaired processing in the other. Dissociations across task at this point cannot be explained by differences in familiarity, age of acquisition, imageability or language dominance. The RH model can explain dissociations across script if TGX sustained more damage to an independent Mongolian lexicon, allowing performance on tasks in Mongolian to be worse than tasks presented in Chinese. Impairment to the Mongolian lexicon should however, also translate to impaired performance on oral reading and written word comprehension tasks, although lexical decision may be a more difficult task. Overall, the effects of script and different patterns across tasks in level of performance across scripts are problematic for BIA models.

The explanatory power of the BIA model may be remedied by a more recent version called the BIA+ model (Dijsktra & Van Heuven, 2002). The BIA+ model assumes that orthography and phonology are represented at independent levels of processing, including sublexical connections between orthography and phonology (O- > P). These additional parameters can account more fully for differential effects of task on performance. Oral reading requires spoken word production and may require sublexical O- > P mappings. If brain damage impacts on these representations but not orthographic or semantic representations, then task effects are possible in the model. The BIA+ model could explain greater impairment to reading in L2 than L1 by assuming that brain damage results in inhibition of spoken word forms. Greater inhibition of spoken word production would be expected in the less dominant language, i.e. use of spoken language in daily life (which may be L1 or L2). For all participants, L1 was the dominant language premorbidly, although written word forms are commonly encountered in both L1 and L2 in Inner Mongolia. Oral reading in L2 could also be more impaired than oral reading in L1 if selective inhibition of spoken word forms is 'pathological'. One possibility is for inhibition to be instantiated in the BIA+ model at the level of language nodes connected to lexical phonology. Another possibility is a 'lesion' at the task schema stage leading to pathological language mixing (Brysbaert & Dijkstra, 2006). Our results highlight the desirability of implementing both phonological and semantic representations within the architecture if the BIA+ model to explain impaired oral reading in bilingual aphasia.

Implications for models of reading in Mongolian and Chinese

There is no model of oral reading in Mongolian. However, a model of oral reading in Chinese is described in Figure 16.3. This general framework allows us to compare disorders of oral reading in Mongolian with Chinese. In normal oral reading, if lexical representations of words in two or more languages overlap at the orthographic and phonological levels (as in the BIA+ model) then Chinese characters and Mongolian symbols may be processed by both pathways. This means that a written word form presented in either script will activate abstract orthographic representations, as well as the lexical representations related by meaning via the lexical-semantic pathway and by phonology in the nonsemantic pathway. An oral reading response in either language could be produced. However, errors will not routinely be produced in oral reading of bilingual speakers because input from the nonsemantic pathway can inhibit semantically related (although incorrect) responses and input from the lexical-semantic pathway can inhibit phonologically related errors. Damage to the nonsemantic pathway may, however, result

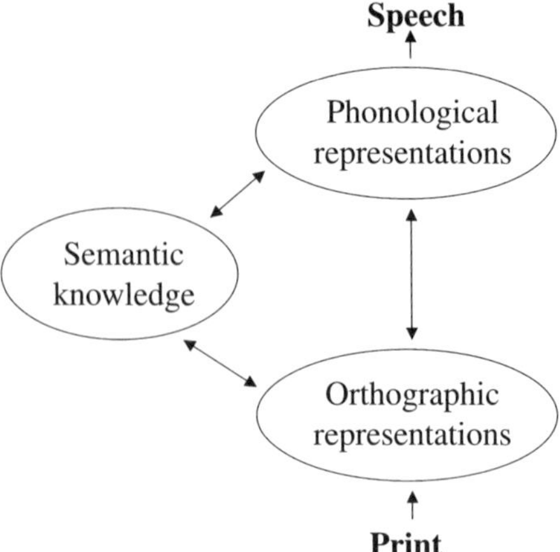

Figure 16.3 A functional model of reading and writing in Chinese adapted from Weekes *et al.* (1997).

in over-reliance on lexical-semantic reading, leading to cross-linguistic and semantic reading errors. Evidence of interactions between pathways in monolingual Chinese speakers is plentiful, e.g. Law (2004) who reported that participant KCM produced more semantic errors in picture naming than reading, suggesting semantic reading errors can be inhibited with sufficient input from the nonsemantic reading pathway. In biscriptal Chinese–Mongolian participants, damage to the nonsemantic pathway will lead to reliance on lexical-semantic reading, resulting in cross-script errors as we observed for individuals TGX, SL and LH (see also Raman & Weekes, 2005). The framework in Figure 16.3 also allows for a division of labor in oral reading across scripts for bilingual speakers, without assuming separate lexica for word forms in Mongolian and Chinese.

We have argued that reading aloud correctly in Mongolian might require understanding of word context. The model in Figure 16.3 assumes this is not necessary given a nonsemantic route to reading which bypasses knowledge of word context. We found some data to suggest that oral reading in Mongolian might proceed without access to word meaning, as WT could read aloud words in Mongolian that he could not identify on word-picture matching tasks. However, given that words map onto a small number of possible phonological forms, WT could correctly pronounce a phonologically ambiguous word by chance. We note here that evidence of preserved Mongolian reading with impaired written word comprehension is necessary before it could be concluded that access to word meaning is not required to read aloud correctly in Mongolian.

A different possibility is that reading aloud in Mongolian requires an interaction between the semantic and nonsemantic routes, unlike reading aloud in Chinese. The data in Table 16.2 show that oral reading performance in Mongolian is always inferior to written word-picture matching in Chinese in those cases that show a reliable difference between tasks, i.e. for participants TGX, SL and LH. This suggests that, when there is damage to the lexical-semantic route, impairment to oral reading is inevitable. On the other hand, participant WT shows the opposite pattern of better oral reading than written-picture matching. As reading in Chinese can proceed via the nonsemantic route alone (in the majority of cases), but reading Mongolian relies on both reading routes, the combination of acquired bilingual dyslexia in Mongolian and Chinese raises an issue about oral reading that has been ignored by current models. This suggests that data from cases of reading in bilingual speakers can be informative to the question of underlying mechanisms for reading relevant scripts when explaining patterns of impaired or intact performance across script.

Implications for understanding bilingual language aphasia

We found little evidence of language mixing. Brain activation of control circuits in the anterior cingulate and basal ganglia are used to account for alternating antagonistic recovery (Green, 2006). The majority of our participants had damage to perisylvian regions. These areas are necessary for processing language representations rather than switching or control. Damage to occipital regions that are important for written word recognition in L1 and L2, or to frontal brain regions, e.g. the anterior cingulate, basal ganglia or caudate nucleus that are necessary for the control of behavior (Crinion *et al.*, 2006), may result in more effects of script in participants with bilingual aphasia.

Conclusion

Communication disorders are a problem for people all over the world. However, language disorders are rarely studied in the context of bilingualism and research in this field is minimal (Fabbro, 1999; Roberts, 1998). This is despite the fact that many individuals with aphasia are multilingual. Studies of polyglot aphasic speakers can reveal important conceptual insights about the cognitive and neurological factors in multilingualism with implications for rehabilitation. For example, training lexical retrieval in one language results in some cross-language generalization as predicted by both the BIA and RH models (Edmonds & Kiran, 2006). Although there is a literature on bilingual aphasia in European languages, the rigorous psycholinguistic methods that are needed to assess language processing in bilingual aphasia are lacking, with no consideration of effects of word frequency, familiarity, imageability and age of acquisition on performance. The focus is on participants with impairments to lexical-retrieval skills such as anomia, which is a common symptom of bilingual aphasia (Stadie *et al.*, 1995), with far less attention to syntactic skills. There are surprisingly few reports of Chinese participants with aphasia who speak another language (though see April & Han, 1980; April & Tse, 1977; Lyman *et al.*, 1938; Reich *et al.*, 2003), considering that bidialectal participants will be affected by aphasia. However, the number of Chinese–English speakers is increasing. These individuals are currently relatively young. In the next generation however, there should be more language-impaired bilingual speakers across East Asia in Hong Kong, Mainland China, Singapore and Taiwan as well as in countries where Chinese-speaking emigrants have learned a second language (including but not limited to English). One question for future studies will be whether therapy is more effective if carried out through a bilingual coworker. In the West, most speech and language therapists are monolingual English speakers.

In sum, we found evidence of bilingual aphasia in Mongolian–Chinese speakers recovering from stroke. The most important finding was a modest effect of script on reading which was better in L1 (Mongolian) than L2 (Chinese), although we also observed impairments to lexical processing that were significantly worse in L1 than L2. Our conclusion is that oral reading of familiar words in Mongolian and Chinese does not necessarily require independent cognitive systems or separate brain regions.

Acknowledgements

This work was supported by research grants from the Royal Society and the Research Grants Council of the Hong Kong Government (HKU7275/03H). We thank Dr Zhang Xihong of the Department of Neurology, Tongliao People's Hospital for help with recruitment and testing of the participants reported.

References

Aglioti, S. and Fabbro, F. (1993) Paradoxical selective recovery in a bilingual aphasic following subcortical lesions. *Neuroreport* 4, 1359–1362.

Albert, M.L. and Obler, L.K. (1978) *The Bilingual Brain: Neuropsychological and Neurolinguistic Aspects of Bilingualism*. New York: Academic Press.

April, R.S. and Han, M. (1980) Crossed aphasia in a right-handed bilingual Chinese man. A second case. *Archives of Neurology* 37, 342–346.

April, R.S. and Tse, P.C. (1977) Crossed aphasia in a Chinese bilingual dextral. *Archives of Neurology* 34, 766–770.

Beauvillain, C. and Grainger, J. (1987) Accessing interlexical homographs: Some limitations of a language-selective access. *Journal of Memory and Language* 26, 658–672.

Beland, R. and Mimouni, Z. (2001) Deep dyslexia in the two languages of an Arabic/French bilingual participant. *Cognition* 82, 77–126.

Benson, D.F. (1985) Aphasia. In K. Heilman and E. Valenstein (eds) *Clinical Neuropsychology* (Vol. 2, pp. 17–32). New York: Oxford University Press.

Bijeljac-Babic, R., Biardeau, A. and Grainger, J. (1997) Masked orthographic priming in bilingual word recognition. *Memory and Cognition* 25, 447–457.

Brysbaert, M. and Dijkstra, T. (2006) Changing views on word recognition in bilinguals. In J. Morais and G. d'Ydewalle (eds) *Bilingualism and Second Language Acquisition* (pp. 25–37). Brussels: KVAB.

Brysbaert, M., Van Dyck, G. and Van de Poel, M. (1999) Visual word recognition in bilinguals: Evidence from masked phonological priming. *Journal of Experimental Psychology: Human Perception and Performance* 25, 137–148.

Byng, S., Coltheart, M., Masterson, J., Prior, M. and Riddoch, M.J. (1984) Bilingual biscriptal deep dyslexia. *Quarterly Journal of Experimental Psychology* 36A, 417–433.

Caramazza, A. and Brones, I. (1979) Lexical access in bilinguals. *Bulletin of the Psychonomic Society* 13, 212–214.

Caramelli, P., Parente, M.A.M.P., Hosogi, M.L., Bois, M. and Lecours, A.R. (1994) Unexpected reading dissociation in a Brazilian Nisei with crossed aphasia. *Behavioural Neurology* 7, 156–164.

Chee, M., Caplan, D., Soon, C., Sriram, N., Tan, E., Thiel, T. *et al.* (1999) Processing of visually presented sentences in Mandarin and English studied with fMRI. *Neuron* 23, 127–137.

Chee, M.W.L., Weekes, B.S., Lee, K.M., Soon, C.S., Schreiber, A., Hoon, J.J. *et al.* (2000) Overlap and dissociation of semantic processing of characters English words and pictures: Evidence from fMRI. *NeuroImage* 12, 392–403.

Chen, Y.P., Fu, S.M. and Iversen, S.D. (2002) Testing for dual brain processing routes in reading: A direct contrast of Chinese character and Pinyin reading using fMRI. *Journal of Cognitive Neuroscience* 14, 1088–1098.

Cremaschi, F. and Dujovny, E. (1996) Japanese language and brain localization. *Neurological Research* 18, 212–216.

Crinion, J., Turner, R., Grogan, A., Hanakawa, T., Noppeney, U., Devlin, J.T. *et al.* (2006) Language control in the bilingual brain. *Science* 312, 1537–1540.

Dijkstra, A. and van Heuven, W.J.B. (1998) The BIA model and bilingual word recognition. In J. Grainger and A. Jacobs (eds) *Localist Connectionist Approaches to Human Cognition* (pp. 189–225). Mahwah, NJ: Lawrence Erlbaum.

Dijkstra, T. and van Heuven, W.J.B. (2002) The architecture of the bilingual word recognition system: From identification to decision. *Bilingualism: Language and Cognition* 5, 175–197.

Dijkstra, A.F.J. and Van Hell, J.G. (2003) Testing the language mode hypothesis using trilinguals. *International Journal of Bilingual Education and Bilingualism* 6, 2–16.

Doctor, E.A. and Klein, D. (1992) Phonological processing in bilingual word recognition. In R.J. Harris (ed.) *Cognitive Processes in Bilinguals* (pp. 237–252). Amsterdam: Elsevier.

Edmonds, L. and Kiran, S. (2006) Effect of semantic based treatment on cross linguistic generalization in bilingual aphasia. *Journal of Speech, Language and Hearing Research* 49, 729–748.

Edmonds, L.A. and Kiran, S. (2004) Confrontation naming and semantic relatedness judgments in Spanish/English bilinguals. *Aphasiology* 18, 567–579.

Eng, N. and Obler, L.K. (2002) Acquired dyslexia in a biscript reader following traumatic brain injury: A second case. *Topics in Language Disorders* 22, 5–19.

Fabbro, F. (1999) *The Neurolinguistics of Bilingualism: An Introduction.* Hove: Psychology Press.

Fabbro, F. (2001) The bilingual brain: Cerebral representation of languages. *Brain and Language* 79, 211–222.

Ferguson, G.A. (1966) *Statistical Analysis in Psychology and Education* (2nd edn). New York: McGraw-Hill.

Ferrand, L. and Humphreys, G.W. (1996) Transfer of refractory states across languages in a global aphasic participant. *Cognitive Neuropsychology* 13, 1163–1119.

Francis, W.S. (1999) Cognitive integration of language and memory in bilinguals: Semantic representation. *Psychological Bulletin* 125, 193–222.

Gollan, T.H., Forster, K.I. and Frost, R. (1997) Translation priming with different scripts: Masked priming with cognates and noncognates in Hebrew-English bilinguals. *Journal of Experimental Psychology: Learning, Memory, and Cognition* 23, 1122–1139.

Gollan, T.H. and Kroll, J.F. (2001) Lexical access in bilinguals. In B. Rapp (ed.) *A Handbook of Cognitive Neuropsychology: What Deficits Reveal about the Human Mind* (pp. 321–345). New York: Psychology Press.

Green, D. (2006) The neurocognition of recovery patterns in bilingual aphasics. In J.F. Kroll and A.M.B. de Groot (eds) *Handbook of Bilingualism: Psycholinguistic Perspectives* (pp. 516–530). Oxford: Oxford University Press.

Grosjean, F. (1998) Studying bilinguals: Methodological and conceptual issues. *Bilingualism: Language and Cognition* 1, 131–149.

Grosjean, F. (2001) The bilingual's language modes. In J. Nicol (ed.) *One Mind, Two Languages: Bilingual Language Processing* (pp. 1–22). Oxford: Blackwell.

Havelka, J. and Rastle, K. (2005) The assembly of phonology from print is serial and subject to strategic control: Evidence from Serbian. *Journal of Experimental Psychology: Learning, Memory and Cognition* 31, 148–158.

Iwata, M. (1984) Kanji versus kana: Neuropsychological correlates of the Japanese writing system. *Trends in Neuroscience* 7, 290–293.

Jared, D. and Kroll, J. (2001) Do bilinguals activate phonological representations in one or both of their languages when naming words? *Journal of Memory and Language* 44, 2–31.

Kapaj, L. (2001) The silver horde. On WWW at http://www.viahistoria.com/SilverHorde/main.html. Accessed 31.1.2007.

Karanth, P. (2002) The search for deep dyslexia in syllabic writing systems. *Journal of Neurolinguistics* 15, 143–155.

Kiran, S. and Tuchtenhagen, J. (2005) Imageability effects in normal Spanish–English bilingual adults and in aphasia: Evidence from naming to definition and semantic priming tasks. *Aphasiology* 19, 315–327.

Kroll, J.F. and de Groot, A.M.B. (1997) Lexical and conceptual memory in bilinguals: Mapping form to meaning in two languages. In A.M.B. de Groot and J.F. Kroll (eds) *Tutorials in Bilingualism: Psycholinguistic Perspectives* (pp. 169–199). Mahwah, NJ: Lawrence Erlbaum.

Kroll, J.F. and Stewart, E. (1994) Category interference in translation and picture naming: Evidence for asymmetric connections between bilingual memory representations. *Journal of Memory and Language* 33, 149–174.

Law, S.P. (2004) A morphological analysis of object naming and reading errors by a Cantonese dyslexic participant. *Language and Cognitive Processes* 19, 473–501.
Lebrun, Y. (1971) The neurology of bilingualism. *Word* 27, 179–186.
Lyman, R.S., Kwan, S.T. and Chao, W.H. (1938) Left occipito-parietal brain tumor with observations on alexia and agraphia in Chinese and in English. *The Chinese Medical Journal* 54, 491–516.
Masterson, J., Coltheart, M. and Meara, P. (1985) Surface dyslexia in a language without irregularly spelled words. In K. Patterson, J.C. Marshall and M. Coltheart (eds) *Surface Dyslexia: Neuropsychological and Cognitive Studies of Phonological Reading* (pp. 215–223). Hove: Lawrence Erlbaum.
McClelland, J.L. and Rumelhart, D.E. (1981) An interactive-activation model of context effects in better perception, Part 1: An account of basic findings. *Psychological Review* 88, 375–405.
McNemar, Q. (1947) Note on the sampling error of the difference between correlated proportions or percentages. *Psychometrika* 12, 153–157.
Nilipour, R. and Ashayeri, H. (1989) Alternating antagonism between two languages with successive recovery of a third in a trilingual aphasic participant. *Brain and Language* 36, 23–48.
Nilipour, R. and Paradis, M. (1995) Breakdown of functional categories in three Farsi-English bilingual aphasic participants. In M. Paradis (ed.) *Aspects of Bilingual Aphasia* (pp. 123–138). Oxford: Pergamon Press.
Paradis, M. (1977) Bilingualism and aphasia. In H. Whitaker and H.A. Whitaker (eds) *Studies in Neurolinguistics* (Vol. 3, pp. 65–121). Academic Press: New York.
Paradis, M. (1995) *Aspects of Bilingual Aphasia*. Oxford: Pergamon Press.
Paradis, M. (2001) Bilingual and polyglot aphasia. In R.S. Berndt (ed.) *Handbook of Neuropsychology (Vol. 3) Language and Aphasia* (2nd edn, pp. 69–91). Amsterdam: Elsevier Science.
Paradis, M. and Goldblum, M.C. (1989) Selected crossed aphasia in a trilingual participant followed by reciprocal antagonism. *Brain and Language* 36, 62–75.
Paradis, M., Goldblum, M.C. and Abidi, R. (1982) Alternate antagonism with paradoxical translation behaviour in two bilingual aphasic participants. *Brain and Language* 15, 55–69.
Paulesu, E., McCrory, E., Fazio, F., Menoncello, L., Brunswick, N., Cappa, S.F. *et al.* (2000) A cultural effect on brain function. *Nature NeuroScience* 3, 91–96.
Poppe, N. (1970) *Mongolian Language Handbook*. Washington, DC: Center for Applied Linguistics.
Potter, M.C., So, K.F., Von Eckardt, B. and Feldman, L. (1984) Lexical and conceptual representation in beginning and proficient bilinguals. *Journal of Verbal Learning and Verbal Behavior* 23, 23–38.
Raman, I. and Weekes, B.S. (2005) Acquired dyslexia and dysgraphia in a biscriptal Turkish-English Reader. *Annals of Dyslexia* 55, 71–96.
Reich, S., Chou, T-L. and Patterson, K. (2003) Acquired dysgraphia in Chinese: Further evidence on the links between phonology and orthography. *Aphasiology* 17, 585–604.
Roberts, P.M. (1998) Clinical research needs in bilingual aphasia. *Aphasiology* 12, 119–130.
Sakurai, Y., Momose, T., Iwata, M., Sudo, Y., Ohtomo, K. and Kanazawa, I. (2000) Different cortical activity in reading of Kanji words, Kana words and Kana nonwords. *Cognitive Brain Research* 9, 111–115.
Sasanuma, S. (1975) Kana and Kanji processing in Japanese aphasics. *Brain and Language* 2, 369–383.

Sasanuma, S. and Monoi, H. (1975) The syndrome of Gogi (word meaning) aphasia. *Neurology* 25, 627–632.

Scarborough, D., Gerard, L. and Cortese, C. (1984) Independence of lexical access in bilingual word recognition. *Journal of Verbal Learning and Verbal Behavior* 23, 84–99.

Smith, M.C. (1997) How do bilinguals access lexical information? In A.M. De Groot and J.F. Kroll (eds) *Tutorials in Bilingualism: Psycholinguistic Perspectives* (pp. 145–168). Hillsdale, NJ: Erlbaum.

Stadie, N., Springer, L., de Bleser, R. and Bürk, F. (1995) Oral and written naming in a multilingual aphasic participant. In M. Paradis (ed.) *Aspects of Bilingual Aphasia* (pp. 85–99). Oxford: Pergamon.

Sugishita, M., Otomo, K., Kabe, S. and Yunoki, K. (1992) A critical appraisal of neuropsychological correlates of Japanese ideogram (kanji) and phonogram (kana) reading. *Brain* 115, 1563–1585.

Vaid, J. and Hull, R. (2002) Re-envisioning the bilingual brain using functional neuroimaging: Methodological and interpretive issues. In F. Fabbro (ed.) *Advances in Neurolinguistics of Bilingualism* (pp. 315–355). Udine: Forum.

Van Heuven, W.J.B., Dijkstra, T. and Grainger, J. (1998) Orthographic neighborhood effects in bilingual word recognition. *Journal of Memory and Language* 39, 458–483.

Wang, X.D., Gao, S.R. and Hu, C.Q. (1988) Chinese aphasia examination scale. *Chinese Journal of Neurology* 21, 252–253.

Weekes, B.S., Chen, M.J. and Yin, W-G. (1997a) Anomia without dyslexia in Chinese. *Neurocase* 3, 51–60.

Yiu, E.M.L. and Worrall, L.E. (1996) Agrammatic production: a cross-linguistic comparison of English and Cantonese. *Aphasiology* 10, 623–647.

Zhou, Y.G. (1978) To what degree are the 'phonetics' of present day Chinese characters still phonetic? *Zhingguo Yuwen* 156, 172–177.

Appendix

Oral reading responses in Mongolian of three dyslexic participants SL, TGX and LH

Stimulus		***SL***	***TGX***	***LH***
Star	[illegible]	√	√	[illegible] tree
Cat	[illegible]	√	√	√
Eye	[illegible]	Nr	√	Nr
Ship	[illegible]	√	[illegible] hunter	Nr
Table	[illegible]	√	[illegible] square	[illegible] stool
Ox	[illegible]	√	√	Nr
Square	[illegible]	√	√	[illegible] table
Grandmother	[illegible]	√	[illegible] ship	Nr
Skirt	[illegible]	[illegible] teacher	√	Nr
Egg	[illegible]	Nr	[illegible] stand	√
Elephant	[illegible]	√	√	Nr
Bowl	[illegible]	Nr	√	[illegible] male
Fish	[illegible]	魚 *yu2* 'fish' (in Chinese)	√	√
Woman	[illegible]	Nr	[illegible] teacher	√

Note. Nr = no response

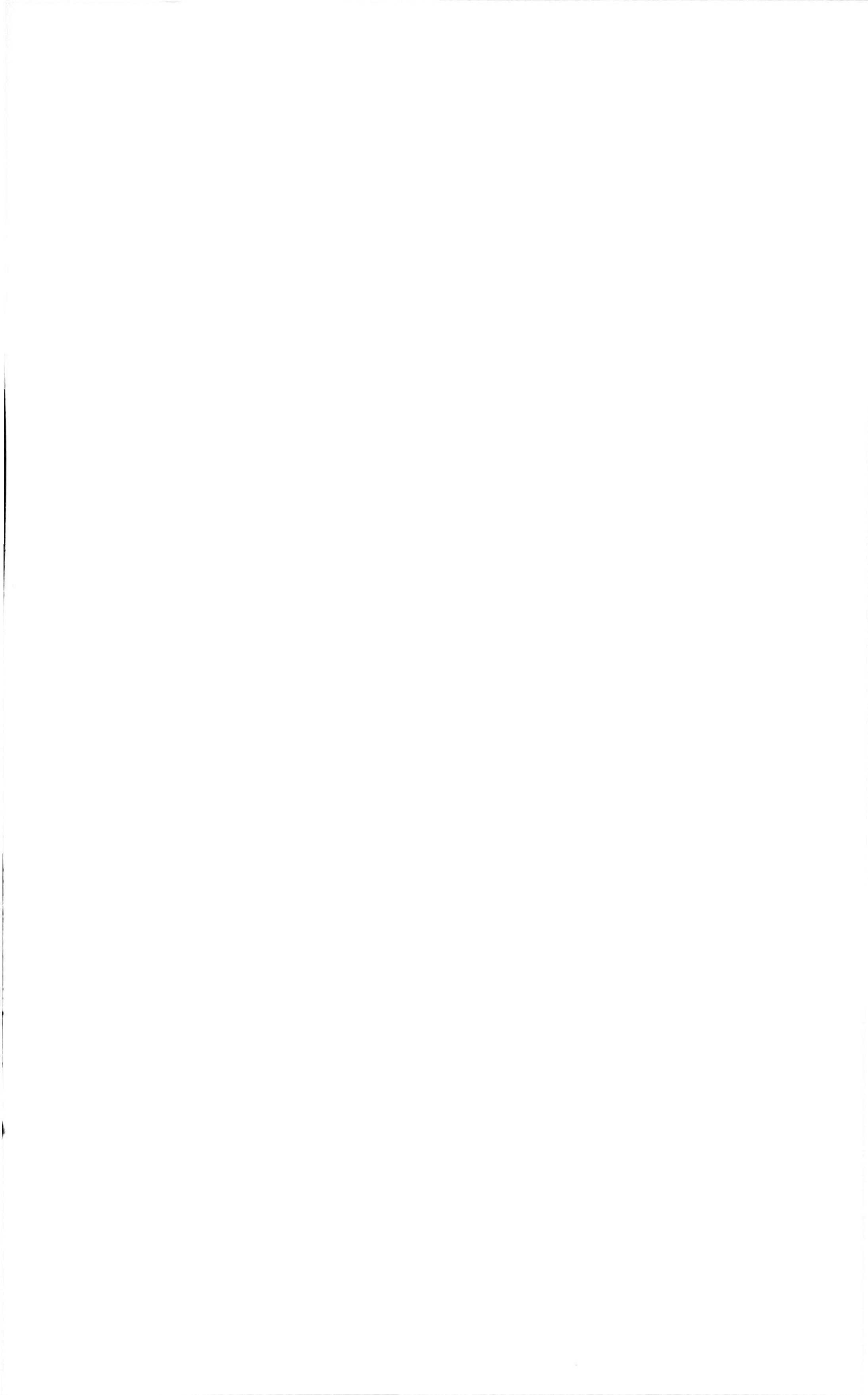